DATE DUE

Sidney J. Winawer, M.D., and Moshe Shike, M.D.

PHYSICIANS AT MEMORIAL
SLOAN-KETTERING CANCER CENTER

and Philip Bashe and Genell Subak-Sharpe

CANCER FREE

The Comprehensive Cancer Prevention Program

Introduction by Paul A. Marks, M.D.,
PRESIDENT, MEMORIAL SLOAN-KETTERING CANCER CENTER

Simon & Schuster
NEW YORK   LONDON   TORONTO   SYDNEY
TOKYO   SINGAPORE

SIMON & SCHUSTER
Rockefeller Center
1230 Avenue of the Americas
New York, New York 10020

Designed by Carla Weise/Levavi & Levavi
Manufactured in the United States of America

1   3   5   7   9   10   8   6   4   2

Library of Congress Cataloging-in-Publication Data
Cancer free : the comprehensive cancer prevention program /
Sidney J. Winawer and Moshe Shike ;
and Philip Bashe and Genell Subak-Sharpe ;
introduction by Paul A. Marks.
p.   cm.
Includes bibliographical references and index.
1. Cancer—Prevention.   I. Winawer, Sidney J.   II. Shike, Moshe.
RC268.C356   1995
616.99'4052—dc20   94-37680
CIP
ISBN: 0-671-79967-3

Acknowledgments

D r. Sidney J. Winawer would like to acknowledge the support and love given so generously by his wife, Andrea, and his children, Daniel, Jonathan and Joanna.

Dr. Moshe Shike would like to thank his wife, Sherry, and his children, Nathan and Naomi, for their encouragement and their love.

Philip Bashe would like to thank his agent, Jed Mattes; Rochelle and Robert Bashe; the late Evelyn Bashe; Justin Bashe; and, as always, Patty Romanowski Bashe.

Together, the authors would like to thank the following for providing print materials and/or general assistance: Action on Smoking and Health, American Academy of Dermatology, American Cancer Center, American Cancer Society, American College of Obstetricians and Gynecologists, American College of Physicians, American Institute for Cancer Research, American Institute of Stress, American Lung Association, American College of Physicians, Cancer Research Institute, Martha Casey, Centers for Disease Control, Stacy Charney, Food and Drug Administration, GASP, Health Insurance Association of America, Hereditary Cancer Institute at Creighton University School of Medicine, Leukemia Society of America, Livingston Foundation Medical Center, Metropolitan Life Insurance Company, National Cancer Cytology Center, National Cancer Institute, National Clearinghouse for Alcohol and Drug Information, National Council on Alcoholism and Drug Dependence, National Foundation for Cancer Research, National Pesticide Telecommunications Network, People Against Cancer, Skin Cancer Foundation, U.S. Department of Labor Occupational Safety and Health Administration, U.S. Environmental Protection Agency Information Access Branch and U.S. General Accounting Office.

Very special thanks to our editor, Rebecca Saletan, for her guidance; her assistant, Denise Roy; copy editors Isolde Sauer and Philip James; and designer Carla Weise/Levavi & Levavi; Catherine Dold, who cowrote Chapter 5 on nutrition; John Fried, who cowrote Chapter 10 on prostate cancer; Stephanie Denmark, for her assistance on Chapter 2; and Susan Carleton, for her assistance on Chapter 13 on colorectal cancer; and Sassona Norton, for helping to develop the menus. Finally, an expression of gratitude to Genell Subak-Sharpe, who directed the entire project.

We greatly appreciate the contributions and critical reviews of chapters by the following Memorial Sloan-Kettering Cancer Center staff: Chapter 4—Dr. Kenneth Offit, Dr. Hans Gerdes; Chapter 8—Dr. Jimmie Holland; Chapter 10—Dr. Willet F. Whitmore Jr., Dr. William Fair; Chapter 11—Dr. Michael Moore; Chapter 12—Dr. Diane Stover; Chapter 14—Dr. William Hoskins; Chapter 15—Dr. Robert Kurtz, Dr. Murray Brennan; Chapter 16—Dr. Bijan Safai.

Contents

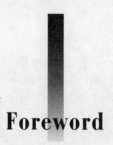

Foreword

When I was graduated from medical school in 1949, the field of cancer research was largely perceived to be a "black box." There was almost no knowledge of the way genes or the environment were involved in causing cancers. Attempts to cure cancer patients, other than by surgery for localized tumors, were usually frustrating and of generally limited value to the patient.

By the late 1950s, this situation began to change. The transformation accelerated with the focused effort to conquer cancer launched under the National Cancer Act of 1971. There was a marked increase in funding of studies aimed at elucidating the causes of cancer, as well as the search for cures. Ironically, at that time, there was relatively little enthusiasm for cancer prevention, and, consequently, few studies addressed it. Over the two decades since then, we have made impressive progress in our understanding of the causes of cancer and have significantly improved our ability to control and cure the disease—substantial achievements indeed. Perhaps of even more importance in the long run are the various new strategies that have been developed for the prevention of cancer.

Today, a patient diagnosed with cancer has about a 50 percent chance of having the disease cured or controlled. For certain cancers, the outlook for patients is considerably better than 50 percent; these include cancers of the breast, testis, colon, cervix, larynx, uterus, prostate, thyroid and bladder, along with melanoma, lymphomas and a number of childhood cancers. However, definitive effective therapy for several of the more common cancers such as lung, pancreatic and liver, and almost all metastatic cancer, has not yet been achieved. Indeed, despite intensive efforts, over the past decade relatively little progress has been made in developing more effective drugs to cure these cancers. Our greatest hope for further reducing the burden of cancer for individuals and for society *lies in cancer prevention.*

It is now established that to a greater or lesser extent, genetics

—that is, heredity—plays a role in the development of almost all human cancers. We are rapidly developing tools to identify genes that place people at increased risk for cancer; indeed, to identify persons at increased risk before they actually develop the disease. In turn, we may be able to intervene in a targeted way to prevent progression to clinical cancer or detect the disease at its earliest stages, when it is most likely to be curable. This is a rapidly evolving field. Many challenges remain before we can bring the full potential of genetic diagnosis to bear on strategies for cancer prevention. Although we have already identified certain genes that place people at increased risk for some common cancers such as that of the colon and a number of relatively rare cancers such as tumor of the eye, specific gene probes for most cancers are yet to be developed. In the meantime, through the use of careful analysis of family and personal histories, it is possible to estimate a particular individual's risk for many major cancers. In a number of instances, this permits us to design a practical program that has the potential to decrease that individual's risk of developing cancer and to increase the chance that cancer, if it develops, can be detected at an early stage when it is curable. The promise of these new strategies for prevention of cancer can, to an important extent, be realized today. This book is a comprehensive review of the current practical, available strategies for prevention of cancers, laid out in a clear and useful fashion. The challenges to a broad program of cancer prevention—scientific, psychological and social —are also discussed.

Through the practical approaches to applying currently available knowledge and techniques described in this book, the risk for developing cancers may be reduced. Drs. Winawer and Shike have drawn upon their extensive experience and strong commitment to prevention and have enlisted the help of many other experts. The result is an outstanding, informative and comprehensive book that is a *must* for individuals and families seeking to prevent cancer. Cancer prevention is a dynamic field, and we can look forward to further progress as new technologies—for genetic diagnosis and for intervention to prevent cancers—are developed for clinical use.

—PAUL A. MARKS, M.D.,
PRESIDENT, MEMORIAL SLOAN-KETTERING CANCER CENTER

PART ONE

Cancer:
The Facts

CHAPTER

1

Cancer Is Preventable

Cancer Facts • Primary and Secondary
Prevention • The Importance of
Early Detection

Life is not merely to be alive, but to be well.

—*Martial, first-century
Roman epigrammatist*

A recent Gallup poll found that 6 out of 10 Americans surveyed believed they would develop cancer in their lifetime, when in reality the actual odds are only about half that. Maybe you count yourself among that group. For so long, the origins and mechanisms of cancer were so enigmatic, and the treatments so harsh, that the disease assumed an aura of dread and terrible capriciousness. Only recently has the public become aware that cancer is gradually yielding up its secrets, including the secrets of prevention. But the barrage of information is so confusing and seemingly contradictory that it leaves people feeling uncertain what to do—and doubtful that anything they can do will make a difference anyway.

Nothing could be further from the truth. It is estimated that most men and women can reduce their odds of getting cancer *by half*. This book will show you how.

CAUSE	PERCENTAGE OF CANCER DEATHS
Diet	35 percent
Tobacco use	30 percent
Reproductive and sexual behavior	7 percent
Occupational hazards	4 percent
Excessive alcohol use	3 percent
Excessive sun exposure	3 percent
Environmental pollution	2 percent
Industrial products	1 percent
Food additives	1 percent
Medicines and medical procedures	1 percent

To be sure, cancer is a devastating disease, one that currently claims over half a million American lives each year. Despite advances in research that have enabled us to chip away steadily at the mortality rate, the incidence continues to climb. It is projected that by the year 2000, cancer will surpass heart disease as America's number-one killer.

As longtime physicians at New York City's Memorial Sloan-Kettering Cancer Center, designated a comprehensive cancer center by the National Cancer Institute in Bethesda, Maryland, we've seen firsthand the agony this disease inflicts on patients and loved ones. Even the many success stories contain their share of heartbreak, for cancer treatment can be a grueling ordeal that depletes finances and severely strains even the closest of families.

But the biggest tragedy by far is that most of the cancer cases we see daily could have been prevented. Only 10 percent to 15 percent of all cancers are of obscure or completely unknown origin, which includes factors of heredity, environmental radioactivity and other environmental hazards. As you can see from the following table, many cancers are caused by our own behavior, *something we each have the power to control.*

With this in mind, consider the following:

- Each year 165,000 Americans die from cancers brought on by tobacco use. The vast majority of those premature deaths could be avoided. The same is true of the 17,000 cancer deaths attributed to excessive alcohol use.
- Reducing fat consumption to 20 percent of total calories and increasing fiber intake to 25 to 30 grams a day, levels recom-

mended by a number of authorities on cancer nutrition, could prevent more than 150,000 cancer fatalities per year.
- Safe sunning habits could slash the incidence of melanoma and other skin cancers by 90 percent, saving more than 8,000 lives annually.

HOW TO USE THIS BOOK

Why, then, do people often feel helpless to avert cancer? One reason may be that information on prevention is extremely fragmented. Visit your local library or book store, and you'll likely find a few titles on breast cancer prevention, others on preventing prostate cancer, and some on diet as it relates to cancer. But the vast majority of cancer books are intended specifically for cancer patients.

It was recognizing the need for a clear, concise, comprehensive book outlining preventive action against cancer that inspired us to write *Cancer Free*. In it we will explain step by step how to design your personal, practical and surprisingly simple cancer prevention program, using the guidelines developed by physicians at Memorial Sloan-Kettering. We'll also decipher for you the latest research on the relationship between cancer and nutrition, genetics, exercise—minus the scientific jargon that tends to confuse rather than enlighten—and explain what these studies mean to *you*.

Part One provides a basic understanding of cancer: what it is, how and why it occurs, and how it is detected and treated. Part Two, The Building Blocks of a Cancer Prevention Program, is devoted to what we call *primary* prevention: identifying, then modifying or eliminating those environmental and lifestyle risk factors that can cause cancer. In these chapters you'll learn:

- How to draw your family tree, a valuable tool in determining your inherited cancer risk and the steps you must take to reduce it.
- The dangers of tobacco and other substances, and proven methods for quitting smoking.
- How to follow a low-fat, high-fiber diet with relative ease, with a week's sample menus to get you started.
- Steps for protecting yourself and your family from *carcinogens* (cancer-causing agents) commonly found at home and on the job.

- How stress and emotions may influence cancer, and techniques for reducing stress.
- The benefits of physical activity, which may lower cancer risk.

Does practicing cancer prevention require revamping your entire way of life? Only if you're a beer-swilling, fat-consuming, chain-smoking couch potato who exercises nothing other than your TV-remote-control trigger finger and hasn't seen a doctor since the days of house calls. Chances are that you already practice some preventive measures, but you need to develop a comprehensive game plan. These lifestyle recommendations apply to everyone, regardless of individual risk of developing cancer. In addition, they offer protection against heart disease, diabetes, emphysema and other deadly disorders, and in general help to promote vital, active, healthy living.

We advocate a total approach to prevention. However, because readers may be more vulnerable to particular cancers, Part Three presents specific strategies to combat the major adult cancers:

- Prostate cancer
- Breast cancer
- Lung cancer
- Colorectal cancer (colon and rectum)
- Gynecologic cancers
- Stomach cancer
- Esophageal cancer (cancer of the esophagus)
- Skin cancers

TYPES OF CANCER

Cancer	Estimated Annual Number of New Cases (1994)	Cancer	Estimated Annual Number of Deaths (1994)
Skin (including melanoma)	732,000	Lung	153,000
Prostate	200,000	Colon and rectum	56,000
Breast	183,000	Breast	46,300
Lung	172,000	All other and unspecified	
Colon and rectum	149,000	sites	41,000
Gynecologic	75,300		

Urinary bladder	51,200	Prostate	38,000
Non-Hodgkin's lymphomas	45,000	Pancreas	25,900
All other and unspecified sites	43,000	Stomach and esophageal	24,400
Stomach and esophageal	35,000	Gynecologic	24,100
Oral (mouth, lip, tongue, pharanyx)	29,600	Non-Hodgkin's lymphoma	21,200
Leukemia	28,600	Leukemia	19,100
Kidney	27,600	Liver	13,200
Pancreas	27,000	Brain and central nervous system	12,600
Brain and central nervous system	17,500	Kidney	11,300
Liver	16,100	Urinary bladder	10,600
Endocrine glands	14,450	Multiple myeloma	9,800
Multiple myeloma	12,700	Skin (includes melanoma)	9,200
Larynx	12,500	Oral (mouth, lip, tongue, pharanyx)	7,925
Hodgkin's disease	7,900	Larynx	3,800
Testis	6,800	Soft-tissue sarcomas	3,300
Soft-tissue sarcomas	6,000	Endocrine glands	1,725
Other and unspecified respiratory organs	4,500	Hodgkin's disease	1,550
Small intestine	3,600	Other and unspecified respiratory	1,400
Other and unspecified digestive organs	2,600	Bone	1,075
Bone	2,000	Other and unspecified digestive organs	1,000
Eye	1,750	Small intestine	950
Other and unspecified genital, male	1,300	Testis	325
		Eye	250
		Other and unspecified genital, male	200

SOURCE: American Cancer Society

These chapters on specific cancers incorporate the recommendations of a number of specialists at Memorial Sloan-Kettering. (Other, less common or less fatal forms of cancer, while not covered in detail, are referred to throughout as they relate to nutrition, smoking and other factors that can fasten cancer.) Besides offering suggestions for primary prevention, Part Three will describe in detail the *screening* procedures used to discover a cancerous or precancerous growth before a person shows symptoms.

We can't emphasize enough the importance of these tests, which comprise *secondary* prevention. Early detection can spell the difference between life and death or spare a patient rigorous treatment, as Adele H., a mother and grandmother from Long Island, will vouch. In 1991, during her annual gynecologic exam at Memorial Sloan-Kettering, Dr. William Hoskins, chief of the gynecology service, studied the 56-year-old woman's medical records and noted that she was due for a routine breast x-ray called a mammogram.

"He set up the appointment for that day," recalls Adele, "and the x-ray turned up something suspicious," even though Dr. Hoskins had been unable to feel anything when he'd examined her breasts. Subsequent laboratory analysis of a tissue sample taken from the area in question confirmed a tiny malignancy.

The cancer was caught so early that the breast surgeon was able to perform a lumpectomy, the least invasive surgical method for removing a breast tumor. Normally after a lumpectomy, patients are treated with radiation therapy or chemotherapy. "But the doctor told me that the cancer was so small," says Adele, "no further treatment was necessary."

According to the American Cancer Society and the National Cancer Institute, most cancers are about 90 percent curable if found early, when the disease is still *localized,* or confined to the original (primary) site, and has not yet invaded the tissues or spread to other organs:

CANCER	CURE RATE FOR LOCALIZED DISEASE
Basal-cell carcinoma (skin)	99 percent
Squamous-cell carcinoma (skin)	95 percent
Uterine cancer	94 percent
Female breast cancer	93 percent
Prostate cancer	92 percent
Melanoma (skin)	92 percent
Urinary bladder cancer	91 percent
Cervical cancer	90 percent
Colorectal cancer	89 percent
Ovarian cancer	88 percent
Kidney cancer	86 percent

Finally, Part Four looks ahead to the promising cancer-prevention methods of the future, while an appendix lists names, addresses and telephone numbers of organizations and institutions that provide informative free booklets and helpful referrals. We urge you to make use of these resources and to consult the glossary of terms at the end of each chapter.

Throughout *Cancer Free* you will meet a number of patients, like Adele, from Memorial Sloan-Kettering Cancer Center. For the sake of privacy, we've given each a pseudonym. But their experiences with cancer and its prevention are real.

Henry M., a vigorous 68-year-old attorney and avid golfer from New Jersey, is another living testament to the benefits of cancer screening. Ironically, the father of two used to avoid doctors the way moles shun sunlight.

"My philosophy on life was that I was the rock of Gibraltar," he says. He came in for a general checkup in 1977 only because a friend had insisted on making appointments for both of them. "Otherwise," Henry admits, "I probably wouldn't have gone. The last thing on my mind was that I might have any physical ailment of significance." But a routine test detected blood in the stool, a finding that eventually led to a diagnosis of early colon cancer. Fortunately the growth was localized and could be removed surgically.

"I was stunned, because I'd had no symptoms," Henry remembers. "Dr. Winawer told me, 'Your chance for a cure is excellent.' When I walked out into the hall, I must have looked somewhat dazed. I saw a priest there, who asked, 'What seems to be the problem?'

"I said, 'I was just told I have cancer and need an operation.'

"He said, 'Let me tell you something: I've been visiting patients for many years. In my experience, many times patients are told the outcome looks bleak, only to succeed; and some are told the outlook is good, and they don't make it.' "

Henry replied numbly, "Thank you, Father," and walked away.

"Little did the priest realize," he says, laughing, "I'd gotten the *good* news, that I would be all right. He thought I was on the other end."

Henry required no additional treatment. More than 15 years later, he visits Memorial Sloan-Kettering annually for a series of followup tests, boards an exercise treadmill every morning before work, and shuns his once favorite fried and fatty foods. "I said to myself, *Now it's time to follow a straight course. I've got to do what I've got to do.* And I will continue to do it." Henry's case raises an important point: that practicing cancer prevention is no less essential if you've had a brush with the disease, for cancer survivors are at the same risk as other members of the population.

A medical scare likewise compelled Brian D., a successful New York businessman, to give up tobacco after 30 years. "I'd had occasional girlfriends, dates and office mates try to get me to quit," he recalls. "But that wasn't useful."

Then in 1992 the 52-year-old divorced father of two went to his doctor complaining of general malaise. "I just felt like hell," he says. "I couldn't be more specific than that." A CT scan indicated an unusual growth on one lung. Although it turned out to be nothing more than scar tissue from earlier bouts of bronchitis, the scar was what it took to jolt Brian into action. "I said to myself, *You are not going to smoke anymore.*" With the help of a nicotine patch to ease withdrawal, Brian quit in a matter of weeks.

Another patient of ours, Judith K., surely qualifies as a role model for conscientious cancer prevention. We first met her in 1981, when her elderly mother, Rose, was diagnosed with advanced colon cancer. Sadly, Rose died the following year. So had Judith's maternal grandmother at age 55, also from colon cancer. It was news to Judith, then 37, that her family history put her at increased risk for the disease.

"One of the nurses told me it could be hereditary and said, 'You should go for the colon cancer screening,' " she remembers. "She gave me Dr. Winawer's name and number, and I called immediately. He considered me to be at high risk of having colon cancer." She underwent her first colonoscopy shortly thereafter and has had the screening procedure repeated every three years.

In addition, the New Jersey mother of three gets tested annually for breast and gynecologic cancers. She notes with a laugh, "A nurse at work said she thought I was 'a fanatic.' " But Judith, a chemist for a major oil corporation, doesn't think of herself that way at all. "I have young children," she reflects. "I'm doing everything I can to make sure I live a long time. I don't know if I can beat the odds, but I feel like if I give it my best shot, if I do end up with a cancer, then at least I won't have any regrets."

Rather than living in fear of the disease, taking these precautions affords Judith peace of mind. It's a good feeling, she says, to know that you can exert a degree of control over your health. "You can't put your life in the hands of a doctor," she adds. "You really have to take responsibility for your own life."

CHANGING ATTITUDES

If only more men and women had the same attitude as Judith. But as Dr. Daniel Nixon of the American Cancer Society observes, "It's very difficult to get people to change their habits, which are hard to break. I think there's something about human nature where people may be fatalistic, on the one hand, but they're omnipotent-thinking, on the other: 'Cancer can't happen to me; therefore I'll go ahead and smoke and drink and eat fat.' There are many psychologic factors involved here that we don't understand."

In 1986 the National Cancer Institute issued a detailed report entitled "Cancer Control Objectives for the Nation: 1985–2000." Its goal: to halve the number of cancer deaths in the United States. To accomplish this would require trimming the average American's fat intake to less than 30 percent of total calories and increasing the fiber to 20 to 30 grams a day, and reducing the percentage of adult smokers to 15 percent.

As of 1994, how close were we? According to Dr. Peter Greenwald, director of cancer prevention and control for the National Cancer Institute, the 50 percent reduction is not yet in sight. But the figures he cites, while higher than we would like to see, represent progress nonetheless:

"We've seen the smoking rate drop since the nineteen sixties," he points out. From 30 percent at the time of the NCI report, "Now we're down to 25 percent of the adult population. In diet, we've seen some decrease in fat, from 40 percent of calories to 36 percent."

Both Dr. Greenwald and Dr. Nixon believe we may be entering an era of increased awareness of cancer prevention. The country simply can no longer afford *not* to take note, as the current health-care crisis has made painfully clear. It is estimated that in addition to causing suffering and death, cancer costs the economy $104 billion annually. We believe that practicing cancer prevention, in addition to saving lives, will ultimately help keep medical costs down.

To do so entails changing our notions about the purpose of medicine. "Neither the medical profession nor the public has taken prevention completely seriously," comments Dr. Joseph Simone, Memorial Sloan-Kettering's physician-in-chief. "A lot of it's inertia, and a lot of it's vested interest. There are not well-oiled systems in place for undertaking preventive medicine strategies. We just haven't invested the time and energy into that as much as we have into taking care of the disease once it has happened."

Many people view their doctor as someone to be called upon only when something breaks down. Often, the same person who faithfully brings in his car for its yearly inspection will avoid going for a checkup as long as possible. We feel strongly that it is in everyone's best interest to view medicine as a complement to sustaining good health rather than solely a means for curing illness— in other words, not just intervention, but prevention. We've long advocated this philosophy, presenting scientific papers and giving lectures on the subject both to medical professionals and the public. The growing acceptance of the importance of cancer prevention methods has us excited and optimistic that the ravages of cancer can be significantly reduced.

Can we guarantee readers that they will never contract cancer? Of course not. The disease's origins are still somewhat mysterious. Even "healthy" people—nonsmoking, teetotaling, top physical specimens—can get cancer. But we can show you ways to improve your odds. The encouraging news is that because cancer typically lurks in the human body for between 10 and 30 years before it is diagnosed, time is on your side.

Now let's get to work.

KEY WORDS

Carcinogen: Any agent in food or the environment that causes cancer.

Localized: A cancerous growth found only in the original (primary) site.

Primary prevention: Identifying, then modifying or eliminating dietary, environmental and lifestyle factors that can cause cancer, such as tobacco, fat consumption or exposure to asbestos.

Screening test: A procedure used for early detection of cancer or precancerous growths in people who have not yet developed symptoms.

Secondary prevention: Finding, identifying and eliminating a cancer or precancerous growth when it is still curable, through the use of screening examinations.

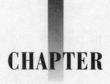

CHAPTER

2

What Is Cancer?

How Cancer Develops · Cancer
Treatment · Cancer Studies

enes. Neoplasm. Metastasis. We know from experience that
people's eyes sometimes glaze over at these and other scientific terms. But learning the basics of cancer's origins and progression is really quite easy, and it will help you to understand how
the preventive measures outlined in this book work. Don't let
the subject matter intimidate you; you needn't be a physician to
comprehend cancer any more than you have to be a mechanic to
drive a car.

Cancer, named by the Greek physician Hippocrates around 400
B.C., encompasses a group of approximately 150 diseases that can
arise anywhere on or within the body. All cancers share a critical
characteristic, however: uncontrolled cell growth.

A BRIEF (WE PROMISE) BIOLOGY LESSON

Cells are the basic units of biologic growth and development for
all living organisms. Virtually all cells contain thousands of
genes, imprints that determine every physical, biochemical and
physiologic trait, from the color of your eyes to your ability to
resist disease. These genes, made up of DNA (deoxyribonucleic
acid), precisely program and control cell division. You inherit

them from your parents and, in turn, pass them on to your children.

Normally cells replicate themselves constantly: One cell becomes two, each with an identical genetic code; two become four; four, eight; eight, sixteen; and so on. As the new cells arise, the old ones die out. For reasons that are still not fully understood, about once every one million divisions, a daughter cell departs with an altered genetic code, or misprint.

Dr. Peter Greenwald of the National Cancer Institute compares it to "copying an encyclopedia, which is more or less what's happening: You have all these DNAs replicating themselves. Mistakes can happen, and if they happen at a critical point that's severe enough to damage the DNA but not kill the cell, you've got a mutation."

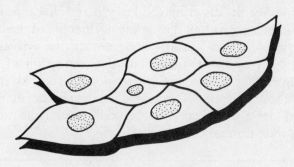

normal cells

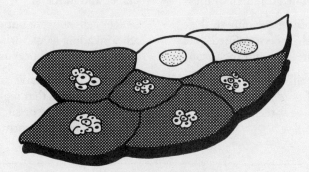

malignant transformation

How Cancer Starts. Normally, cells replicate themselves in an orderly fashion. A malignant tumor develops when something goes awry, and poorly differentiated cells, such as those with disorganized nuclei in the lower illustration, grow without control.

A defective gene doesn't necessarily lead to cancer; it increases vulnerability. The process that creates the defective gene is called an *initiation,* and the cause is called an *initiator.* Examples of initiators include cigarette smoking, x-rays and certain chemicals. A second element, a *promoter,* must act upon the initiated gene in order for the disease to occur.

"Promoters," explains Dr. Daniel Nixon of the American Cancer Society, "make the cell-division process more active and disruptive, so that an initiated cell grows into a tumor." Alcohol, for instance, compounds the increased risk of mouth and throat cancers when combined with tobacco.

Cancer develops when the tightly orchestrated structure and function of cell replication are disrupted by changes (mutations) that occur in the genetic material. Most normal cells carry several genes known as *proto-oncogenes,* a name derived from the Greek word *onco,* meaning mass or tumor. Usually they are considered allies of good health, fostering cell growth and division. Or they may exert no influence at all during the normal life of the cell. But under certain conditions, proto-oncogenes can be activated and changed into *oncogenes* that mediate the conversion of normal cells to cancer cells. Once again, carcinogens such as the ones mentioned above are often responsible for the transformation.

Viewed under a microscope, cancer cells appear distinctly different from their normal counterparts:

Normal cells are round and have clearly defined cell membranes.	Cancer cells possess irregular shapes and borders.
Normal cells grow only to the limits of their own defined space and architecture and then stop.	Cancer cells squeeze out other cells, invading neighboring and distant tissues and organs.
Normal cells have a nucleus with 23 sets of *chromosomes,* biologic units that bear the DNA.	Cancer cells often have an enlarged nucleus that may contain a shortage or surplus of chromosomes or abnormal genes.

What's more, whereas a healthy cell grows and divides systematically, a cancer cell multiplies rapidly and recklessly until the errant cells infiltrate and destroy the normal cells and tissues. Unless apprehended, the cancer will continue to spread, damaging healthy organs, interfering with body systems and possibly causing death.

Even after the initial events produce a cancerous cell, the disease must still elude various defense and repair mechanisms to gain a foothold. The body's *immune system* is usually able to ferret out and dispose of roving cancer cells before they can spread or form a tumor. There are also defenses that prevent one or a few cancerous cells from developing into a significant cancer, although little is known about them at present.

"We know of situations where people have occult cancers that never become clinically significant," says Dr. Peter Greenwald of the National Cancer Institute. (An occult cancer is one too tiny to produce symptoms or to be seen without microscopically examining the tissue.) "That's very common in the prostate, for example, and it undoubtedly occurs in the breast and other organs as well." Except for extremely rare cancers, it takes more than one mutation, or change, in one gene for a normal cell to progress all the way into a cancer cell.

From scientific studies, it appears that the immune response to cancer may generally resemble the assault against bacteria and viruses, although the specific mechanism in cancer is unknown, and may, in fact, be quite different.

- First a white blood cell called a *macrophage* consumes and digests one of the invaders, then displays fragments of its prey on its surface.
- A *helper T cell,* another type of white blood cell, recognizes the fragments, or *antigens,* a process which induces the macrophage and helper T cell to produce chemicals called cytokines which allow for intercellular communication.
- The cytokines signal the helper T cells to proliferate. As the helper T cells reproduce, they release substances that stimulate *B cells* to multiply and manufacture *antibodies,* molecules that adhere to and interact only with specific antigens.
- At the same time another type of white blood cells, the natural killer cells, attack the antigen or invading microbes directly.
- Mission accomplished: The infection is eradicated. Yet another class of T cells, *suppressor T cells,* deactivate the B and T cells, while "memory" T cells and B cells stay.

This remarkably complex, intricate system functions normally most of the time. However, a number of factors—excess dietary fat, stress and depression, diseases such as AIDS, medical treatments involving radiation therapy or immunosuppressive drugs—can impair immune response, permitting cancer cells to evade this critical line of defense. As Dr. Nixon notes, even when the immune system is functioning at its peak, "the cancer can be much stronger."

Other natural safeguards can also go awry. Cells have systems that correct genes with mutations throughout each cell's lifetime. People who get cancer seem to have irreparable mutations, too many mutations or mutations that the repair mechanism somehow overlooked.

All cells in the body produce *free radicals,* highly active oxygen molecules that contain unpaired electrons. Normally, neutralizing substances known as antioxidants thwart the unpaired electrons from damaging healthy cells in their hunt for a mate. But sometimes free radicals get out of control, a process believed to heighten the risk of cancer.

Yet another natural defense system: proteins that stop cells with defective DNA from dividing. These molecular traffic cops can either program a damaged cell to self-destruct or shut down the growth cycle long enough to allow the cell to repair its damaged DNA before it divides. However, another type of protein somehow prevents cells from manufacturing these useful proteins. Its "brakes" having malfunctioned, the mutant cell is free to hurtle down the pathway to cancer.

CANCER: A MULTISTEP PROCESS

Cancer most commonly afflicts men and women over 50, although, we hasten to emphasize, the disease by no means excludes younger people. You are more likely to contract cancer as you age because of various events that unfold over many years, such as exposure to carcinogens. Even after cancer develops, it usually progresses very slowly and can take as long as 10 to 30 years before symptoms emerge. Hence the importance of screening tests, for detecting the disease in its earliest, most curable state.

Some cancers, but not all, enter a precancerous stage known as *dysplasia,* characterized by abnormal cell structure and organization. Dysplastic cells sometimes reverse course spontaneously, without medical intervention.

The next step, *carcinoma in situ,* can be likened to a calm before the storm. Cancerous cells exist but remain confined to the microscopic site in which they formed. Cervical cancer typically lingers in this noninvasive state for 8 to 30 years before finally penetrating the outer layer of the cervix.

Eventually cancer cells will form a small expanding mass called a *tumor*. A *benign* growth is noncancerous and cannot spread, or *metastasize*, to other parts of the body. A *malignant* tumor, on the other hand, is cancerous, and can invade other tissues and organs. Either it infiltrates adjacent healthy tissue as a single mass, or a cluster of malignant cells breaks off from the original mass and migrates to a neighboring part of the body. It may also travel through the bloodstream or circulatory system to form *secondary* tumor deposits at distant sites. A woman whose breast cancer has spread to her bones is said to have metastatic breast cancer of the bones. At this advanced stage, the cancer becomes much harder to cure.

Although there are over 150 different types of cancer, we classify the disease according to four major groups:

1. Nine in ten cancers are *carcinomas,* which form in the epithelial cells that cover the skin and line the mouth, throat, lungs, gastrointestinal tract and other organs.
2. *Sarcomas* affect the bones and soft tissue that connect, support or surround other tissues and organs. Hard-tissue sarcomas surface in bones and cartilage; soft-tissue sarcomas, in muscles, tendons, fibrous tissues, fat and the linings of the lungs, abdomen, heart, central nervous system and blood vessels.
3. *Leukemias* develop in blood and blood-forming tissues such as the bone marrow and the spleen.
4. *Lymphomas,* classified as either Hodgkin's disease or non-Hodgkin's lymphomas, strike the lymphatic system, a network of vessels and nodes that bathe body tissues with lymph and help combat infection by filtering out bacteria, viruses, dead cells and other harmful agents.

HOW WE TREAT CANCER

Cancer is typically treated through surgery, chemotherapy or radiation therapy, or a combination of these approaches. In the past, surgery was our only effective means of combating the disease. But today, according to the National Cancer Institute, 25 percent of cancer survivors owe their lives to radiation, and 15 percent, to chemotherapy.

In determining which therapy will work best, physicians take into account the type, location and stage of disease, as well as the patient's overall health. Will the body tolerate the potential side effects of radiation and chemotherapy? Or is surgery a more appropriate choice? Although we observe standard therapeutic protocols for the different forms of cancer, each patient is unique and must be treated as such.

Staging is the system used to describe the extent of disease, with stage 0 considered the most curable and stage IV the least. It provides physicians with a common language. Classifications are redefined periodically, as we learn more about the disease and how it spreads.

In addition, the classifications vary from cancer to cancer. To give you an example, stage II colon cancer, 50 percent to 75 percent curable, is limited to the colon and adjacent tissues; the lymph nodes remain unaffected. Contrast that with lung cancer, which by the time it reaches stage II has infiltrated nearby lymph nodes and is only 30 percent curable.

Five years is the yardstick generally used to measure a cure. With most cancers, if a patient survives for that amount of time, he or she is likely to be a long-term survivor. As with every rule, there are exceptions: For lung cancer patients, the first two to three years are most critical, whereas with breast cancer 20 years may pass before a woman can be pronounced fully cured.

SURGERY

Surgery remains the most common method of cancer treatment, credited with saving the lives of 6 in 10 survivors. Most cancer operations involve removing primary cancers. However, in recent years it has become common practice to take out metastases from organs other than the one in which the tumor originated.

RADIATION THERAPY

External *radiation* therapy aims high-energy x-ray beams directly at rapidly dividing cancerous cells, damaging or destroying them and, when effective, shrinking or eliminating the tumor. Physicians have employed radiation in cancer therapy since the beginning of the twentieth century, though until the 1950s its drawbacks nearly outweighed its advantages. Equipment was primitive, and little was known initially about the hazards of overexposure. This led to patients' receiving excessive doses that damaged healthy cells and organs as well as cancerous ones.

Several innovations have improved radiation's effectiveness and reduced its risks. Powerful megavolt radiation from sophisticated new machines penetrates the body's densest tissues. And the vivid computerized pictures generated by computed tomography (CT) scans and magnetic resonance imaging (MRI) enable specially trained *radiation oncologists* to pinpoint the tumor's location and target the beams more precisely, sparing vital organs. Inevitably healthy cells come under fire, but these usually recover faster than cancer cells, which sustain greater damage because they divide more rapidly and are therefore more vulnerable. Radiation is delivered in small, exact dosages over a period of weeks, so that damaged normal cells have a chance to mend or be replaced.

With internal radiation treatment, a radioactive substance is implanted near the tumor, usually temporarily. Unlike patients exposed to external radiation—which, contrary to popular misconception, does not make them radioactive—those with implants do in fact emit some radiation briefly.

Radiation has provided new treatment benefits to patients. Often it is the only way to manage a local or regional cancer that's deeply embedded or in an organ that can't be reached without destroying adjacent tissue—certain brain tumors, for instance. And in many cases, radiation is used to shrink large tumors so that they can then be removed surgically.

CHEMOTHERAPY

Chemotherapy literally means chemical treatment. Whereas physicians typically apply radiation to local or regional disease, chemotherapy is used to eradicate cancer that has spread throughout the entire body.

As with radiation, these highly toxic drugs cannot distinguish between normal and cancerous cells. Therefore chemotherapy is dispensed in series called courses, with periods off in between to allow the healthy cells to renew themselves.

The first, and most intensive, course lasts weeks or months and is designed to wipe out as many malignant cells as possible. Because the drugs' effectiveness eventually wanes, for the next round, a new drug or combination of drugs is often prescribed. Maintenance, the final and mildest phase, is for obliterating any stragglers over a period of months or sometimes years.

Oncologists have gradually refined the dosages to mitigate complications such as vomiting, diarrhea and hair loss. While chemotherapy can certainly be unpleasant, most cancer survivors regard the temporary discomfort in return for a cure an acceptable exchange. In addition, we have new drugs at our disposal that reduce many of the side effects.

Many chemotherapeutic drugs are available in ingestible liquid, capsule or tablet form. Those that cannot be taken orally (because they either damage the stomach lining or aren't readily absorbed that way) must be injected or administered via an intravenous drip.

History shows that physicians used plant extracts to dissolve tumors over 2,000 years ago. To date, more than 250,000 agents have been studied for their chemotherapeutic value, but only 50 or so have been deemed safe enough to give to patients. Interestingly, some of these are derived from plants used in folk remedies. For example, vinblastine, a drug used to treat a number of cancers, is derived from tropical periwinkle.

The longtime public perception was that doctors resorted to chemotherapy only in hopeless cases. Today it is an integral part of cancer treatment, saving approximately 50,000 lives annually.

STUDYING THE CAUSES AND PREVENTION OF CANCER

Now and then throughout this book we will be referring to scientific studies, which researchers rely on to help answer the many riddles related to cancer's causes and prevention. A brief explanation of the different types of studies will make this information more meaningful to you.

CLINICAL TRIALS

Clinical trials study the efficacy of a certain treatment or diagnostic test. The participants in the trial are generally assigned at random to either the study group or the control group. The former receive the treatment or diagnostic test under investigation, while the latter do not. At the end of the study, researchers analyze the outcome in the two groups to determine whether the treatment or the diagnostic test was effective.

To give you an example, the National Cancer Institute is currently sponsoring dozens of clinical trials to test cancer-preventive compounds. A study group receives the agent under investigation, while a control group is administered a sugar pill, or *placebo*. Neither group—nor the physicians assessing the results—knows which subjects are getting the compound and which are getting the placebo. At the conclusion of the study, researchers analyze the participants' medical records. Fewer premalignant or malignant lesions among the study group would support the hypothesis that the agent helps ward off the disease.

ANIMAL STUDIES

As the name implies, *animal studies* use animals rather than human volunteers. Here researchers have strict control over all variables: the food the animals consume, their exposure to cancer-causing agents, even their genetic predisposition to cancer.

The results of these studies can provide important clues. When studying the effects of chemicals believed to cause cancer, scientists expose the animals to far larger doses than any human could conceivably ingest. What's more, tumors are sometimes chemically induced, so that researchers can observe the impact of factors such as diet or drugs on cancer's progression. Obviously, tumors deliberately produced in rats are quite different from those that occur in humans, so the comparison value is limited. Nevertheless, we can learn a great deal from animal studies, which the National Academy of Sciences recently reaffirmed as a sound means for identifying potential cancer risks to humans.

POPULATION STUDIES

Population studies, also referred to as *epidemiologic studies,* fall into several categories, listed below. To explain the differences, let's look at diet as it pertains to cancer.

• *Ecologic studies* compare populations with low and high cancer rates, seeking to identify other differences that could influence the development of cancer. Ecologic studies, especially those comparing residents of different countries, suggest links between high-fat diets and colorectal, breast, prostate and uterine cancers. The major disadvantage of these studies is that their comparisons are between population averages, not individuals, so they cannot be used to draw firm conclusions about any particular food in relation to cancer.

• *Migrant studies* look at what happens when men and women

from geographic areas where cancer is relatively rare migrate to areas plagued by higher rates of cancer. Japanese who relocate to the United States and adopt American eating habits see their incidence of colorectal, prostate and breast cancers rise.

• *Case-control studies* compare the habits of cancer patients (the *cases*) with those of cancer-free men and women similar in age, gender and ethnic background (the *controls*). The goal, as in ecologic studies, is to identify differences that could explain why cases developed cancer and controls did not. These studies provide more specific and reliable evidence than ecologic studies, but they can be hard to conduct because it is difficult to find cases and control subjects who are similar in all respects except the suspected cause under investigation.

• For *cohort studies,* researchers enlist healthy volunteers who are generally alike except for their dietary habits. After a fixed amount of time—typically several years—cancer rates between the groups are compared to see if they correlate to any specific dietary factors.

SUGGESTED READING ABOUT CANCER

From the National Cancer Institute (800-4-CANCER):

• "Cancer Prevention"
• "What You Need to Know About Cancer"
• "Everything Doesn't Cause Cancer"

KEY WORDS

Cancer: Not one but approximately 150 diseases caused by abnormal cells that develop and divide uncontrollably. The four major types of cancer are *carcinoma, sarcoma, leukemia* and *lymphoma.*

Carcinoma in situ: A brief calm before the storm, when malignant cancer has yet to invade healthy tissue. In situ tumors are more curable than invasive or metastatic tumors.

Cells: The basic units of biologic growth and development for all living organisms.

Chemotherapy: Systemic cancer treatment through powerful anticancer drugs that are administered orally or intravenously. Often two or more medications are used in what is called combination chemotherapy.

Chromosomes: Twig-shaped structures that contain genes made up of linear threads of deoxyribonucleic acid, or DNA. Each cell's nucleus contains 23 pairs of chromosomes. Numbers 1 through 22 are *autosomes;* pair 23, labeled X and Y, determines a baby's sex.

Free radicals: Oxygen molecules that contain unpaired electrons. Sometimes the electrons' search for a mate disrupts normal cell functions, increasing the risk of cancer.

Genes: Biologic units, composed of DNA, that control all physical, biochemical and physiologic traits.

Immune system: A network of cells, cell products and cell tissues that defends the body against disease-causing agents such as bacteria, viruses and cancer.

Initiation: An event that causes a genetic mutation, predisposing a person to cancer.

Malignancy: A cancerous tumor capable of spreading, or *metastasizing.*

Metastasis: The process by which a colony of malignant cells separates from the primary site and travels to another site not adjacent or connected to it.

Oncogenes: Genes that promote the conversion of normal cells to cancer cells.

Placebo: A sugar pill or injection of sterile water given to a subject taking part in an experiment to test a drug's efficacy.

Promotion: An event that follows initiation to cause cancer.

Proto-oncogenes: The neutral or inactive stage that precedes the oncogene.

Radiation therapy: Treatment of disease by means of ionizing radiation from x-ray machines, cobalt, radium and other sources.

Staging: A classification system for identifying the extent of disease.

Tumor: A benign or malignant mass of tissue containing rapidly dividing cells.

PART TWO

The Building Blocks of a Cancer Prevention Program

CHAPTER

3

Assessing Your Cancer Risk

How Heredity, Personal Health History,
and Environmental and Lifestyle Factors
Influence Your Cancer Risk

The first step in tailoring a personal cancer-prevention program is to evaluate the factors that form your cancer risk profile, which in turn determines any modifications you may need to make in your lifestyle and the regimen of screening tests you may need to follow. We've divided these factors into "building blocks": *heredity, or family history, personal health history, environment* and *lifestyle*.

HEREDITARY FACTORS

Although most cancers are related to lifestyle and environmental factors—diet, tobacco and alcohol use, overexposure to the sun and so on—it is believed that an inherited genetic susceptibility increases a person's vulnerability to such factors.

Furthermore, a family history of certain cancers is in itself a risk factor. At present, we can clearly detect direct hereditary factors in but a small segment of cancer patients because only a handful of cancer-inducing genes have yet been identified. However, science has pegged more than 200 hereditary cancer patterns, in which a high incidence of cancer is woven through generations of some families, predisposing relatives to one or more malignancies. Examples include:

- Having a parent or sibling with colorectal cancer triples your risk of getting the disease.
- A woman's chances of being diagnosed with breast cancer double if her mother or sister had the disease.
- A man whose father or brother had prostate cancer has more than twice the risk of contracting the disease himself.
- A mother's or sister's history of ovarian cancer more than doubles a woman's risk.

Let us draw an important distinction: A familial pattern of cancer does not necessarily denote a hereditary component but could be due to common environmental or lifestyle factors. A high incidence of lung cancer may plague family A because a number of members smoke tobacco or perhaps live in a radon-contaminated home. Likewise, cervical cancer may appear to run in family B because successive generations of daughters repeat high-risk behavior such as early sexual activity and having multiple sexual partners.

Nevertheless, anyone whose family has been touched by cancer or an inherited syndrome (see accompanying box) should draw a family tree—something we show you how to do in Chapter 4— and bring it to his or her physician's attention, to determine whether genetic counseling and early cancer surveillance are appropriate.

HEREDITARY DISEASES AND SYNDROMES THAT MAY INDICATE A HEIGHTENED CANCER RISK

PROSTATE CANCER

Family history of
- prostate cancer

BREAST CANCER

Family history of
- breast cancer
- breast-ovarian cancer syndrome

LUNG CANCER

Family history of
- lung cancer

COLORECTAL CANCER

Family history of
- colorectal cancer
- adenomatous polyps

- hereditary nonpolyposis colorectal cancer (HNPCC), also known as Lynch syndrome II
- familial adenomatous polyposis (FAP)
- Gardner's syndrome

CERVICAL CANCER

None identified at present

UTERINE CANCER

Family history of
- Lynch syndrome II

OVARIAN CANCER

Family history of
- site-specific ovarian cancer syndrome
- Lynch syndrome II
- breast-ovarian cancer syndrome

ESOPHAGEAL CANCER

None identified at present

GASTRIC CANCER

- type A blood

Family history of
- gastric cancer

SKIN CANCERS

Any of the following traits:
- fair complexion
- red or blond hair
- many freckles
- blue, green or gray eyes
- a greater-than-average number of moles
- atypical moles
- an unusually large congenital mole (one present at birth)

Family history of
- xeroderma pigmentosum
- albinism
- basal-cell nevus syndrome
- dysplastic nevus syndrome
- familial atypical multiple mole melanoma (FAMMM) syndrome
- melanoma

PERSONAL HEALTH HISTORY FACTORS

A personal history of cancer elevates risk, as do certain nonmalignant conditions. The inflammatory bowel disease ulcerative colitis, for example, escalates the possibility of developing colorectal cancer, while diabetes places women at higher-than-average risk for malignancies of the uterus and ovaries. Reproductive history, too, influences risk: Women who've given birth are less likely to get uterine cancer than those who've never been mothers; having a first baby after age 30 is considered a risk factor for ovarian cancer.

Just as knowing your family pedigree can yield important clues as to your vulnerability to cancer, it's important to take stock of your personal medical history. Read the following list. Alert your doctor if you've had any of these conditions, so that the two of you can discuss whether or not you're a candidate for any preventive screening procedures.

DISEASES AND CONDITIONS THAT MAY INDICATE A HEIGHTENED CANCER RISK

PROSTATE CANCER

None identified at present

BREAST CANCER

Personal history of
- breast cancer
- moderate hyperplasia
- papilloma with a fibrovascular core (a benign tumor)
- atypical hyperplasia
- any medical condition that required large doses of radiation to the chest
- early menarche (beginning menstruation before age 12)
- late menopause (ending menstruation after age 50)
- no children
- first child born after age 30
- taking hormone replacement therapy
- using oral contraceptives (only for women at increased risk due to other factors)

LUNG CANCER

Personal history of
- chronic obstructive pulmonary disease, such as emphysema or chronic bronchitis
- lung scarring
- Hodgkin's disease
- any medical condition that required large doses of radiation to the chest
- lung cancer

COLORECTAL CANCER

Personal history of
- inflammatory bowel diseases (IBD) such as ulcerative colitis or Crohn's disease
- breast cancer
- ovarian cancer
- uterine cancer
- adenomatous colorectal polyps or cancer

CERVICAL CANCER

Personal history of
- sexually transmitted diseases such as genital herpes, gonorrhea, syphilis and genital warts (human papillomavirus, or HPV)
- vulvar dysplasia or cancer
- vaginal dysplasia or cancer
- cervical dysplasia or cancer
- exposure to the drug diethylstilbestrol (DES) before birth (taken by the mother during pregnancy)

UTERINE CANCER

Personal history of
- diabetes
- high blood pressure
- estrogen replacement therapy
- fibroid tumors that are still present
- uterine polyps
- adenomatous uterine hyperplasia
- colorectal cancer
- ovarian cancer
- breast cancer
- uterine cancer
- early menarche (beginning menstruation before age 12)
- late menopause (ending menstruation after age 50)
- no children

OVARIAN CANCER

Personal history of
- diabetes
- high blood pressure
- estrogen replacement therapy
- ovarian cysts or tumors
- colorectal cancer
- uterine cancer
- breast cancer
- first child born after age 30
- no children
- early menarche (beginning menstruation before age 12)
- late menopause (ending menstruation after age 50)

ESOPHAGEAL CANCER

Personal history of
- severe persistent heartburn
- Barrett's esophagus
- untreated achalasia
- caustic trauma to the esophagus (for example, from swallowing a corrosive substance)

GASTRIC CANCER

Personal history of
- pernicious anemia
- chronic atrophic gastritis
- achlorhydria or hypochlorhydria (lack of or reduced acid in the stomach)
- the microorganism *Helicobacter pylori*
- partial gastrectomy (the surgical removal of all or part of the stomach) as treatment for a noncancerous condition

SKIN CANCERS

Personal history of
- being pregnant
- leukemia
- lymphoma
- any medical condition that required chemotherapy or radiation therapy
- kidney transplant
- exposure to medical x-rays or treatments utilizing artificial ultraviolet radiation
- skin cancer

ENVIRONMENTAL FACTORS

In the field of cancer study, environmental factors traditionally encompass anything in our surroundings that influences the development of cancer, including lifestyle factors such as diet, tobacco and alcohol use, physical fitness and other personal habits. For the purposes of this book, we've separated these factors, limiting environmental factors specifically to carcinogens found in and around the home, the workplace and elsewhere. Examples include excessive exposure to various chemicals, pesticides and natural poisons that can lead to cancer. Workers who come into prolonged, unsafe contact with the gas vinyl chloride have comparatively higher concentrations of urinary bladder cancer; radon, a naturally occurring radioactive gas that can seep undetected into homes, is the number-two cause of lung cancer. Taking precautions against these environmental hazards, a subject discussed at length in Chapter 7, constitutes an important facet of primary prevention.

LIFESTYLE FACTORS

Lifestyle factors refer to personal behavior, the fuse that ignites approximately *four in five* cancers. Thirty-five percent of all cancer deaths can be traced to dietary factors, and tobacco use accounts for 30 percent of cancer mortalities. Reproductive and sexual behavior? Excessive alcohol use? Tack on another 7 percent and 3 percent, respectively. Overexposure to the sun's ultraviolet rays contributes an additional 3 percent of cancer deaths. No one knows for sure what effect the mind has on cancer, but we include this discussion under the heading of lifestyle.

Nothing can be done to reverse your genetic makeup or past medical history, and environmental factors, while alterable, contribute to relatively few cancers. Ultimately, the most effective way to avert this disease is to integrate cancer prevention into your daily life.

Heredity. Personal health history. Environment. Lifestyle.

These building blocks are intertwined, and all are vitally important to warding off cancer even if your family pedigree reveals a genetic predisposition to the disease. In most instances, you can counterbalance susceptibility by reducing or, ideally, eliminating other risk factors—cancer triggers—such as a high-fat diet, tobacco smoke, stress, and your exposure to radon, asbestos and other environmental carcinogens. The Building Blocks of a Cancer Prevention Program will demonstrate how.

KEY WORDS

Environmental factor: Exposure to environmental carcinogens that heighten the chances of getting cancer.

Health history factor: A personal medical condition that enhances cancer risk.

Hereditary factor: A genetically inherited predisposition to cancer.

Lifestyle factor: Refers to diet, body weight, personal habits such as tobacco and alcohol use, and so on, all of which can influence cancer risk.

CHAPTER

4

Heredity and Family History

How to Draw Your Family Tree •
The Benefits of Genetic Screening

The news that their mother had inoperable ovarian cancer hit Mary V. and her three sisters hard. "We were a very close family," says Mary, the second youngest, "and it was just devastating." In 1971 no cure existed for Caroline V.'s cancer, which had spread throughout the abdomen. In desperation, her doctors put the 54-year-old woman on a chemotherapeutic drug, "one they don't even use anymore," says Mary.

Caroline survived more than a year. Refusing to wallow in self-pity, she insisted her husband and daughters go on with their lives. But it was also a time to treasure the past.

"When my mother was dying," Mary says, "my older sister Kathy started recording a family history, because information can be lost forever after someone passes on." In compiling fascinating anecdotes from family members about relatives both deceased and living, Kathy stumbled upon fragments of medical information.

Their father, Edward, produced a death certificate for his own father, a victim of colon cancer at just 33 years of age. He also recalled how stomach cancer had ended the life of his only sister, Edna, in 1942. Caroline's mother had died at age 62 of uterine cancer. At the time, the significance of these details escaped everyone, for as Mary explains, "Nobody thought that colon cancer, uterine cancer and ovarian cancer in a family might be related somehow."

Following their mother's death, Kathy stored the half-bare family tree inside a drawer, taking it out now and then to add a detail gleaned from a distant relative. Over the next decade and a half she, Mary and the youngest sister, Susan, all flourished in their careers, while Margaret, the eldest, raised four children.

Two developments compelled Kathy to begin updating the family pedigree in earnest. In 1986 comedienne Gilda Radner focused public attention on ovarian cancer when she disclosed her battle with the disease. Around the same time, their father developed tumors of both the prostate and ureter.

Other cancers began to fill the family tree like so many spring leaves. Mary, by then a television reporter and anchorwoman with a husband and young son, wondered if ovarian cancer would stalk her and her sisters once they reached their fifties, as it had their mother.

Edward V., 75, died in August 1989, three months after Gilda Radner's death. While in California for the funeral, Susan, a 38-year-old government banking economist, complained of a pain in her side.

"She had just gotten married and was trying to start a family," Mary recalls. Her gynecologist initially diagnosed an ovarian cyst. But to everyone's shock—perhaps most of all the doctor's—exploratory surgery revealed a tumor on an ovary and another in the uterus. Susan began chemotherapy and radiation therapy at once. Meanwhile, says Mary, "the oncologist said the rest of us had to be checked."

That Christmas, everyone gathered in Los Angeles. Margaret flew in from Thailand, where her husband, a member of the foreign service, was stationed. The sisters conferred with several genetics specialists. "They all said that each of us had a fifty-fifty chance of getting ovarian cancer," says Mary, "because our mother and sister were first-degree relatives." *First degree* refers to a sibling, parent or child; *second degree,* a grandparent, maternal or paternal aunt or uncle, or grandchild; *third degree,* a great-grandparent, maternal or paternal great-aunt or great-uncle, or first cousin.

"One of the doctors went on to say, 'You should have your colons fully checked as well, because your family also has a risk of colon cancer at a young age. And that can be connected to ovarian *and* uterine cancers.' " Mary immediately thought back to her maternal grandmother, who'd died of uterine cancer. "I should also point out that while my mother was diagnosed with ovarian cancer, it's unclear whether she'd also had uterine cancer; the disease was too advanced for them to know at the time." This *syndrome,* or pattern of *familial* cancers, had a name: Lynch syndrome II. A familial disease is one that strikes relatives more often than would be expected by chance.

The doctor informed them that all three should undergo colonoscopies, a viewing procedure of the colon, as well as mammograms of the breasts, for yet another multiple cancer syndrome caused early tumors of the breasts and ovaries. And, he added, the sisters should consider having their ovaries and uteruses removed as a precautionary measure.

"It was so devastating," Mary recalls, "like the loss of innocence; the realization that at age 40 my days could really be numbered. I was looking at a 3-year-old child and trying to have a second. I didn't sleep and didn't stop crying for weeks."

Margaret and Kathy proceeded with their surgeries at once. The oldest sister was found to be cancer free. But Kathy, despite having exhibited no symptoms, had precancerous cells in her uterus and an early-stage ovarian tumor. "It was so tiny," says Mary, "they're lucky they found it."

The same day as her sisters' operations, Mary was en route to New York, her new home. Once settled there, she scheduled an appointment with Dr. William Hoskins, chief of the gynecology service at Memorial Sloan-Kettering. He confirmed the earlier recommendation for gynecologic surgery.

"Just before the operation," Mary recalls, "they wanted to do the colonoscopy as a routine check. That way if they did find anything, they could take care of it at the same time." Her siblings' colonoscopies had not revealed any evidence of colorectal cancer, and the family had wondered if the invasive exam had truly been necessary.

"But when Dr. Shike performed the colonoscopy on me, he discovered a tiny malignant tumor." Eerily, the lesion occupied the same section of the colon as the tumor that had killed her paternal grandfather as a young man. So in addition to the already scheduled surgery, doctors removed a section of Mary's colon. Nothing suspicious was discovered in either her ovaries or her uterus.

The V. family's extraordinary story doesn't end there, unfortunately. No sooner had Mary recovered from her surgery than

Kathy's cancer, thought to be fully cured, returned in the lining of the pelvic cavity, or peritoneum. The initial prognosis was not encouraging, but Kathy responded extremely well to intensive chemotherapy. Two years later doctors pronounced her in *remission;* that is, showing no signs of cancer.

What might have happened had Kathy not chronicled the family's medical history? Or had physicians not known enough about cancer and heredity to recommend aggressive treatment? Mary V. shudders at the thought.

"If I didn't know my family history," she says bluntly, "I would be dead or close to it. Because I had no symptoms at all. None. I was very, very lucky."

Heredity plays a role in many major adult cancers. Therefore assessing your family's medical history is a valuable tool in combating cancer. We can put family members deemed susceptible under aggressive surveillance, which—as the case of Mary V. and her sisters dramatically illustrates—can be a lifesaving measure. What's more, by following the primary prevention steps outlined in this section, even men and women who are at high risk because of the genes they carry can help to trim their odds of getting cancer.

GENES: HUMAN PROGRAMMING

Since we live in the computer age, it seems appropriate to compare genes to a software program, one that creates, maintains and repairs all aspects of the human body. It is no exaggeration to say genes make up the blueprint of our existence.

Imagine you're looking at a human cell under a microscope. In the middle sits the *nucleus,* the spheroid body that houses all genetic material. Enlarging the image with one of today's superpower microscopes reveals within the nucleus 23 pairs of twig-shaped structures called *chromosomes.* Pairs 1 through 22 are referred to by number. The remaining twosome, the sex chromosomes, are labeled X and Y. Women's cells possess two X chromosomes; men's, one X and one Y.

Each chromosome is a collection of genes, strings of chemical material called DNA that control every physical, biochemical and physiologic trait, from hair color to intellect to the level of cholesterol in the bloodstream.

When a cell divides, a process known as *mitosis,* each new

daughter cell formed departs with an exact copy of its parents' chromosomes. However, a man's sperm and a woman's egg, or ovum, form through *meiosis,* with each receiving only one of each pair of the chromosomes found in all the cells. Should conception take place, and the sperm penetrate the ovum, the fertilized egg is left with a new full set of 46, or 23 pairs. It then divides over and over, developing eventually into an embryo.

But which 46 chromosomes? A sperm bearing an X chromosome produces a girl; a Y chromosome, a boy. The process that determines our genetic composition is a lot like a lottery drawing: A man can produce 8 million genetically different sperm; and a woman, the same number of genetically different ova. That's 64 million potential combinations.

Thus we are products of our parents in the most literal sense. However, although your mother and father each bequeathed you half your genes, heredity is truly a multigenerational affair. After all, your parents inherited their genetic programming from *their* parents, who inherited their genetic programming from *their* parents, and on and on. In reality, we share 50 percent of our genes with each parent and sibling; 25 percent with each grandparent, aunt and uncle; and 12.5 percent with each great-grandparent, great-aunt and great-uncle and first cousin. Identical twins share 100 percent of their genes.

When you consider the endless variables that shape a person's genetic structure, it's a miracle that family members even remotely resemble one another at all:

- Depending on the blend of chromosomes, genes can express themselves in one generation but not another.
- Most traits are fashioned not by a single gene but by a combination of several.
- Genes are described as being either dominant or recessive. A dominant gene—brown eyes, for example—will take precedence over a recessive gene, such as blue eyes. Therefore, only two blue-eye genes will produce a blue-eyed child. (This baby's parents need not have blue eyes themselves, but each must carry the trait.)
- Finally, genes sometimes mutate, so that a trait mysteriously appears or disappears in a family.

Just as genes determine eye color and the shape of a nose, they can predispose offspring to cancer, either directly or indirectly.

One person may inherit a cancer gene that in time results in a malignancy, while another may inherit a genetic susceptibility to the disease that is later triggered by an environmental factor.

Understanding the association between cancer and heredity dates back to A.D. 100, when Roman physicians observed with great interest a familial clustering of breast cancer. But the first major breakthrough in this field would be nearly two millennia in coming, and then only due to a chance conversation between a pathologist and a seamstress.

In 1895 Dr. Aldred Scott Warthin, today regarded as the father of cancer genetics, had just been appointed a demonstrator of pathology at the University of Michigan. One day he noticed his seamstress looking troubled. "What seems to be the matter?" he inquired.

She replied that she expected to die of cancer, as had virtually all her relatives. Intrigued, Warthin began to study two generations of her family, which would become known as "Warthin's Family G." As of 1913, the year he published his groundbreaking paper, "Heredity with Reference to Carcinoma as Shown by the Study of the Cases Examined in the Pathological Laboratory of the University of Michigan, 1895–1913," the preponderance of cancer in this family was truly extraordinary: Of 48 members, 17 died or had to be treated for cancer. Sadly, the seamstress's prophecy came true; she succumbed to carcinoma of the uterus. The same study tracked three more cancer-ravaged families, two of which were rendered extinct by the disease. Warthin, a virtuoso musician as well as a brilliant physician, concluded, "A marked susceptibility to carcinoma exists in the case of certain family generations and family groups." The doctor died in 1931, probably never imagining the extent to which cancer and heredity would be correlated.

CANCER PREDISPOSITION GENES

Of the handful of cancer predisposition genes that have been identified, cloned and named to date, most are associated with children's cancers. The best studied are retinoblastoma and Wilms' tumor. Four in ten cases of retinoblastoma, a cancer of the eye found primarily in children under age 4, are caused by an abnormal retinoblastoma gene (Rb), which has been localized to chromosome 13. It is generally passed down from parent to child. A defective gene on chromosome 11, called *WT1*, touches off Wilms' tumor, a congenital (meaning present at birth) pediatric cancer of the kidneys.

With respect to adult cancers, much progress has been made in identifying specific genes that cause a variety of familial cancer syndromes. A 1993 study published in the *New England Journal of Medicine* cited a mutant *HRAS1* gene in more than 50,000 cancers a year, of the breast, colon and bladder, leukemia, and possibly the lung and prostate as well, while in 1994 a group of Utah researchers announced their discovery of yet another mutant gene: *MTS1*. This multiple tumor suppressor appeared in more than half the tumors they examined, including those of the lung, ovary, kidney, brain, breast, blood, bladder, bone and skin.

There are more than 200 hereditary cancer syndromes that cast ominous shadows over certain families' futures. Some examples:

• *Hereditary breast and ovarian cancer syndrome.* A number of families have been studied in areas around the world where there is a high prevalence of either breast cancer alone or breast and ovarian cancer. This syndrome is characterized by the early onset of cancer and the inheritance of a gene on chromosome 17, *BRCA1*, which is responsible for the syndrome.

What's more, a defective *BRCA1* gene is responsible for about half of all inherited cases of breast cancer. The more than 600,000 women who may carry this defective gene see their chances of developing breast cancer during their lifetime rise to 85 percent. (The average risk is approximately 11 percent.) A second gene, *BRCA2*, located on chromosome 13, has yet to be isolated, but scientists believe that it too genetically predisposes to breast cancer.

• *Basal-cell nevus syndrome.* A genetic propensity to develop malignancies of the skin in unusual areas of the body, such as the palms of the hands and the soles of the feet.

• *Familial atypical multiple-mole melanoma syndrome.* FAMMM, a dominant genetic disorder, leaves family members prone to malignant melanoma as well as cancers of the eye, breast, respiratory tract, gastrointestinal tract and lymphatic system. One in twenty offspring will inherit the disease.

• *Li-Fraumeni syndrome.* Named for the two doctors who discovered it, this syndrome is as pernicious as it is rare. Only 100 families the world over have been diagnosed with Li-Fraumeni syndrome, which heightens their vulnerability to seven cancers (including breast cancer, leukemia, osteosarcoma and soft-tissue sarcoma) at an unusually early age. National Cancer Institute scientists recently linked the syndrome to a mutant p53 tumor-suppressor gene that, instead of destroying cancer cells, permits them to thrive.

• *Familial adenomatous polyposis.* FAP accounts for about 1 percent of colorectal cancer cases in the United States. As Dr. Hans Gerdes of Memorial Sloan-Kettering explains, "Men and women with FAP develop thousands of potentially cancerous polyps in their large intestine, usually starting around puberty. Their risk of colorectal cancer is so high that doctors recommend what's called prophylactic colectomy, in which the colon is surgically removed, usually in the early twenties, before cancer develops.

"The syndrome FAP," he continues, "is usually transmitted from an affected parent to half of the children. However, as many as one third of cases are new mutations, meaning that the two parents of such a person were not affected, though the individual may have developed the gene for the syndrome prior to birth."

The gene for familial adenomatous polyposis has been localized to chromosome 5 and been named *APC,* for adenomatous polyposis coli. Those who have FAP possess one normal and one abnormal *APC* gene, but the abnormal gene appears to result in the full syndrome (a dominant gene). A blood test to identify the abnormal *APC* gene has recently been developed and is undergoing clinical trials. Using this test, all other family members could be tested to determine their risk for the disease.

• *Lynch syndrome I.* Families beset by Lynch I, also known as hereditary nonpolyposis colorectal cancer (HNPCC), exhibit unusually high rates of colorectal cancer, and at a relatively young age: under 50. Unlike FAP, people with Lynch syndrome I have only a few colorectal polyps that progress into cancer, so it is a much more difficult condition to diagnose.

• *Lynch syndrome II,* the type of HNPCC that has ravaged Mary V.'s family, exemplifies what cancer geneticists call variable expression. Lynch II sufferers are in danger of an array of cancers: primarily early-onset colorectal, uterine and ovarian, but also cancers of the ureter, small bowel, stomach and pancreas.

The story of the syndrome's discovery recalls Dr. Aldred Warthin and the seamstress. In 1962 a medical resident at the University of Nebraska Medical Center, Dr. Henry T. Lynch, encountered a patient diagnosed as psychologically disturbed.

"He had a great fear that he was going to die of cancer," Dr. Lynch recalls. "He said that everybody in his family had died of cancer of the colon or the gynecologic system. This cancer pattern seemed quite unusual at the time. I was really interested in cardiology and was going to be a cardiologist. But I had been a geneticist before I went to medical school.

"I worked up his pedigree, and lo and behold, about half of his first-degree relatives had colon cancer, and a number of them had gynecologic cancer, just as he'd said. I became fascinated with the family, a huge one from Missouri and Nebraska. So I studied them, and I grew so fascinated with cancer in general, I pursued the family for years throughout my residency and then when I elected to go into oncology.

"Finally, through some colleagues at the University of Michigan, I found another family"—which turned out to be none other than Warthin's Family G. "We immediately studied that family, because we thought it had some similarities." Dr. Lynch's quest for death certificates and other evidence took him to Germany, where the family originated.

"We know now," he says, "that it was the same syndrome." In his 1966 paper on this multiple-cancer pattern, Dr. Lynch referred to it as "cancer family syndrome"; it was later renamed in his honor.

The study of cancer genetics became such a passion for Dr. Lynch that in the early 1970s he established the Hereditary Cancer Institute in Omaha, Nebraska. There he studies and screens high-risk relatives in cancer-prone families. Among those under study: the family of Mary V.

The ongoing efforts of physicians like Dr. Lynch to help people with a familial predisposition to cancer has brought about a greater understanding of these conditions and has also led to the development of better methods of diagnosis. In 1993 the gene responsible for Lynch syndrome was located on chromosome 2 by a group of investigators from Finland, Canada, New Zealand and the United States. These researchers found that men and women who had inherited the abnormal gene *(MSH2)* developed cancers that contained multiple abnormalities in their chromosomes. They termed it "the mutator gene." Additional genes have been implicated.

HOW GENETIC SCREENING WORKS

The V. family's experience illustrates the practical application of genetic screening: first, to identify families at risk of hereditary cancer, then to direct them to appropriate surveillance programs, so that should they one day develop cancer, it can be halted while still at a curable stage.

It is not routine in this country to offer patients genetic screening for cancer. Awareness and appreciation of family history are not uniform among physicians, even among oncologists.

We envision the role of genetic screening in cancer prevention this way:

A fictional patient we'll call Suzanne F., 37, visits Memorial Sloan-Kettering's Evelyn Lauder Breast Center for her first mammogram. In the course of taking Suzanne's medical and family histories, her physician learns that one grandmother died of breast cancer at age 78, while an older sister had the disease in her early forties but was treated successfully. Before Suzanne was born, uterine cancer took the life of her other grandmother. And her 67-year-old father, diagnosed with both prostate and bladder cancers over the last seven years, is in remission and doing well.

The doctor passes along this information to Karen Brown, a genetic counselor at Memorial Sloan-Kettering. One look at the family's history raises concern, for the F. family meets all the basic criteria of hereditary cancer:

1. Cancer that develops 15 to 20 years earlier than normal.
2. Cancer that affects more than one close relative.
3. One or more close relatives with more than one form of cancer.
4. Cancer that spans more than one generation.

In cases where inheritance appears likely, a note is sent to the doctor saying that the patient's family history demonstrates that she and her family might benefit from genetic counseling. We ask the doctor's permission to contact the patient.

Ultimately, it is the patient's decision whether or not to make an appointment.

Suzanne, anxious to learn what she can do to protect herself from cancer, agrees to attend a counseling session. Her two sisters would like to accompany her, but both live out of state, so it is agreed that Suzanne will go and report back to them.

"F" FAMILY HISTORY

Name   Suzanne F.

Address   794 Sawyer Ct.

             Mahwah, NJ

Date of birth   4-13-57

Please list all family members including those without cancer. This information will be used to develop a family tree.

RELATIVE	NAME	DATE OF BIRTH	HISTORY OF CANCER	TYPE OF CANCER	AGE AT DIAGNOSIS	ALIVE OR DEAD	DATE OF DEATH
MOTHER	Evelyn	5-18-28	None			Alive	
FATHER	John	8-28-26	Yes	Prostate Bladder	63 60	Alive	
SISTERS	Johnetta	1-2-47	Yes	Breast	41	Alive	
	Danielle	5-2-59	None			Alive	
BROTHERS	Richard	8-15-51	None			Alive	
DAUGHTERS	Chelsea	1-16-86	None			Alive	
SONS	Joshua	12-21-91	None			Alive	

	Name	Birth Date		Cause	Age	Status	Death Date
MOTHER'S MOTHER	Dora	2-23-08	Yes	Breast	76	Dead	4-13-86
MOTHER'S FATHER	Charles	9-11-02	None			Dead	3-14-84
FATHER'S MOTHER	Matilda	5-18-05	Yes	Uterine	43	Dead	7-2-49
FATHER'S FATHER	Paul	10-30-04	None			Alive	
MATERNAL AUNTS (Your mother's sisters)	Peggy	6-10-26	None			Alive	
PATERNAL AUNTS (Your father's sisters)	Elise	11-4-29	None			Alive	
	Alice	2-17-31	None			Alive	
MATERNAL UNCLES (Your mother's brothers)	Alfred	6-10-25	None			Dead	2-26-45
	Michael	7-23-30	None			Alive	
PATERNAL UNCLES (Your father's brothers)	Robert	9-9-33	None			Alive	
ANY ADDITIONAL RELATIVES NOT LISTED ABOVE (Ex. Half Brothers & Sisters, Cousins, etc.)							

FAMILY HISTORY

Name _____

Address _____

Date of birth _____

Please list all family members including those without cancer. This information will be used to develop a family tree.

RELATIVE	NAME	DATE OF BIRTH	HISTORY OF CANCER	TYPE OF CANCER	AGE AT DIAGNOSIS	ALIVE OR DEAD	DATE OF DEATH
MOTHER							
FATHER							
SISTERS							
BROTHERS							
DAUGHTERS							
SONS							

MOTHER'S MOTHER							
MOTHER'S FATHER							
FATHER'S MOTHER							
FATHER'S FATHER							
MATERNAL AUNTS (Your mother's sisters)							
PATERNAL AUNTS (Your father's sisters)							
MATERNAL UNCLES (Your mother's brothers)							
PATERNAL UNCLES (Your father's brothers)							
ANY ADDITIONAL RELATIVES NOT LISTED ABOVE (Ex. Half Brothers & Sisters, Cousins, etc.)							

First she is asked to fill out a confidential family history questionnaire, similar to the one reproduced here. It gives you an idea of the type of information patients are asked to supply:

- The names of parents, siblings, paternal and maternal aunts and uncles, grandparents, first cousins and children
- Whether the relative is alive or deceased
- The relative's current age or age at death
- Any history of cancer, and if so:
- Which type(s) of cancer(s)
- The relative's age at the time of diagnosis

From this we diagram the main branches of the F. family tree. But ideally, still others need to be added. "We like to go back as far as we can," explains Dr. Kenneth Offit, director of Memorial Sloan-Kettering's clinical genetics service. "Usually you can get back to the great-grandparents, then things become cloudy. "Each generation of information is critically important, because it tells you about a gene's pattern of movement through the family. Very often that becomes our only guidepost to an inherited syndrome."

Given the crucial decisions that may be made based on a patient's family history, all information must be verified through death certificates, medical records and hospital discharge summaries, for people are often mistaken about the details. They may think, for example, that a relative had breast cancer, when in fact she never did. Or they'll note as "liver cancer" what was actually breast cancer that metastasized to the liver.

At Memorial Sloan-Kettering's clinical genetics service, a data manager assists patients in tracking down these and other records. Once Mary V. recovered from the tidal wave of cancer that engulfed her and her sisters, she took it upon herself to complete the family tree. Being a reporter, digging up information came naturally to her. But anyone, she assures us, can do the same.

"The very first thing that you do is to ask a lot of questions, particularly of elderly relatives in your family," says Mary, author of a book on how to construct a family pedigree. "Some of the matters they're talking about might be very sensitive, so you have to be patient and kind and assure them that there are reasons for knowing it. Approach it from the standpoint that this could help the entire family.

"Then you want to get your hands on the medical records of anybody who's still living and has gone through a medical situation. Designate somebody the family librarian, to gather up all the medical materials and keep a confidential file that doctors can have access to."

Next, send away for copies of family members' death certificates. You can obtain them through the vital records division for the state in which the relative died. In New York, for example, it is called the vital records section and operates under the state department of health. Just dial information for the state capital and ask for the phone number of the vital records branch. The staff there or a recording will give you the mailing address and other pertinent information, such as cost. Most states charge a nominal fee of $10 to $15 per copy, payable by check or money order.

Be sure to include the following in your written request:

- The deceased's full name as it would have appeared on the certificate
- The city, town or village in which he/she died
- The exact date of death (if you don't know, you must at least pinpoint the year)
- Your relationship to this person
- Your reason for requesting a copy of the death certificate

Should the department be unable to locate the certificate, it will advise you of this by mail. You may be referred to the vital records bureau of the county, city or town in which the person died. Don't be surprised if your investigation runs into the occasional roadblock. Genetic counselor Karen Brown recalls one family that had an entire generation wiped out during the Russian Revolution. Other dead ends are shrouded in mystery, with the deceased's records seeming to have vanished without a trace. In such instances, double-check with relatives the date and place of death.

It's remarkable what that single sheet of paper can tell you— not only the date and cause of death, but the onset of illness, so crucial in determining whether a disease may be genetically inherited. While Mary V. knew that her maternal grandmother had died of uterine cancer at age 62, the death certificate disclosed that Selma had been diagnosed five years before, "so it became a much more significant piece of information."

Another invaluable detail: the hospital in which the person died. "This can lead you to medical records," says Mary, "if you're really persistent." Contact the hospital's medical records branch and inquire, "How do I obtain the medical records for _____, who died there on _____? I am his/her _____ and am researching a medical family tree."

"Some states have privacy laws that make it very difficult to get medical records," Mary explains, "but in others it's easy for family members." If you meet resistance, your physician may be able to intervene on your behalf, stating in a letter that these documents are needed to make a proper diagnosis.

Mary learned firsthand how the passage of time sometimes distorts memories. "My father had always said that his sister died when she was 32 of stomach cancer," she recalls. "I sent away for her death certificate and found out that she'd had *ovarian* cancer. Had we known when my sister Susan was having problems with her ovaries that ovarian cancer existed at such a young age on my father's side of the family, we might have been much more aggressive in getting her treated earlier." Mary's father had kept letters from his sister, then recently married and living a distance away.

"I discovered that his sister's husband had told him in a letter that it was ovarian cancer. But it just didn't seem very significant to him at the time." Fifty years later the news came as a revelation. "It helped confirm the syndrome for us," she says, "that we had ovarian, colon and uterine cancers on that side of the family."

DRAWING YOUR FAMILY PEDIGREE

Once you have assembled as much information as possible, you can construct your family tree. Take a large piece of paper and in the middle draw your generation of the family, using circles for women and squares for men. Write the person's name below each, and denote any cancers by shading the shape, as we've done in charting the fictitious F. family. Furnish additional details such as whether the relative is living or deceased, the type or types of cancers, and the age of onset and/or death.

Connect these with a horizontal line, then extend a vertical line upward and start to work on your parents' generation. Then your grandparents'. And so on. Children's and grandchildren's generations, if applicable, would go below yours, also joined by a vertical line. Indicate the *proband*, the original person whose symptoms or disease prompted the genetic study, with an arrow. For reference, compare the written information on Suzanne F.'s family history questionnaire with her family pedigree.

"F" Family Pedigree

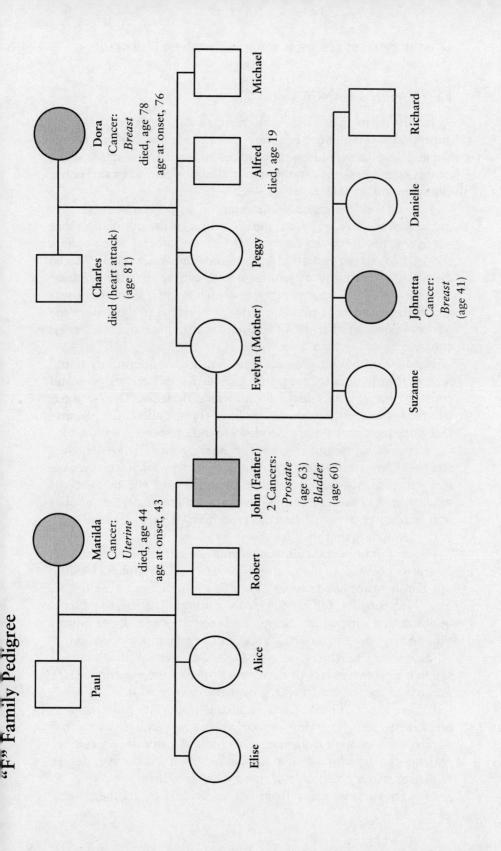

ESTIMATING CANCER RISK

A family deemed at risk for hereditary cancer is routed to an appropriate surveillance program. Suzanne F. and her cancer-free sister, Danielle, would be encouraged to have yearly gynecologic exams encompassing a mammogram, clinical breast exam, pelvic exam and a Pap smear.

The flip side of genetic counseling is to prevent unnecessary medical procedures. There's a great subset of the population that perceives they're at extremely high risk for cancer, when in fact they're not. Karen Brown offers as an example a woman who so dreads the possibility of getting breast cancer that she contemplates prophylactic mastectomy, in which healthy breasts are surgically removed as a preventive measure. This is done only for patients considered to be at *extraordinarily* high risk for breast cancer.

Needless to say, a woman considering this operation should receive thorough counseling that carefully spells out its pros and cons, so that she may make an informed decision. The National Cancer Institute urges anyone thinking about undergoing prophylactic mastectomy to *always* seek a second opinion.

"Genetic counseling is generally nondirective," Karen Brown stresses. "So we take the stance that although prophylactic mastectomy is certainly not a mainstream option for the majority of women, it may well be suitable for women coming from families with strong patterns of hereditary cancer, who really can't live with the anxiety that they feel."

Hence the importance of conveying a patient's cancer risk as clearly as possible, in plain language. "It's not as simple as looking at a family history and saying, 'Your risk is high, low or intermediate,' " explains Dr. Offit. "We try to communicate risk to patients in absolute terms, which means the percentage of risk per unit of time. As opposed to saying, 'Your risk is four times increased,' " an assessment that may be meaningless to some patients, "we'll say that a woman's risk of developing breast cancer before age 25 is equal to the risk of drowning over the next year.

"These kinds of numbers are critically important for most people, because they're trying to figure out what these risks mean." Armed with enough information to make an informed decision, patients choose which course to take based on whether the degree of cancer risk is acceptable or unacceptable to them.

"It varies dramatically from one individual to another," says

Dr. Offit. "This is made vividly clear when counseling women with family histories of breast cancer who are considering hormone replacement therapy." Hormone pills, given to postmenopausal women to counteract symptoms of menopause, may heighten slightly the risk of breast cancer. But they are also a great aid in preventing cardiovascular disease and osteoporosis, a thinning of the bones in elderly women.

"We've given the same types of statistical results to women with very similar histories," Dr. Offit continues, "and in one case a woman will find any increased risk of breast cancer totally unacceptable, even though her risk for heart disease and bone fracture would be dramatically decreased; whereas another woman will see the same figures and say she had no idea that her risk for developing significant cardiac disease was in the range of 20 percent to 30 percent over the next ten years, or *double* her risk of developing breast cancer."

The next frontier in cancer genetics is DNA testing, something now being conducted on an experimental basis in major cancer centers such as ours. By drawing a patient's blood and analyzing the DNA, cancer geneticists can determine whether seemingly healthy individuals carry genes that will cause disease later in life or predispose them to a specific disorder.

At present we don't screen routinely for cancer predisposition genes, so that an accurately constructed family tree remains our most useful predictor of hereditary cancer risk. But genetic testing may soon become a clinical reality for cancers such as colorectal and breast.

Dr. Hans Gerdes uses the example of a family afflicted with familial adenomatous polyposis to explain the dual benefits of genetic testing. "In FAP families, identifying individuals with the disease requires endoscopic examinations for polyps and cancers. The children of someone with FAP are usually examined with sigmoidoscopy to identify those who have inherited the FAP gene and will develop the disease. But," he notes, "only half these children will actually inherit this gene. The other half may not, and therefore will be examined by sigmoidoscopy needlessly." Sigmoidoscopy involves inserting a flexible viewing instrument up the anus and into the colon and requires consuming a clear-liquid diet and cleansing the bowel beforehand.

"A genetic blood test has recently been developed for FAP families to help identify those children who have the gene and will require surveillance and treatment, as well as those children who have *not* inherited the gene, will not develop the syndrome, and thus do not require surveillance and treatment."

Dr. Gerdes cautions that this type of potential genetic testing may be useful only to families affected with FAP and the inherited syndromes described earlier in this chapter, such as Lynch syndrome II and hereditary breast and ovarian cancer syndrome. (Genetic testing to identify the transmission of the *BRCA1* gene responsible for the latter syndrome and hereditary breast cancer is currently being offered at a number of cancer centers, and a similar blood test to screen for Lynch syndrome is expected soon.)

TRYING TO ENSURE THAT HISTORY NEVER REPEATS

No one wants to be told that a lethal disease may be pursuing them, all because of a toss of the genetic dice. You might think

Anyone can research his or her own family tree, but to properly analyze this information requires the expertise of a genetic counselor. The Cancer Information Service (800-4-CANCER), sponsored by the National Cancer Institute, can refer you to medical centers in your area that have genetic counseling departments.

Dr. Henry Lynch's Hereditary Cancer Institute offers free genetic counseling to those who suspect a pattern of hereditary cancer in their family. You or your physician can contact the institute at (800-648-8133). If there does seem to be a significant enough history, you will be sent a detailed family questionnaire to complete. The institute writes to family members for permission to obtain their medical records for verifying reported cancers, then its health-care team reviews the family history and recommends appropriate surveillance measures. For more information contact the Hereditary Cancer Institute, Creighton University, Department of Preventive Medicine, 2500 California Plaza, Omaha, NE 68178.

Memorial Sloan-Kettering Cancer Center's clinical genetics service recently established a similar program, which you can contact at 1275 York Avenue, New York, NY 10021, (212-639-7099).

SUGGESTED READING ABOUT HOW TO RESEARCH AND
DRAW YOUR FAMILY TREE

- *How Healthy Is Your Family Tree? A Complete Guide to Tracing Your Family's Medical and Behavioral History,* by Carol Krause (Fireside, New York, 1995).

---

that the weight of such distressing news would leave a patient dispirited, defeated, immobilized. That's not at all the effect it had on Mary V. and her sisters.

"The fact that we could take action and do something that might improve our chances for survival was tremendously empowering and lifted us out of our depression," she emphasizes. "That we could actually have some control over our medical destiny really helped.

"Knowledge empowers you. I am a living, breathing example of that."

KEY WORDS

Congenital: Present at birth.

Familial cancer syndrome: A pattern of cancer that strikes family members more than would be expected by chance.

First-degree relative: Parent, sibling or child.

Proband: The original person whose symptoms or disease prompts a genetic study.

Second-degree relative: Grandparent, aunt, uncle or grandchild.

Third-degree relative: Great-grandparent, great-aunt, great-uncle or first cousin.

CHAPTER
5

Diet and Nutrition

Cutting Down on Fat · Increasing
Fruits and Vegetables, Grains and
Fiber · Antioxidants · Chemoprevention

It seems every time you open a newspaper you encounter yet
another "groundbreaking" report that some food or nutrient
either causes or prevents cancer. One day everyone is talking
about fiber, the next day it's carrots or broccoli. You know you
should pay attention to these reports, but trying to keep up with
the onslaught of information—not to mention trying to adjust
your eating habits to the newest findings—is confusing enough to
make anyone give up in exasperation.

We hear this from our patients time and again. But as we tell
them, before you mutter, "The heck with it all!" and reach for the
chocolate cake, take heart. With just a little effort, you can eat a
diet that significantly reduces your risk of developing several types
of cancer, improves your general health and still allows you to
enjoy your food.

Consider this: Scientists now believe that at least one third of
all cancers are related to what we eat. Some think that as many as
40 percent of men's cancers and *60 percent* of women's are linked
to diet. That's enough to make anyone take a second look at what
is on his or her plate! In this chapter we'll show you what to look
for and how to make some changes.

Nutrition is a complex subject, and one we still have a lot to learn about. No single food or nutrient can be thought of as a "magic bullet" that will protect you from cancer. Taken together, however, the years of research on a variety of foods and types of cancer have yielded enough information to enable us to offer broad guidelines on what your overall dietary plan should look like, guidelines that you can follow *right now*.

Adjusting your diet will require effort. You'll need to consider everything you eat and learn about the many components that make up your diet: fats, calories, vitamins, minerals, fiber and naturally occurring chemicals. You'll probably have to change habits developed over many years.

You will not, however, have to carry around a calculator and a food scale. We'll give you the basic guidelines to follow, the reasons why, and plenty of food choices. Before you know it, eating healthily will become a routine part of your life, rather like getting dressed in the morning. Just like getting dressed, on some days you'll get it right, while on others you may not put it together perfectly. But all in all you'll have it figured out.

We also want to assure you that you won't have to give up the foods you love for a bland, unappealing diet. (But no, you won't be able to eat steak and chocolate cake every day.) What we propose is not a rigid "diet" at all, but guidelines for healthy, enjoyable eating that adjust to your life—and your taste buds. As a bonus, an anticancer diet may help you avoid other health problems, such as heart disease, and you'll look and feel better than you have in years.

THE CANCER PREVENTION DIET

Surveys show that in the past few years, about one third of Americans have modified their diets for health reasons, so you may already be following principles of an anticancer diet without realizing it. On the other hand, nearly everyone has some room for improvement.

Let's start by looking at what you're eating now. Because what we *say* we eat and what we actually put in our mouth are often quite different, we suggest you write down everything you eat for at least four days, including one weekend day. This should give you a good idea of your typical diet.

Also, complete the accompanying "Eating Smart Quiz," prepared by the American Cancer Society. Be honest! The more truth-

EATING SMART QUIZ

Oils & Fats		Points
butter, margarine, shortening, mayonnaise, sour cream, lard, oil, salad dressing	I always add these to foods in cooking and/or at the table.	0
	I occasionally add these to foods in cooking and/or at the table.	1
	I rarely add these to foods in cooking and/or at the table.	2
	I eat fried foods 3 or more times a week.	0
	I eat fried foods 1–2 times a week.	1
	I rarely eat fried foods.	2

Dairy Products		
	I drink whole milk.	0
	I drink 1%–2% fat milk.	1
	I seldom eat frozen desserts or ice cream.	2
	I eat ice cream almost every day.	0
	Instead of ice cream, I eat ice milk, low-fat frozen yogurt & sherbet.	1
	I eat only fruit ices, seldom eat frozen dairy dessert.	2
	I eat mostly high-fat cheese (jack, cheddar, colby, Swiss, cream).	0
	I eat both low- and high-fat cheeses.	1
	I eat mostly low-fat cheeses (pot, 2% cottage, skim milk mozzarella).	2

Snacks		
potato/corn chips, nuts, buttered popcorn, candy bars	I eat these every day.	0
	I eat some occasionally.	1
	I seldom or never eat these snacks.	2

Baked Goods		
pies, cakes, cookies, sweet rolls, doughnuts	I eat them 5 or more times a week.	0
	I eat them 2–4 times a week.	1
	I seldom eat baked goods or eat only low-fat baked goods.	2

Poultry & Fish *

I rarely eat these foods.	0	☐
I eat them 1–2 times a week.	1	
I eat them 3 or more times a week.	2	

Low-Fat Meats

extralean hamburger, round steak, pork loin roast, tenderloin, chuck roast

I rarely eat these foods.	0	☐
I eat these foods occasionally.	1	
I eat mostly fat-trimmed red meats.	2	

High-Fat Meat *

luncheon meats, bacon, hot dogs, sausage, steak, regular & lean ground beef

I eat these every day.	0	☐
I eat these foods occasionally.	1	
I rarely eat these foods.	2	

Cured & Smoked Meat & Fish *

luncheon meats, hot dogs, bacon, ham & other smoked or pickled meats and fish

I eat these foods 4 or more times a week.	0	☐
I eat some 1–3 times a week.	1	
I seldom eat these foods.	2	

Legumes

dried beans & peas: kidney, navy, lima, pinto, garbanzo, split-pea, lentil

I eat legumes less than once a week.	0	☐
I eat these foods 1–2 times a week.	1	
I eat them 3 or more times a week.	2	

Whole Grains & Cereals

whole-grain breads, brown rice, pasta, whole-grain cereals

I seldom eat such foods.	0	☐
I eat them 2–3 times a day.	1	
I eat them 4 or more times daily.	2	

Vitamin C–Rich Fruits & Vegetables

citrus fruits and juices, green peppers, strawberries, tomatoes

I seldom eat them.	0	☐
I eat them 3–5 times a week.	1	
I eat them 1–2 times a day.	2	

Dark Green & Deep Yellow Fruits & Vegetables **

broccoli, greens, carrots, peaches, etc.

I seldom eat them.	0	☐
I eat them 3–5 times a week.	1	
I eat them daily.	2	

Vegetables of the Cabbage Family			
broccoli, cabbage, brussels sprouts, cauliflower, etc.	I seldom eat them.	0	☐
	I eat them 1–2 times a week.	1	
	I eat them 3–4 times a week.	2	

Alcohol			
	I drink more than 2 oz. daily.	0	☐
	I drink alcohol every week but not daily.	1	
	I occasionally or never drink alcohol.	2	

Personal Weight (see Chapter 6 for ideal weight)			
	I'm more than 20 lbs. over my ideal weight.	0	☐
	I'm 10–20 lbs. over my ideal weight.	1	
	I am within 10 lbs. of my ideal weight.	2	
	Total Score		☐

* If you do not eat meat, fish or poultry, give yourself a 2 for each meat category.
** Dark green and yellow fruits and vegetables contain beta carotene. Your body can turn beta carotene into vitamin A, which helps protect you against certain types of cancer-causing substances.

How Do You Rate?

0–12: A Warning Signal
Your diet is too high in fat and too low in fiber-rich foods. It would be wise to assess your eating habits to see where you could make improvements.

13–17: Not Bad! You're Partway There
You still have a way to go.

18–36: Good For You! You're Eating Smart
You should feel very good about yourself. You have been careful to limit your fats and eat a varied diet. Keep up the good habits and continue to look for ways to improve.

ful you are, the more motivated you may be to make some healthy changes.

We are presenting samples of "healthy" and "unhealthy" diets (developed by Abby Bloch, coordinator of clinical nutrition research at Memorial Sloan-Kettering, and Lori Cohen, our research nutritionist), to illustrate the difference between the two.

You may be surprised by the foods in these diets. The unhealthy diet certainly doesn't seem loaded with ice cream and fatty deserts, yet it is much too high in fat and too low in fiber. And the healthy diet certainly would be considered fulfilling and delicious.

THE CANCER PREVENTION DIET

- Lower your dietary fat intake to no more than 20 percent of your total daily calories.
- Increase your dietary fiber intake to at least 25 grams per day.
- Eat five to nine servings of fruits and vegetables daily.
- Eat foods rich in vitamins A, C and E.
- Cut down on charred, salt-cured, nitrate-cured or smoked foods such as hotdogs, ham and bacon.
- Try to maintain your ideal weight by avoiding overeating and incorporating physical activity into your daily life.

KEEPING A FOOD LOG

Use a food log to keep track of what you eat for several days. Be sure to carry it with you and write down everything you eat *immediately after each meal or snack*, noting the time.

1. Write down all foods and beverages you consume throughout the day. Indicate whether the food is eaten raw or cooked. Note quantity in terms of measuring cups and spoons, weights or serving sizes as listed on food labels or estimated from package volume, if available.

2. Don't forget all the items you might add to your cereal, vegetables, meat or other foods: milk, sugar, fruit, butter, sauces, toppings, margarine, oil, cheeses, spices, condiments, gravies.

3. Note the following:
   - ingredients of salad dressings
   - the fat percentage in milk and dairy products
   - whether poultry skin is eaten or removed, and whether meats are trimmed of visible fat
   - each of the ingredients in mixed dishes and casseroles
   - types of bread: white, whole wheat, rye, pumpernickel
   - types of cooked and dry cereals, or ingredients of homemade cereals

(continued)

- snacks, candies, gum
- vitamins or other supplements taken
- method of preparation: breaded, fried, baked, broiled, poached

4. If you eat in a restaurant, ask the waiter the size of the cooked portion of your entree. If it is not available, make an estimate. A three-ounce cooked portion of meat or fish is about the size of a deck of cards. An average chicken leg or split breast has approximately three ounces of meat. One ounce of cheese is about ¼ cup diced or 4 tablespoons grated.

TYPICAL LOW-FAT MENU

BREAKFAST:

Buckwheat pancakes	2 med.
Maple syrup	1 Tbs.
Fresh raspberries	½ cup
Skim milk	⅓ cup
Coffee or tea	1 cup

LUNCH:

Cracked wheat bread	2 slices
Roast chicken breast	3 oz.
Low-fat Swiss cheese	1 oz.
Lettuce	1 leaf
Tomato	¼ med.
Mustard	1 Tbs.
Fresh peach	1 med.
Iced tea with lemon wedge	1 cup

DINNER:

Broiled swordfish	4 oz.
Brown rice	1 cup
Steamed broccoli	½ cup
Steamed carrots	½ cup
Fresh fruit	2 med.
Club soda	1 cup

SNACK:

Fig cookies	4 items
Skim milk	1 cup

NOTE: 18 percent of calories in this menu are from fat.

TYPICAL HIGH-FAT MENU

BREAKFAST:	
Fried egg	1 whole
White bread	2 slices
Bacon, broiled	1 slice
Whole milk	1 Tbs.
Coffee or tea	1 cup
LUNCH:	
Peanut butter, smooth	2 Tbs.
White bread	2 slices
Jam	2 Tbs.
Vanilla wafers	2 items
Whole milk	1 cup
DINNER:	
Fried chicken breast	1 med.
Mashed potato	½ cup
Green salad	½ cup
Italian dressing	1 Tbs.
Chocolate chip cookies	2 items
Presweetened iced tea	1 cup

NOTE: 41 percent of calories in this menu are from fat.

At first glance, these one-day menus might not seem all that different from each other. Each provides three full meals, including a meat entree at dinner, that should satisfy anyone's appetite. But take a look at the extreme differences in the amounts of nutrients:

- The unhealthy diet's fat content, at 41 percent of the total calories, is much too high; the healthy diet gets only 18 percent of its calories from fat.
- The unhealthy diet's fiber content is much too low: only 9 grams, compared with 27 grams for the healthy diet.
- The unhealthy diet includes far fewer fruits and vegetables, and is also low in several vitamins and minerals. One green salad does not compose a diet rich in fruits and vegetables.

Unfortunately, the unhealthy diet reflects what the typical American eats. For example, most people get up to 40 percent of their calories from fat. For healthy living, *limit it to 20 percent or less of calories.* (Important: This guideline applies to adults only; children need more fat.)

Most men and women average 10 to 11 grams of fiber per day, when they should consume at least twice that. *We recommend that you include a minimum of 25 grams daily.* A diet high in fiber, incidentally, tends to be lower in fat and calories.

And more than 90 percent of the U.S. population does not eat the recommended *five to nine daily servings of fruits and vegetables;* most eat only 1.7 servings each day. Consequently, they are getting less than the recommended levels of antioxidants, vitamins and other cancer-fighting compounds that fruits and vegetables contain.

If this sounds like your usual diet, just look at what a few simple changes can do:

- Substituting bran flakes with skim milk for that fried egg trims 10 grams of fat and adds 6 grams of fiber.
- Enjoying a skinless roasted breast of chicken instead of the fried chicken breast saves 274 calories and a whopping 27.1 grams of fat.
- Adding an afternoon snack of a Bartlett pear increases the fiber load by 4.3 grams and adds vitamins and minerals.
- Drinking skim milk instead of whole milk eliminates 75 calories and 10 grams of fat.

FATS

You'll note that in analyzing these two diets, we have focused our attention on fats, and with good reason. The effect of excess fat on your circulatory system (not to mention your waistline) is well known: A high-fat diet can raise cholesterol levels and lead to coronary heart disease, the number-one killer of Americans. Perhaps less recognized by most men and women is the fact that a high-fat diet may well increase the risk for many cancers, including those of the colon, breast, prostate, ovary, uterus and skin.

There are three types of fats. *Saturated* fats, found in meat, fish, poultry, eggs, nuts, whole-fat dairy products, and palm and coconut oils, are the largest source of fat in the typical American diet, and also the least desirable. Studies have associated those fats with a variety of cancers, including colon, prostate, lung, and breast (and other types of breast disease as well).

Polyunsaturated fats, such as corn, safflower, sesame, sun-flower, soybean and cottonseed oils, are not as risky but should be kept to a minimum, while *monounsaturated* fats (olive oil, canola oil, peanut oil) are generally considered the healthiest choice in the fats menu.

There are several theories as to the mechanisms by which fats might instigate or assist in the growth of tumors:

- In the process of using fats, the body produces free radicals, which can damage DNA.
- Increasing the secretion of bile into the intestines. Bile acids, produced by the liver to help the body digest fats, might then be converted into carcinogenic compounds in the colon.
- Interfering with the body's signals to cells to stop dividing.
- Interfering with the immune system, which can destroy some cancer cells.
- Making cells less able to defend against invaders.

An ongoing study conducted by the Harvard University School of Public Health added some compelling evidence to the story on fat and colon cancer in 1990. In following the health and diets of more than 88,000 U.S. nurses, scientists found a clear correlation between animal fat and colon cancer. The more red meat—beef, lamb or pork—the women consumed, the higher their risk of colon cancer. Those who ate red meat every day were found to be two to three times more likely to get the disease than those who ate it less than once a month. Eating vegetable fat or fat from dairy foods did not appear to increase the risk.

FIBER

The idea that a diet high in fiber might offer protection from colon cancer first arose in the mid-1970s. Scientists compared the diet of African villagers, who rarely developed colon cancer, with that of the people at an English school in Africa who exhibited much higher rates of the disease. The difference was clear: The Africans had a very high fiber intake, while the English people ate very little fiber.

In 1989 researchers at New York Hospital–Cornell Medical Center discovered that adding fiber to the diet could shrink pre-cancerous polyps that had already begun to form in the colon. This study was the first to show that an ordinary food—in this case, a cereal rich in bran—could reverse a progression toward cancer.

The word *fiber* has been tossed around a great deal in recent years, yet few people could probably tell you what it is. Fiber is nothing more than a common structural part of plants that humans cannot digest: celery strings, corn-kernel skins, the membranes that separate the sections of an orange, the bran that surrounds grains, and numerous other familiar materials in the food we eat.

There are two basic types of fiber: *soluble* and *insoluble*. Soluble fiber, found in oat bran, rice bran, fruit pectin and barley, is noted for its ability to lower blood cholesterol. On the other hand, insoluble fiber—the kind in wheat bran and the woody parts of vegetables and fruits—is thought to provide the greatest protection against colon cancer. It does this in several ways: sweeping carcinogens through the intestines; preventing chemicals from harming the colon's delicate lining; and discouraging growth of harmful bacteria that could lead to cancer and bolstering growth of beneficial bacteria.

Fiber's role in preventing other types of cancer has not been studied very extensively. In two studies, however, diets high in fiber were believed to decrease the risks of stomach cancer and breast cancer. It has been postulated that fiber binds up and helps rid the body of estrogen, a hormone known to raise a woman's risk of breast cancer.

CALORIES

Another dietary goal is reducing your caloric intake to a level that provides the energy needed for daily activities while maintaining a desirable body weight. In the 1940s, scientists discovered that laboratory animals on restricted-calorie diets were less likely to develop many types of cancer. Thirty years later, scientists studying the average number of calories consumed in various countries noticed a similar effect: Higher calorie consumption seemed to coincide with higher rates of cancers of the breast, colorectum, uterus and kidney.

Of course, a very active person—for example, a competitive athlete—can burn a large number of calories without gaining weight. But for most people, a high-calorie diet adds extra body fat. And being overweight increases the risk of cancers of the breast, kidneys, colorectum, gallbladder, cervix, uterus, ovaries and prostate.

Excess body fat increases a woman's risk of breast, uterine and possibly ovarian cancer because it metabolizes the hormone estrogen, which stimulates cell growth in those organs. There are a couple of hypotheses on how body fat and high-calorie diets affect other cancers. One is that chemical carcinogens are stored in body fat, rather than being expelled from the body. Another is that the energy supply from calories exerts some control over the rate of cell multiplication.

LIMIT YOUR TOTAL DAILY FAT INTAKE TO NO MORE THAN 20 PERCENT OF TOTAL CALORIES

Keeping track of your fat intake doesn't require complicated mathematics at every meal. First, calculate how many calories you need per day (see box for a simple formula). Suppose it is about 2,000 calories; you want to limit your fat consumption to 20 percent of those calories, or 400.

Next, since most food labels and recipes list fats by number of grams, not calories, you need to figure out how many grams 400 calories equals. One gram of any fat contains 9 calories. So divide

---

CALCULATING HOW MANY CALORIES YOU NEED

If you are a healthy adult, use this formula:
1. Basic metabolic needs and normal daily activities: 13 calories per pound of body weight
2. Add to this the number of calories burned during exercise
3. Subtract 2 percent of total calories for each decade after age 30

Example: If you are a 45-year-old woman who weighs 130 pounds and walks 4 miles per day:

Basic needs	$13 \times 130 = 1,690$
4-mile walk	$4 \times 100 = 400$
Subtotal	2,090
Age adjustment	4% of $2,090 - 80$ (round to nearest ten)
Total calories	2,010

400 by 9, for a daily allowance of 44.5 grams of fat. *This is the total grams of fat, from all foods, that you should eat in one day.*

Use this simple formula to compute your fat allowance:

1. _____ total calories per day x .20 (percent) = _____ calories of fat per day.
2. _____ calories of fat per day divided by 9 calories per gram of fat = _____ grams of fat per day.

Many people are confused by claims on food labels, such as "98 percent fat-free," or "only 2 percent fat," assuming that these figures refer to the percentage of calories from fat. Not so. For example, whole milk is 3.5 percent to 4 percent fat, leading many people to assume that only 4 percent or less of its calories come from fat. In reality, a cup of whole milk typically contains 8 or 9 grams of fat; thus 72 to 81 calories, out of a total of 160, come from fat. In other words, about half the calories are from fat—a far cry from 4 percent. The difference lies in the fact that milk (and many other foods) are mostly water, and the 4 percent refers to total volume, water and all.

Another point some people find confusing: the fat content of various foods. We advocate an overall diet that is 20 percent fat or less, but this does not mean every item you eat must be 20 percent fat or less. To give you an example, 100 percent of the calories in a pat of butter or margarine are from fat. It's all right to include a limited amount of these products in your diet, as long as your *total* daily fat intake does not exceed your fat allowance. Of course, include them too often, and you will exceed your fat limit.

The trick is to keep that 44.5 grams (or whatever amount your calculation allows you) of fat in mind as you make your food choices throughout the day. Keep a running tally for several days on a small index card that you can carry with you. You'll discover how far over the limit you are, and with the help of the charts and tips below, you'll discover where you can cut back.

Keep a close watch especially on your consumption of salad dressings, margarine, cheese, ground beef, luncheon meats and dairy products. Studies show that these products are where we get most of our fats.

Not All Fats Are the Same

- Limit especially your intake of saturated fats. Polyunsaturated fats should also be consumed only sparingly. Your best option is to select mostly monounsaturated fats.

Cut Back on Meat Consumption

- Cut down your portions of meat, poultry and other animal products. Use them as garnishes rather than as the main course. For example, use a small amount of meat or chicken to add texture and flavor to a vegetable dish or starch-based meals (pasta, rice, potatoes, etc.).
- Eat a meatless or low-meat meal several times a week.
- Choose skinless white-meat chicken or turkey rather than dark.
- Select only the leanest cuts of beef, pork, veal, lamb, poultry and fish. Choice and good grades of meat usually contain less fat than prime cuts.
- Trim away all visible fat from meat, and remove skin and visible fat from poultry before cooking. Refrigerate gravies, soups and stews, and remove congealed fat before reheating and serving. A gravy strainer—available in housewares and kitchen supply stores—is handy for defatting small quantities of broth and gravy.
- Another reason for reducing the amount of meat you eat: It is one of the greatest sources of dioxin, a toxic chemical that a 1994 Environmental Protection Agency study found may be responsible for anywhere from 26,500 to 265,000 cases of cancer. Dioxin, produced by incinerators, chemical processing, chlorine bleaching of paper and pulp and the burning of diesel fuel, usually gets released into the atmosphere by smokestacks. The particles then settle on crops and vegetation and are consumed by livestock and poultry.

Select Foods Low in Fat

- These include fruits, vegetables and most grains, breads and starches such as rice, potatoes and pasta.
- Select reduced-fat luncheon and variety meats.
- Buy fish packed in water, not oil.

LOW-FAT FOODS

Some low-fat foods to choose more often are:

ITEM	SERVING	CALORIES	GRAMS OF FAT
Dairy Products			
Cheese:			
Low-fat cottage (2%)	½ cup	100	2
Mozzarella, part skim	1 oz.	80	5
Parmesan	1 Tbs.	25	2
Milk:			
Low-fat (2%)	1 cup	125	5
Nonfat, skim	1 cup	85	trace
Ice milk	1 cup	185	6
Yogurt, low-fat, fruit flavored	1 cup	230	2
Meats			
Beef:			
Lean cuts, such as trimmed bottom round, braised or pot-roasted	3 oz.	190	8
Lean ground beef, broiled	3 oz.	230	16
Lean cuts, such as eye of round, roasted	3 oz.	155	6
Lean and trimmed sirloin steak, broiled	3 oz.	185	8
Lamb:			
Loin chops, lean and trimmed, broiled	3 oz.	185	8
Leg, lean and trimmed, roasted	3 oz.	160	7
Pork:			
Cured, cooked ham, lean and trimmed, baked	3 oz.	135	5
Center loin chop, lean and trimmed, broiled	3 oz.	195	9
Rib, lean and trimmed, roasted	3 oz.	210	12
Shoulder, lean and trimmed, braised	3 oz.	210	10
Veal:			
Cutlet, braised or broiled	3 oz.	185	9
Poultry Products			
Chicken, roasted:			
Dark meat without skin	3 oz.	175	8

Light meat without skin	3 oz.	145	4
Turkey, roasted:			
Dark meat without skin	3 oz.	160	6
Light meat without skin	3 oz.	135	3
Egg, hard cooked	1 lge.	80	6
Seafood			
Flounder, baked, no butter or margarine	3 oz.	85	1
Oysters, raw	3 oz.	55	2
Shrimp, boiled or steamed	3 oz.	100	1
Tuna, packed in water, drained	3 oz.	135	1
Other Foods			
Salad dressing, low calorie	1 Tbs.	20	1

Low-Fat Crackers/Snack Foods

Fresh and dried fruits	Pretzels
Fresh vegetables	Rusks
Breadsticks	Rye Krisp
Finn Crisp	Popcorn (no added fat)
Flatbread	Saltines
Graham crackers	Soda crackers
Hardtack	Swedish crispbread
Matzo	Wasa Brod
Oyster crackers	Zwieback toast

SOURCE: U.S. Department of Agriculture

SOME HIGH-FAT FOODS

Many foods contain large amounts of fat and should be used with special care. These include foods that provide important nutrients, such as meat, dairy products, nuts and seeds, etc. So make new choices from their leaner counterparts, or choose them less often and in smaller portions. Examples of high-fat foods you can cut down on are listed below.

ITEM	AMOUNT	GRAMS OF FAT
Fats and Oils		
Butter, margarine	1 Tbs.	12
Mayonnaise, regular	1 Tbs.	11
Salad dressing, regular	1 Tbs.	7

(continued)

ITEM	AMOUNT	GRAMS OF FAT
Seeds (sunflower, sesame, pumpkin)	2 Tbs.	8
Vegetable oil	1 Tbs.	14
Nuts: walnuts	¼ cup	20
almonds	¼ cup	32
pecans	¼ cup	48
peanuts	¼ cup	48
cashews	¼ cup	32
Peanut butter	2 Tbs.	14
Avocado	½	15
Bacon fat or lard	1 Tbs.	10
Coconut (shredded, unsweetened)	1 oz.	5
Cream cheese	1 oz.	10
Olives	4	5
Sour cream	2 Tbs.	6
Whole egg or yolk	1 lge.	6
Half and half	¼ cup	7
Whipped cream	¼ cup	11

Dairy Group

Whole milk	1 cup	9
Condensed sweet milk	¼ cup	6
Evaporated whole milk	½ cup	10
Whole milk yogurt	1 cup	8

Frozen Desserts

Ice cream, regular	1 cup	14
Ice cream, rich	1 cup	24
Tofutti	1 cup	28

Cheeses

American, blue, cheddar, colby, fontina, Gjetost, Gruyère, Monterey Jack, muenster, Roquefort	1 oz.	10
Brie, Edam, Gouda, Jarlsberg, Limburger, provolone, Romano, Swiss	1 oz.	8
Camembert	1 oz.	7
Ricotta (whole milk)	½ cup	16
Ricotta (part skim)	½ cup	10

Canned Soups

Cream of: Celery	1 cup	6
Chicken	1 cup	7
Mushroom	1 cup	9
Cheese	1 cup	10
New England clam chowder	1 cup	10

Meat and Poultry

Bacon	3 slices	21
Cold cuts: corned beef, bologna, liverwurst, pastrami, pepperoni, salami	2½ oz.	21
Sausages: bratwurst, frankfurter sausages, Thuringer	1 link (2 oz.)	22
Porterhouse steak	10-oz. serving	89
Pork spareribs	7-oz. serving	77
Prime rib	12-oz. serving	140

Snack/Desserts

Brownies	1 med.	15
Chocolate cake	1 piece	11
Cookies, commercial cream-filled sandwich types, shortbreads, sugar, chocolate chip, oatmeal, peanut butter	4	12
Chips: corn	10	10
potato, taco	1 small bag (1 oz.)	12
Crackers: Ritz, Triscuits, Wheat Thins	10	10
Croissant	1 average	13
Danish	1 med.	15
Doughnut	1 med.	10
French fries	21 (small order)	15
Onion rings	6	22
Pancakes, French toast, waffles	2 lge.	10
Milk chocolate candy bar	2¼ oz.	20
Chocolate-covered almonds/nuts	1 oz.	15
Fruit pie with crust: apple, blueberry, cherry	⅛ pie	15
Pie: pecan	⅛ pie	20
pumpkin, plain	⅛ pie	17
fried pies	1	20
Poptart	1	5
Muffin	1 med.	9

SOURCE: American Cancer Society

FISH AND SHELLFISH
FAT AND CHOLESTEROL COMPARISON CHART

When following a cholesterol-lowering diet, you may want to eat more fish and shellfish, which in general have a lot less saturated fat (i.e., saturated fatty acids) and cholesterol than meat and poultry. However, some shellfish is relatively high in cholesterol and should be eaten less often. Fish and shellfish also contain less total fat and calories than meat and poultry. Use the information on total fat, percent calories from fat, and calories to help you lose weight.

This table ranks fish and shellfish within each category (finfish, crustaceans, mollusks) from low to high saturated fat. You will want to select the lower fat and cholesterol fish and shellfish from the upper portion of the table. To reduce the amount of saturated fat in your diet even more, eat smaller portions (no more than 6 ounces a day).

Omega-3 fatty acid (fish oil) is a type of polyunsaturated fat found in the greatest amounts in fatter fish. Evidence is mounting that omega-3 fatty acids in the diet may help lower high blood cholesterol and guard against cancers of the breast, ovary, uterus and prostate. Since their potential benefit is not fully understood, the use of fish oil supplements is not recommended. However, eating fish is beneficial because it not only contains omega-3 fatty acids but, more importantly, it is low in saturated fat.

Product (3½ Ounces Cooked)*	Saturated Fatty Acids (Grams)	Cholesterol (Milligrams)	Omega-3 Fatty Acids (Grams)	Total Fat[1] (Grams)	Calories from Fat[2] (%)	Total Calories
Finfish						
Haddock, dry heat	0.2	74	0.2	0.9	7	112
Cod, Atlantic, dry heat	0.2	55	0.2	0.9	7	105
Pollock, walleye, dry heat	0.2	96	1.5	1.1	9	113
Perch, mixed species, dry heat	0.2	42	0.3	1.2	9	117
Grouper, mixed species, dry heat	0.3	47	—	1.3	10	118

Whiting, mixed, species, dry heat	0.3	84	0.9	1.7	13	115
Snapper, mixed species, dry heat	0.4	47	—	1.7	12	128
Halibut, Atlantic and Pacific, dry heat	0.4	41	0.6	2.9	19	140
Rockfish, Pacific, dry heat	0.5	44	0.5	2.0	15	121
Sea bass, mixed species, dry heat	0.7	53	—	2.5	19	124
Trout, rainbow, dry heat	0.8	73	0.9	4.3	26	151
Swordfish, dry heat	1.4	50	1.1	5.1	30	155
Tuna, bluefin, dry heat	1.6	49	—	6.3	31	184
Salmon, sockeye, dry heat	1.9	87	1.3	11.0	46	216
Anchovy, European, canned	2.2	—	2.1	9.7	42	210
Herring, Atlantic, dry heat	2.6	77	2.1	11.5	51	203
Eel, dry heat	3.0	161	0.7	15.0	57	236
Mackerel, Atlantic, dry heat	4.2	75	1.3	17.8	61	262
Pompano, Florida, dry heat	4.5	64	—	12.1	52	211
Crustaceans						
Lobster, northern	0.1	72	0.1	0.6	6	98

(continued)

Product (3½ Ounces Cooked)*	Saturated Fatty Acids (Grams)	Cholesterol (Milligrams)	Omega-3 Fatty Acids (Grams)	Total Fat[1] (Grams)	Calories from Fat[2] (%)	Total Calories
Crab, blue, moist heat	0.2	100	0.5	1.8	16	102
Shrimp, mixed species, moist heat	0.3	195	0.3	1.1	10	99
Mollusks						
Whelk, moist heat	0.1	130	—	0.8	3	275
Clam, mixed species, moist heat	0.2	67	0.3	2.0	12	148
Mussel, blue, moist heat	0.9	56	0.8	4.5	23	172
Oyster, Eastern, moist heat	1.3	109	1.0	5.0	33	137

* 3½ ozs = 100 grams (approximately).

[1] Total fat = saturated fatty acids plus monounsaturated fatty acids plus polyunsaturated fatty acids.

[2] Percent calories from fat = (total fat calories divided by total calories) multiplied by 100; total fat calories = total fat (grams) multiplied by 9.

— = Information not available in sources used.

SOURCE: *Composition of Foods: Finfish and Shellfish Products—Raw • Processed • Prepared, Agriculture Handbook 8–15.* United States Department of Agriculture (in press).

Use Low-fat or Nonfat Dairy and Sauce Products

- Choose skim or 1 percent rather than whole milk. Opt for low-fat or nonfat cheeses, yogurts and frozen desserts.
- If you have a hard time getting used to low-fat milk, mix it with whole milk for a while, then gradually increase the proportion of skim milk.

- Cut down on salad dressings and rich sauces you use in cooking or at the table. Opt for tomato-, broth- or vegetable-based preparations rather than cream-based recipes.
- Use butter or margarine sparingly. One pat contains 4 grams of fat.
- Choose lower-fat cheeses like part-skim mozzarella, skim-milk cottage cheese and other skim-milk products.

Use Low-Fat Cooking Methods

- Broiling, baking, steaming, poaching, microwaving, roasting and stir-frying all help you avoid fatty cooking oils.
- Substitute broth for grease.
- Use vegetable cooking sprays or nonstick cookware instead of cooking in fat.
- Eat fried foods sparingly, if at all.

Beware of Fatty Food Add-ons

- Butter, cheese, sour cream, sauces and gravies can be high in fat.
- Commercially or deli-prepared salads such as tuna, chicken, egg, potato and coleslaw are usually very high in fat. Try mixing your own, using a dressing made from low-fat yogurt and mustard or vinegar instead of mayonnaise or sour cream.
- Use fats such as butter, margarine, oil and mayonnaise sparingly and, whenever possible, use low-fat or reduced-fat mayonnaise, salad dressing or spreads.
- Season foods with herbs, spices, lemon juice, mustard, salsa and other no- or low-fat condiments.

Snack Foods and Desserts Can Be Loaded with Fat

- Substitute pretzels or unbuttered, air-popped popcorn or fat-free chips for regular potato chips, corn chips, tortilla chips and buttered popcorn.
- Weigh out small portions of those fatty snacks that you just can't live without. Then give yourself a treat from time to time. This way you won't be facing a whole can of peanuts, just a small, relatively guilt-free bagful.
- Choose low-fat frozen desserts such as frozen yogurt or ice milk, and avoid the fat-laden premium ice creams.

- Snack on fresh fruits and vegetables and, in small quantities, dried fruits.
- Limit consumption of baked products such as Danish, donuts, croissants, scones, muffins, pies, cakes and cookies. Look for the increasingly popular low-fat alternatives, but be sure to read the labels to see how "low" they really are.
- When baking, use applesauce or other fruit purees in place of butter, shortening or oil.

While changing your food habits regarding meat consumption, remember to limit your intake of barbecued, salt-cured and smoked meats, including anchovies, bacon, beef jerky, corned beef, dried chipped beef, herring, pastrami, pickled pigs' feet, processed meats (bologna, hotdogs, luncheon meats), salted and dried venison, sausage (liverwurst, pepperoni, salami, Polish, bratwurst, pork), smoked cheeses, smoked and cured pork, smoked seafood (cod, salmon, oysters, white fish), smoked hams and poultry. Such foods are processed with nitrates and nitrites, which have been linked to an increased risk of stomach cancer.

By the same token, limit your intake of meats and other foods barbecued over charcoal, wood and other fires. When you cook over a grill, a powerful carcinogen known as benzo(a)pyrene forms from fat dropping onto the hot coals. The rising smoke then deposits this chemical onto the meat. To be safe, wrap meat or other foods in foil and keep it as far away from the flame as possible.

INCREASE FIBER INTAKE TO AT LEAST 25 GRAMS PER DAY

Calculating your daily fiber intake is even simpler than figuring your fat allowance. Keep a running tally of your fiber sources and amounts for a few days. Most food labels list fiber content, but make sure you count only the fiber content for the serving size that you consumed.

FIBER CONTENT OF FOODS

To increase the amount of fiber, choose several servings of foods from this list, especially the rich and moderately rich fiber sources.

The dietary fiber content of many foods is still unknown, so this is not a comprehensive list of the fiber content of foods. (Fiber content for vegetables and fruits that can be eaten with their skins includes fiber content for the skins.)

RICH SOURCES OF FOOD FIBER

4 grams or more per serving
(Foods marked with an * have 6 or more grams of fiber per serving)

	SERVING	CALORIES (ROUNDED TO THE NEAREST 5)
Breads and cereals		
* All Bran	⅓ cup–1 oz.	70
* Bran Buds	⅓ cup–1 oz.	75
Bran Chex	⅔ cup–1 oz.	90
Corn bran	⅔ cup–1 oz.	100
Cracklin' Bran	⅓ cup–1 oz.	110
* 100% Bran	½ cup–1 oz.	75
Raisin bran	¾ cup–1 oz.	85
* Bran, unsweetened	¼ cup	35
Wheat germ, toasted, plain	¼ cup–1 oz.	110
Legumes (cooked portions)		
Kidney beans	½ cup	110
Lima beans	½ cup	130
Navy beans	½ cup	110
Pinto beans	½ cup	110
White beans	½ cup	110
Fruits		
Blackberries	½ cup	35
Dried prunes	3	60

MODERATELY RICH SOURCES OF FOOD FIBER

1 to 3 grams of fiber per serving

	SERVING	CALORIES (ROUNDED TO THE NEAREST 5)
Breads and cereals		
Bran muffins	1 med.	105
Popcorn (air-popped)	1 cup	25
Whole-wheat bread	1 slice	60
Whole-wheat spaghetti	1 cup	120
40% bran flakes	⅔ cup–1 oz.	90

(continued)

	SERVING	CALORIES (ROUNDED TO THE NEAREST 5)
Grape-Nuts	¼ cup–1 oz.	100
Granola-type cereals	¼ cup–1 oz.	125
Cheerio-type cereals	1¼ cup–1 oz.	110
Most	⅓ cup–1 oz.	95
Oatmeal, cooked	¾ cup	110
Shredded wheat	⅔ cup–1 oz.	100
Total	1 cup–1 oz.	100
Wheat Chex	⅔ cup–1 oz.	105
Wheaties	1 cup–1 oz.	100

Legumes (cooked) and Nuts

Chick peas (garbanzo beans)	½ cup	135
Lentils	½ cup	105
Almonds	10 nuts	80
Peanuts	10 nuts	105

Vegetables

Artichoke	1 small	45
Asparagus	½ cup	30
Beans, green	½ cup	15
Brussels sprouts	½ cup	30
Cabbage, red and white	½ cup	15
Carrots	½ cup	25
Cauliflower	½ cup	15
Corn	½ cup	70
Green peas	½ cup	55
Kale	½ cup	20
Parsnip	½ cup	50
Potato	1 med.	95
Spinach, cooked	½ cup	20
Spinach, raw	½ cup	5
Summer squash	½ cup	15
Sweet potato	½ med.	80
Turnip	½ cup	15
Bean sprouts (soy)	½ cup	15
Celery	½ cup	10
Tomato	1 med.	20

Fruits

Apple	1 med.	80
Apricot, fresh	3 med.	50

Apricot, dried	5 halves	40
Banana	1 med.	105
Blueberries	½ cup	40
Cantaloupe	¼ melon	50
Cherries	10	50
Dates, dried	3	70
Figs, dried	1 med.	50
Grapefruit	½	40
Orange	1 med.	60
Peach	1 med.	35
Pear	1 med.	100
Pineapple	½ cup	40
Raisins	¼ cup	110
Strawberries	1 cup	45

SOURCE: National Institutes of Health

- Choose whole-grain varieties of breads, rolls, pastas, pancakes, cereals and flours. These don't discard the fiber-rich bran part of the plant during milling.
- Select high-fiber cereals such as 100 percent bran, raisin bran and oatmeal.
- If you don't like the taste of high-fiber cereals, try mixing them with your favorite cereal.
- Choose whole-wheat, buckwheat, rye, pumpernickel, corn, oat and multigrain breads.
- Add brown rice, white rice, barley, couscous, polenta, buckwheat and bulgur to your diet for variety.
- Eat lots of fruits and vegetables. They contain fiber, although not in very high amounts. And leave the skin on; it's high in fiber.
- Use beans, lentils, peas, tofu and other legumes as meat substitutes for main dishes and in soups, salads and casseroles.
- Nuts and seeds are high in fiber, but they are also high in fat, so use them sparingly.

CHEMOPREVENTION:
VITAMINS AND ANTICANCER CHEMICALS

Some of the most exciting and promising research of the past few years has focused on chemicals in our food, especially those in fruits and vegetables. Every tomato slice, every piece of cauliflower or broccoli, every glass of orange juice, contains hundreds of naturally occurring chemicals, some of which are believed to provide significant protection from many cancers. Some experts estimate that if everyone ate a diet rich in fruits and vegetables, we could eliminate one third of the cancer deaths in the United States. Dr. Peter Greenwald, director of the National Cancer Institute's division of cancer prevention and control, goes even further, saying that men and women who eat lots of fruits and vegetables have about one half the cancer risk of people who eat small amounts of those foods.

As explained earlier, cancer doesn't happen all of a sudden; it is a slow, step-by-step process. And the key to cancer prevention rests in eliminating or short-circuiting one or more of these steps. Increasingly, it appears that fruits and vegetables are loaded with compounds that can do just that.

One set of chemicals that have garnered tremendous attention are *antioxidants,* which include beta-carotene, vitamin C, vitamin E and numerous other compounds. Foods containing antioxidants are believed to protect us from cancer by countering the effect of molecules known as free radicals, highly reactive substances that form as by-products of the normal process of metabolism or as a result of exposure to sunlight, x-rays, tobacco smoke, car exhaust or other outside sources. Because they are unstable, free radicals attack cell membranes as well as damage the cell's DNA and lead to cancer. They can also interact with other substances in the body, turning them into carcinogens.

Normally, free radicals are held in check by the many antioxidants and other substances that our bodies produce or that we consume in foods. Vitamin E, for example, lodges itself in the membranes of a cell and safeguards it from attack. Other antioxidants protect the body by blocking the initial formation of free radicals. Sometimes, however, the balance of power is disturbed, as when environmental causes contribute to the load, and the free radicals get the upper hand. It is thought by some nutritionists that a diet rich in antioxidants can help to keep the free radicals —and their carcinogenic effects—in check.

But antioxidants appear to be only part of the story. Fruits and vegetables contain a number of other chemicals: substances referred to as phytochemicals (*phyto* comes from the Greek word for "plant"). Many of these phytochemicals have evolved as part of a plant's natural defense system against cancers and other diseases—yes, plants also develop cancer!—and it appears that we derive similar benefits when we ingest these substances. How do phytochemicals work in the body?

Take sulforaphane, a cancer-fighting chemical in broccoli and other cruciferous vegetables. (*Cruciferous* refers to foods in the cabbage family—broccoli, cabbage, brussels sprouts, bok choy, collards, kale, kohlrabi, mustard greens, turnip greens, turnips, rutabaga and cauliflower—that have cross-shaped flowers.) Sulforaphane, considered the most powerful anticancer compound found to date, may bolster the body's natural defenses by activating an enzyme that removes carcinogens from cells.

Garlic and onions contain chemicals called allylic sulfides that appear to work in a similar manner; namely, they activate enzymes that neutralize cancer-causing substances. Another strong anticancer compound, genistein, blocks the formation of blood vessels around new tumors. Without these blood vessels, a tumor cannot grow to much more than a speck and certainly cannot grow to life-threatening sizes. It also inhibits uncontrolled cell proliferation and competes with estrogen—one explanation why Japanese women who consume large amounts of genistein have a very low rate of breast cancer. This compound is found in high concentrations in soybeans, and to a lesser degree in cruciferous vegetables.

The mineral selenium is believed to afford some protection from leukemia and cancers of the colorectum, breast, ovary and lung. Calcium, another mineral, possibly safeguards against colon cancer by neutralizing the damaging effects of bile and other cancer promoters. (See the accompanying box for a listing of other protective phytochemicals.)

In addition to their anticancer properties, antioxidants and other phytochemicals appear to safeguard against many other diseases, ranging from cataracts to heart attacks and neurologic disorders such as Parkinson's and Alzheimer's diseases.

OTHER PROTECTIVE CHEMICALS IN FRUITS, VEGETABLES AND NUTS

PROTECTOR	FOUND IN	PROTECTIVE EFFECT AGAINST CANCER
Catechins (tannins)	Green tea Berries	Antioxidant
Flavonoids	Parsley Carrots Citrus fruits Broccoli Cabbage Cucumbers Squash Yams Tomatoes Eggplant Peppers Berries Soy products	Inhibit hormones that promote cancer
Indoles	Cabbage Broccoli Cauliflower Mustard greens and other members of the cabbage family	Destroy the hormone estrogen; induce protective enzymes
Isoflavones	Beans Peas Peanuts and other legumes	Inhibit estrogen and estrogen receptor; destroy cancer-gene enzymes
Isothiocyanates	Mustard Horseradish Radishes	Induce protective enzymes
Lignans	Flaxseed Walnuts	Inhibit the hormone estrogen; block action of cancer-promoting prostaglandins
Limonoids	Citrus fruits	Induce protective enzymes

Lycopene	Tomatoes Red grapefruit	Antioxidant
Monoterpenes	Parsley Carrots Broccoli Cabbage Cucumber Squash Yams Tomatoes Eggplant Peppers Mint Basil Citrus fruits	Some antioxidant properties; aid protective-enzyme activity
Omega-3 polyunsaturated fatty acids	Flaxseed Walnuts	Inhibit the hormone estrogen; block action of cancer-promoting prostaglandins
Phenolic acids	Parsley Carrots Broccoli Cabbage Tomatoes Eggplant Peppers Citrus fruits Whole grains Berries	Some antioxidant properties; inhibit formation of nitrosamines; affect enzyme activity
Plant sterols (vitamin D precursor)	Broccoli Cabbage Cucumbers Squash Yams Tomatoes Eggplant Peppers Soy products Whole grains	Differentiation agents
Polyacetylene	Parsley	Inhibits prostaglandins; destroys the potent carcinogen benzo(a)pyrene

(continued)

PROTECTOR	FOUND IN	PROTECTIVE EFFECT AGAINST CANCER
Protease inhibitors	Soybeans	Destroy enzyme inhibitors that can cause cancer to spread
Quinones	Rosemary	Inhibit carcinogens or cocarcinogens
Sulfur compounds	Garlic	Inhibit carcinogens and tumor development
Terpenes	Citrus fruits	Stimulate enzymes to block the action of carcinogens
Triterpenoids	Licorice root	Inhibit hormones that promote cancer

SOURCES: From *Cancer & Nutrition: A Ten-Point Plan to Reduce Your Risk of Getting Cancer* by Charles B. Simone, MD, © 1992, $12.95. Published by Avery Publishing Group, Inc., Garden City Park, NY (800-548-5757). Reprinted by permission. Also: Copyright © 1991/1993 by The New York Times Company. Reprinted by permission.

BETA-CAROTENE/VITAMIN A

Beta-carotene, a pigmented nutrient that gives carrots and other green and yellow vegetables their color, is a highly efficient neutralizer of free radicals. It is converted to vitamin A in the body, but many researchers believe that it is the beta-carotene, not the resulting vitamin A, that protects against cancer.

More than two dozen studies have concluded that a diet abundant in foods containing beta-carotene can lower rates of lung cancer. Researchers at Johns Hopkins University found that people who had low levels of beta-carotene in their blood were four times more likely to develop the disease than those with higher levels. Conversely, a study conducted in Chicago, which followed 2,100 men from 1958 to 1977, showed that those who ate fewer foods containing beta-carotene were more likely to have died of lung cancer.

Several studies have also shown protection against cancers of the breast, cervix and uterus. The Harvard nurses' study referred to earlier found that women who ate less than one serving a day of foods high in vitamin A had a 20 percent higher-than-normal risk of breast cancer. Eating just one or two daily servings of foods rich in vitamin A appeared to eliminate that additional risk. According to researchers at the University of Alabama, women who consumed large amounts of foods containing beta-carotene exhibited lower incidences of cervical and uterine cancers. Other studies have also discovered that foods containing beta-carotene can provide protection from cancers of the esophagus, stomach, colon and mouth.

In addition to its preventive effects, beta-carotene is also believed to suppress or reverse some cancers. Researchers think that it may quell cancers of the cervix and uterus after they have begun, and may reverse precancerous lesions in the mouth.

Although many of these studies indicate that foods rich in beta-carotene safeguard against cancer, the same may not be true for beta-carotene supplements. A large 1994 Finnish study showed that subjects considered at high risk of lung cancer did not benefit from taking beta-carotene supplements.

FOODS RICH IN BETA-CAROTENE AND VITAMIN A

Carrots	Romaine, red-leaf and green
Spinach	looseleaf lettuces
Broccoli	Whole milk
Sweet potatoes	Egg yolk
Yellow squash	Pumpkin
Apricots	Vegetable-juice cocktail
Cantaloupes	Whole-milk cheese
Mango	Peaches
Papaya	Apricots
Liver	Tomatoes
Turnip greens	Kale
Bok choy	Beet greens

VITAMIN C

Vitamin C, another antioxidant vitamin, is thought to also fend off cancer by enhancing the immune system and detoxifying compounds in the liver, such as potentially cancer-causing pesticides and industrial pollutants. Studies have also demonstrated that vitamin C blocks the formation of nitrosamines in the digestive tract. These cancer-causing compounds form when nitrates and nitrites in foods interact with amines in digestive juices. Nitrites and nitrates are found in many fruits and vegetables, and also in smoked and cured foods.

More than 30 studies have linked the consumption of vitamin C–rich foods with reduced risks of cancer. Vitamin C is believed to afford some protection from cancers of the esophagus, larynx, mouth, pancreas, stomach, rectum, breast, cervix and lung. In animal studies vitamin C has also been shown to protect against sunlight-induced skin cancer.

FOODS RICH IN VITAMIN C

Broccoli	Cantaloupe
Oranges	Grapefruits
Lemons	Limes
Strawberries	Green and red peppers
Cauliflower	Peas
Cherries	Cabbage
Potatoes	Kiwi fruit
Papaya	Brussels sprouts
Apple juice	Blackberries
Tangerines	Tomatoes
Asparagus	Spinach

VITAMIN E

Vitamin E is said to be the antioxidant most effective at eliminating free radicals in the body. And, like vitamin C, it also aids

FOODS RICH IN VITAMIN E

Whole grains	Egg yolks
Nuts	Sunflower seeds
Milk fat	Green, leafy vegetables
Liver	Wheat germ
Corn	Dried beans
Vegetable oils such as soybean, sunflower, peanut, olive and safflower	

immune system function and blocks the production of nitrosa-mines. Several studies have concluded that vitamin E protects against lung and breast cancers. Evidence also exists that eating foods rich in this vitamin can help prevent cancers of the stomach, cervix, pancreas and urinary tract.

VITAMIN D

Although vitamin D is not an antioxidant, it may reduce the risks of breast, colon and prostate cancers. Scientists at the University of California at San Diego noted that these cancers are rare among people living near the equator and become increasingly common the farther you move from the equator. The researchers theorized that vitamin D, which is manufactured by the skin when it is exposed to the sun, protected the inhabitants near the equator from certain cancers. How vitamin D may exert its protective role is unknown, but it may be related to its role in other metabolic processes. For example, vitamin D enables the body to absorb calcium, which is thought to inhibit colon cancer; it also helps cells in the body to mature normally.

FOODS RICH IN VITAMIN D

Milk	Salmon
Tuna	Eggs
Liver	Margarine
Egg yolk	Cod liver oil

Many dairy products and breakfast cereals are also fortified with vitamin D.

EAT FIVE TO NINE SERVINGS OF FRUITS AND VEGETABLES EVERY DAY

There may be hundreds of other potent anticancer compounds in fruits, vegetables and cereals that have not been identified yet—just one more reason why you should eat five to nine servings of fruits and vegetables every day. In addition to providing fiber, most fruits and vegetables are low in calories and fat, and high in vitamins and minerals.

To help preserve the cancer-preventive nutrients in produce, follow these simple recommendations from the American Institute for Cancer Research:

- Select produce that is not damaged, bruised or wilted, as rough handling produces vitamin loss.
- Shop on days when your supermarket receives its produce shipment and eat these fruits and vegetables soon. Vitamins begin to degrade after four to five days.
- Use fresh or frozen products rather than canned.
- Sun-ripening fresh fruit and vegetables, then chilling them immediately, helps preserve vitamins A and C, folate and other nutrients.
- Conserve vitamins B and C by not washing produce until just before cooking and eating.
- Keep frozen vegetables at 0 degrees Fahrenheit or lower; higher temperatures can deplete nutrients.
- If you plan to cut up produce, serve large chunks instead of small chunks, which have more surface area exposed to air and speed the loss of vitamins A, C, E, some B vitamins and selenium.

Be careful how you prepare fruits and vegetables. A dish that has been prepared in lots of fat isn't going to do you much good. Neither is boiling, which can leach out many of the nutrients. Try stir-frying (which uses less oil than conventional frying), steaming, microwaving and baking.

THE QUESTION OF VITAMIN AND MINERAL SUPPLEMENTS

Patients repeatedly ask us whether or not they should take vitamin and mineral pills. The answer is clear: Supplements may be prescribed to treat a specific nutritional deficiency or in special circumstances, such as during pregnancy, when diet alone may not be able to provide the optimum amounts of some nutrients. But if you eat a balanced diet that includes generous amounts of fruits, vegetables and grains, you don't need supplements.

What's more, we don't know the long-term effects of high doses of most vitamins. We do know, however, that some vitamins and minerals, especially vitamins A and D and selenium, can be toxic, even lethal, in high doses; smaller doses, too, may cause damage. Vitamins that are readily excreted from the body can also be harmful in some circumstances. High doses of vitamin C, for example, can adversely affect people with kidney disease or certain blood disorders.

A major study issued in 1994 by the National Cancer Institute and Finland's National Public Health Institute surprised many with its conclusion that vitamin supplements did not guard against cancer and, in fact, could actually *increase* a smoker's chances of getting lung cancer.

Another study showed that taking supplements of beta-carotene, vitamin C and vitamin E did not provide protection against premalignant colon cancer. In this nationwide study, patients who'd had adenomas (polyps in the colon that can develop into cancer) removed from their colon were given either the vitamins or a placebo pill and followed for four years. According to the researchers, the group of patients that received antioxidant vitamins had as many premalignant polyps as those given the placebo. Their conclusion: supplements did not reduce the risk of colon cancer.

These findings only reinforce the recommendation that men and women get their vitamins through a balanced diet, since the benefits shown by previous studies may be due more to the numerous protective compounds described earlier in this chapter.

Perhaps most important, taking supplements tends to give people a false sense of security. They believe they are protected against disease, so they slack off on diet and exercise, and don't make as much of an effort to quit smoking or cut down on alcohol.

THE BAD CHEMICALS: PESTICIDES

Agricultural operations now use millions of pounds of chemical pesticides annually to control pests. Since they are usually sprayed directly on crops, inevitably some residues remain on our food.

While many of these chemicals are known to cause malignancies in humans, the actual risk of developing cancer from eating fruits and vegetables is a matter of debate. Al Heier, a public information officer at the Environmental Protection Agency, says, "We don't believe they pose an unreasonable risk." Yet a 1987 National Academy of Sciences report estimated that pesticide residues on the most common foods might be responsible for 20,000 cancers a year. And in 1993, another NAS report noted that children may be "uniquely sensitive" to pesticides. Furthermore, the NAS expressed concern that youngsters might be ingesting unsafe amounts of the chemicals and recommended that federal agencies improve regulation. The federal government, at the same time, announced that it was moving to reduce pesticide use in American agriculture.

Some scientists believe that naturally occurring pesticides are even more prevalent in our foods than artificial pesticides. Many plants have developed these compounds to ward off attacks by pests. We recommend that you thoroughly wash all fruits and vegetables before eating to remove artificial pesticides. Don't soak, however, which can draw out nutrients into the water.

CHANGING YOUR EATING HABITS

When you begin to change your eating habits, remember that *you are in control* of your diet and your life. Food does not control you. What's more, don't try to do everything at once. Take time to read food labels (more about that later), learn which foods are better for you and allow your body to adjust to a new way of eating. Try a new recipe every four or five days and experiment with new ingredients in your regular recipes. Rachel Barcia-Morse, a research nutritionist at Memorial Sloan-Kettering, recommends you give yourself two to three months to implement significant dietary changes.

If you do most of the cooking for your family, you face a double challenge: making changes in your diet and convincing family members to do the same. "Involve them in the decision making," Rachel advises. Take your spouse along on shopping trips to show him or her the many choices available. Enlist him or her in the cooking, too.

When you see your children making better food choices—snacking on yogurt instead of cookies—praise them and tell them how pleased you are to see everyone working together to change their eating habits. And don't forget to keep an eye on the school lunch program, which tends to be high in fat, and make suggestions for your children's choices. If all else fails, says Rachel, work around your family. Chances are, you can make a number of changes in their diets that they will never notice unless you tell them!

You don't have to give up the foods you love to follow a cancer prevention eating program. Not every meal or food has to be extremely low-fat and high-fiber, but whatever you eat in the course of a day (or two or three days) should total up to a healthy diet that adheres to the principles we have set out.

If you feel that you aren't making much progress, don't be too hard on yourself. Many small changes in your diet will add up to big overall changes in your eating style. Three months after you begin, take the Eating Smart Quiz again and prepare another food log, to see how far you've come. Remember, nobody is perfect.

Mary V., our patient who is at high risk for several cancers, knows well the importance of flexibility in following an anticancer diet. She tries to eat five servings of fruits and vegetables a day and keeps her fat intake below 30 grams a day. But she is also realistic. "If I do much denial of the things that are good to eat," she says, "then my whole eating plan falls apart. You have to balance it."

There are so many things you can do to change your diet that we can't possibly list them all. The tips and lists contained here will get you started, while the food pyramid and the sample menus will help you plan meals. This is an ongoing process, and we expect you will find new and interesting ways to eat healthily for years to come.

TOOLS FOR DIETARY CHANGE

New dietary guidelines and improved nutritional labels on processed food are designed to make it easier for Americans to consume a more healthful diet. Here are ways to use these tools.

THE FOOD GUIDE PYRAMID

In 1993 the U.S. Department of Agriculture unveiled its new Food Pyramid, replacing the former Basic Four Food Groups. The new pyramid divides foods into six groups, emphasizing those that should make up the bulk of your diet. Thus the bread, cereal, rice and pasta group forms the bottom of the pyramid, calling for six to eleven servings per day. Next comes the vegetable group, with three to five servings, and the fruit group, with two to four servings. Nearer the top are the milk, yogurt and cheese group, and the meat, poultry, fish, dry beans, eggs and nuts group, each with two to three servings. At the top is the fats, oils and sweets group, which should be used sparingly.

It may seem that we are asking you to eat a lot of food. Keep in mind that one serving of vegetables, in most cases, is only half a cup and may be smaller than what you consider one serving. The Food Guide Pyramid specifies the serving sizes for various food groups.

HOW TO USE THE FOOD GUIDE PYRAMID

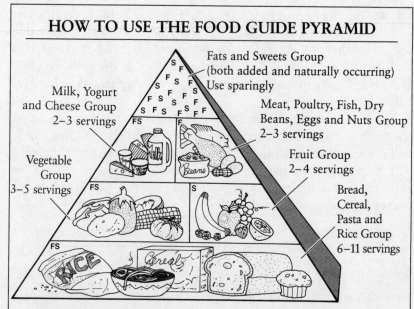

Fats and Sweets Group
(both added and naturally occurring)
Use sparingly

Milk, Yogurt
and Cheese Group
2–3 servings

Meat, Poultry, Fish, Dry
Beans, Eggs and Nuts Group
2–3 servings

Vegetable
Group
3–5 servings

Fruit Group
2–4 servings

Bread,
Cereal,
Pasta and
Rice Group
6–11 servings

The Food Guide Pyramid. This new system divides foods into six groups and recommends the numbers of servings you should get from each every day. The Fats and Sweets Group (F and S) is at the top of the pyramid, indicating that these should be used sparingly. Note also that fats and sugars occur naturally in the other groups. At the bottom of the pyramid is the Bread, Cereal, Rice and Pasta Group, which should be the foundation of your diet.

SOURCE: U.S. Department of Agriculture/U.S. Department of Health and Human Services

Group A: some older adults
Group B: children, teenage girls, active women and men
Group C: teenage boys and active men

Level 1: Bread, Cereal, Pasta and Rice Group
6–11 servings daily (Group A: 6, Group B: 9, Group C: 11)
    One serving = 1 slice of bread, 1 ounce of ready-to-eat cereal,
    ½ cup of cooked rice or pasta, ½ cup of cooked cereal.

Level 2: Vegetable Group
3–5 servings daily (Group A: 3, Group B: 4, Group C: 5)
  One serving = ½ cup of chopped raw or cooked vegetables,
  1 cup of leafy raw vegetables.

Level 2: Fruit Group
2–4 servings daily (Group A: 2, Group B: 3, Group C: 4)
  One serving = 1 piece of fruit or melon wedge, ¾ cup of juice,
  ½ cup of canned fruit, ¼ cup of dried fruit.

Level 3: Milk, Yogurt and Cheese Group
2–3 servings daily (Groups A, B, C: 2–3)
  One serving = 1 cup of milk or yogurt, 1½ to 2 ounces of cheese.

Level 3: Meat, Poultry, Fish, Dry Beans, Eggs and Nuts Group
2–3 servings daily (Group A: 2, total of 5 ounces; Group B: 2,
total of 6 ounces; Group C: 3, total of 7 ounces)
  One serving = 2½ to 3 ounces of cooked lean meat, poultry or
  fish. Count ½ cup of cooked beans, 1 egg or 2 tablespoons of
  peanut butter as one ounce of meat or ⅓ of a serving.

Level 4: Fats, Oils and Sweets Group
Use sparingly.

THE NEW FOOD LABELS

Combined with the guidelines in the new Food Pyramid, the nutritional information on food packages can be one of the most helpful tools in your efforts to eating healthily. These labels used to be unnecessarily confusing, and sometimes misleading, until the Food and Drug Administration simplified and standardized all nutritional labels.

The new labels are called "Nutrition Facts." One of the most important changes is the standardization of serving size. You can now compare the nutritional contents of similar products without having to tote a calculator to the store. The new serving sizes reflect more accurately the usual amount that we eat in a sitting. "One serving" is no longer defined by the manufacturer.

All manufacturers are required to follow the same format for their Nutrition Facts labels, clearly stating the serving size, the number of servings per container and the number of calories per serving. The left-hand column lists the number of calories from fat, the number of grams from all fats, the number of grams from saturated fats and the grams of fiber per serving.

THE NEW FOOD LABEL AT A GLANCE

The new food label carries an up-to-date, easier-to-use nutrition information guide, and is required on almost all packaged foods (compared to about 60 percent of the products previously). The guide serves as a key to help in planning a healthy diet.

Serving sizes are now more consistent across product lines, stated in both household and metric measures, and reflect the amounts people actually eat.

The list of nutrients covers those most important to the health of today's consumers, most of whom need to worry about getting *too much* of certain items (fat, for example), rather than too few vitamins or minerals, as in the past.

The label now tells the number of calories per pgram of fat, carbohydrates and protein.

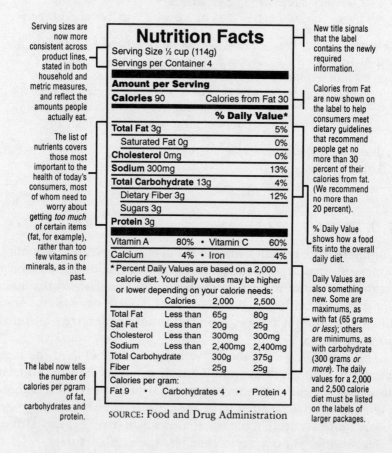

Nutrition Facts

Serving Size ½ cup (114g)
Servings per Container 4

Amount per Serving

Calories 90   Calories from Fat 30

% Daily Value*

Total Fat 3g	5%
Saturated Fat 0g	0%
Cholesterol 0mg	0%
Sodium 300mg	13%
Total Carbohydrate 13g	4%
Dietary Fiber 3g	12%
Sugars 3g	
Protein 3g	

Vitamin A	80%	• Vitamin C	60%
Calcium	4%	• Iron	4%

* Percent Daily Values are based on a 2,000 calorie diet. Your daily values may be higher or lower depending on your calorie needs:

	Calories	2,000	2,500
Total Fat	Less than	65g	80g
Sat Fat	Less than	20g	25g
Cholesterol	Less than	300mg	300mg
Sodium	Less than	2,400mg	2,400mg
Total Carbohydrate		300g	375g
Fiber		25g	25g

Calories per gram:
Fat 9   •   Carbohydrates 4   •   Protein 4

SOURCE: Food and Drug Administration

New title signals that the label contains the newly required information.

Calories from Fat are now shown on the label to help consumers meet dietary guidelines that recommend people get no more than 30 percent of their calories from fat. (We recommend no more than 20 percent).

% Daily Value shows how a food fits into the overall daily diet.

Daily Values are also something new. Some are maximums, as with fat (65 grams *or less*); others are minimums, as with carbohydrate (300 grams *or more*). The daily values for a 2,000 and 2,500 calorie diet must be listed on the labels of larger packages.

The right-hand column shows how those amounts of fat and fiber (and other items) fit into a daily eating plan, as a percentage of Daily Value (or Daily Allowance). In our sample chart, 3 grams of fat is about 5 percent of the Daily Value, and 3 grams of fiber is 12 percent of the Daily Value.

As Abby Bloch points out, "All the information on these labels is based on a diet of 2,000 calories per day." From that the FDA has calculated (see list at bottom of chart) that one can consume 65 grams of fat—including 20 grams of saturated fat—and 25 grams of fiber a day. Thus the 3 grams of fat represent 5 percent of that 65 gram total.

This labeling system has its drawbacks. If you are consuming fewer than 2,000 calories a day, your total fat intake would also be lower. Three grams of fat would then represent a greater portion of your daily fat allowance than the 5 percent listed on the label. What's more, the labels are based on a diet that gets 30 percent of its calories from fat, whereas we recommend an upper limit of 20. So, again, the 3 grams of fat are going to be a larger portion of your fat allowance than the 5 percent listed on the label.

To give you an example: A woman who eats 1,800 calories a day should consume no more than 40 grams (360 calories divided by 9 calories per gram of fat) of fat a day. The food label lists 65 grams of fat as the daily intake. For her, one serving would be 7 percent of her Daily Allowance, not 5 percent.

We suggest using the percentages of Daily Values listed only as a general guide to the role that each food might play in your daily diet. Certainly if the label says a food contributes 75 percent of your daily fat intake, you'll want to avoid it or eat it only in moderation. But rather than relying on the percentages to tell you when you have reached your daily fat limit, simply make note of the actual number of grams of fat in the left-hand column.

The labels also list the amounts of vitamin A, vitamin C, calcium and iron as a percentage of the Reference Daily Intake. This new term, also known as RDI, refers to the federal government's recommendations for daily consumption of nutrients. The levels of the recommendations have not changed, only the name. So on our sample chart, one serving of this food will supply 80 percent of your daily need for vitamin A. These percentages are generally applicable no matter how many calories you consume.

The FDA has also taken steps to regulate manufacturers' nutritional claims. The new rules provide definitions for many terms commonly used on food packages:

Low fat: 3 g or less per serving.

Low saturated fat: 1 g or less per serving.

Low sodium: less than 140 mg per serving.

Low cholesterol: less than 20 mg per serving.

Lean: less than 10 g fat, less than 4 g saturated fat, and less than 95 mg cholesterol per serving and per 100 g (for meat, poultry, seafood and game meats).

Extra lean: less than 5 g fat, less than 2 g saturated fat, and less than 95 mg cholesterol per serving and per 100 g.

High: contains 20 percent or more of the Daily Value for a particular nutrient in one serving.

Good source: one serving contains 10 to 19 percent of the Daily Value for a particular nutrient.

Reduced or *less:* a product where one serving contains 25 percent less of a nutrient or calories than the regular product or a product it is being compared to. *Reduced* is used for two products of a similar nature (for example, two brands of potato chips), while *less* is used for comparing unlike products, such as pretzels and potato chips.

Light: contains one-third fewer calories or half the fat of the comparable food.

SPECIAL SITUATIONS

Of course, not everyone eats every meal at home, where you can control every last ingredient and portion size. But you don't have to throw your best intentions out the window when confronted with business trips, holidays or special occasions. With a little initiative, you can remain in charge of your diet.

When eating out, remember that you have a right to ask for foods that are right for you. Patient Susan S., an artist, revamped her diet after a colonoscopy revealed a precancerous colon polyp. "The better the restaurant," she observes, "the more they are willing to cook something to your order." And it doesn't have to be boring, she adds. "It always has to do with the way it is prepared and presented. I find that if it's presented nicely, if you have the aesthetic pleasure, it makes your juices run."

Here are tips for eating out and other special situations:

- If you go to one restaurant frequently, ask for a copy of the menu to take home with you. Then you can study the food choices when you aren't feeling rushed to order.
- Ask the chef to make some changes in an entree. It may be as simple as leaving the sauce off a dish or putting it on the side. Order fish broiled without fat instead of sauced or sautéed in butter. If your request is a little more complicated, you might want to call the restaurant beforehand.
- Many restaurants offer low-fat meals. These are sometimes indicated on the menu by a small heart or other symbol. Ask your waiter.
- Always ask for salad dressing on the side. That way you can control how much you use.
- If you don't want to make a fuss in a restaurant, eat only a portion of the meal and take the rest home with you.
- Share a dessert! Just a few bites of chocolate cake can be as satisfying as a whole piece. Or order a piece of pie and eat only the filling.
- If you find yourself in a situation where it is impossible or just too difficult to control your diet, don't despair. Enjoy the foods, then compensate by cutting back a little more over the next few days.
- If you are on vacation, you might not want to restrict yourself. After all, part of the fun of visiting new places is sampling new foods. Nutritionist Rachel Barcia-Morse suggests you be extra vigilant at breakfast and lunch. "Then at dinner," she says, "you will have more leeway in your choices."
- Fast-food restaurants have been notorious for the high-fat content of their foods—usually 40 to 55 percent—but that is beginning to change. Most now carry at least a few lower-fat options, such as salads, baked potatoes, plain hamburgers and grilled or baked chicken. Many chains now provide nutritional information for their menus. Pick up a copy so you can plan a low-fat meal in advance.
- Many airlines offer several options for special meals, including low-fat meals. You will probably have to reserve your meal at least a day before your flight.
- Holidays needn't throw a crimp into your new eating plan, either. Analyze your standard holiday menu before you begin preparations, and see where you can make some changes. For instance, leave the sausage out of the stuffing and eliminate the frosting from the carrot cake.

"ALTERNATIVE" DIETS

Numerous alternative diets claim to protect against or to treat cancer. Not only have no benefits been substantiated scientifically, some of these diets are harmful or nutritionally inadequate.

The macrobiotic diet, one of the best known, is based on achieving a balance between *yin* and *yang,* the purported "primary forces in the universe." Yin is believed to be the "expanding" tendency, while yang is the "consolidating" tendency. Illnesses are said to be caused by an excess of either factor. Diseases, including cancer, develop when the forces of yin or yang are out of balance.

NUTRIENT VALUES OF SAMPLE FAST-FOOD MEALS

Sample Meal	% Fat Calories	Calories	Choles-terol (mg)	Sodium (mg)	% U.S. RDA Vitamin A	Vitamin C	Calcium
Double burger with sauce, milk shake, French fries, regular	46	1,275	155	1,190	10	30	80
Chicken nuggets (6), apple pie, coffee with cream	55	655	95	1,115	2	20	9
Fish sandwich with cheese and tartar sauce, soda (12 oz.), French fries, regular	53	885	73	811	2	20	19
Beef tacos (2), low-fat milk (8 oz.)	40	495	60	690	18	3	61
Single burger, tossed salad, low-fat milk	32	445	55	1,005	28	75	50

Baked potato, plain, margarine (1 pat), tossed salad with low-calorie dressing, low-fat milk	18	340	10	620	28	120	45
Cheese pizza (1 slice), tossed salad with low-calorie dressing, orange juice (8 oz.)	30	310	40	500	27	233	26

SOURCE: From *Cancer & Nutrition: A Ten-Point Plan to Reduce Your Risk of Getting Cancer* by Charles B. Simone, MD, © 1992, $12.95. Published by Avery Publishing Group, Inc., Garden City Park, NY (800-548-5757). Reprinted by permission.

To achieve a balance between yin and yang foods, proponents of macrobiotics recommend a diet that is typically 50 to 60 percent whole grains, 20 to 25 percent vegetables, 5 to 10 percent beans and seaweeds, and 5 percent soups. Consumption of meat, poultry, eggs and dairy products and certain other foods is discouraged.

While this is a low-fat, high-fiber diet, we do not recommend macrobiotics. Depending on the practitioner who prescribes it, the diet can be dangerously low in vitamins and minerals, and too high in fiber. And even though it is low in fat, it may supply too few calories. Extreme forms of macrobiotics can cause nutritional deficiencies and starvation.

You should be wary of any diet that relies too heavily on one food or promises to "detoxify" the body with juice fasts, enemas, dietary supplements or enzymes. The Gerson program, to name one, advocates a juice fast that calls only for consumption of one of four juices every hour. Other dietary approaches and remedies include coffee enemas, bee pollen, ginseng, alfalfa tablets, hair analysis, liquid diets and megadose vitamins. We also believe you should not consume herbs in any great quantity, though you certainly may enjoy the many commercially available herbal teas.

Don't get taken in. The American Cancer Society, which publishes a list of unproven practices in the United States and abroad, advises the public to be wary of those who seem isolated from mainstream medicine, claim that organized medicine is prejudiced against them, discourage consultation with reputable physicians, or prohibit you from purchasing the diet or method of treatment from anyone but them. (Beware in particular of "secret" concoctions.)

If you want to consult a professional about your eating plan, take time to find the right one. Unfortunately, anyone can call himself a nutritionist, and many people who have no formal training do just that. In general, your best bet is to stick with a registered dietitian, who has had years of training and has passed state licensing exams. If you are in doubt about the requirements in your state or where to find a dietitian, call the state dietetic association, the department of public health or your local hospital. Or ask your physician for a referral.

RECOMMENDED COOKBOOKS

There are now dozens of cookbooks emphasizing tasty low-fat dishes, so spend some time browsing through the offerings at your local bookstore. Don't overlook ethnic cookbooks—many national cuisines emphasize grains, vegetables and other low-fat ingredients. Remember, too, that you can often reduce the fat in your favorite recipes without sacrificing texture and taste. *Eating Well* magazine, as well as the following cookbooks, tell you how to do this.

- *American Heart Association Cookbook, 5th Edition* (Times Books, New York).
- *Controlling Your Fat Tooth* by Joseph C. Piscatella (Workman Publishing Company, New York).
- *In the Kitchen with Rosie: Oprah's Favorite Recipes* by Rosie Daley (Alfred A. Knopf, New York).
- *Jane Brody's Good Food Book* and *Jane Brody's Good Food Gourmet* by Jane Brody, *The New York Times* health columnist (Bantam Books, New York).
- *Low Fat & Loving It* by Ruth Spear (Warner Books, New York).
- *The Complete Vegetarian Cuisine* by Rose Elliot (Pantheon Books, New York).
- *Weight Watchers Favorite Homestyle Recipes* and *Weight Watchers Meals in Minutes* (Plume/Penguin Books, New York).
- *500 Fat-Free Recipes* by Sarah Schlesinger (Villard Books, New York).

SUGGESTED READING ABOUT
CANCER PREVENTIVE NUTRITION

From the National Cancer Institute (800-4-CANCER):

- "Diet, Nutrition & Cancer Prevention: A Guide for Food Choices"
- "Diet, Nutrition & Cancer Prevention: The Good News"

From the American Institute for Cancer Research, 1759 R Street, N.W., Washington, DC 20069 (800-843-8114):

- "Be Your Best: Nutrition After Fifty"
- "Celebrate Good Health"
- "Cooking Solo"
- "Cook's Day Off"
- "Dietary Fiber to Lower Cancer Risk"
- "Dietary Guidelines to Lower Cancer Risk"
- "Get Fit, Trim Down"
- "Menus and Recipes to Lower Cancer Risk"
- "No Time to Cook"
- "Sneak Health into Your Snacks"

KEY WORDS

Antioxidants: Micronutrients found in fruits and vegetables that are believed to offer protection against cancer by countering the effect of free radicals. Examples of antioxidants: beta-carotene (a precursor of vitamin A), vitamins C and E, and the mineral selenium.

Cruciferous: Refers to members of the cabbage family—broccoli, brussels sprouts, bok choy, cauliflower, turnip greens, turnips, kohlrabi, collards, kale, mustard greens, rutabaga and cabbage—that have cross-shaped flowers.

Fiber: The structural part of plants indigestible by humans; for example, the strings in celery.

Nitrosamines: A potent carcinogen formed in the body when the food preservatives known as nitrates merge with the nitrogen-containing compounds known as amines.

SAMPLE SEVEN-DAY MEAL PLAN

Here's a basic seven-day menu plan designed to give you the kind of balanced diet described in this chapter. It is meant to be a model rather than a rigid diet plan. Feel free to substitute your favorite foods for those suggested here so long as they are from the same pyramid group and of a comparable serving size.

DAY 1

BREAKFAST:

Fresh cantaloupe	³/₄ cup
with fresh berries	*¹/₂ cup*
Raisin bran cereal	1 cup
Skim milk	1 cup
Coffee or tea	1 cup

LUNCH:

Tomato juice with lemon slice	1 cup
Pasta salad	
pasta	*1 cup*
kidney beans	*¹/₄ cup*
mixed vegetables	*1 cup*
fat-free broth	*¹/₄ cup*
olive oil	*1 Tbs.*

DINNER:

Tossed green salad	¹/₂ cup
with low-calorie dressing	*2 Tbs.*
Roast beef, lean	3 oz.
Baked potato, with skin	1 med.
Steamed asparagus with lemon	¹/₂ cup
Pumpernickel rolls	2 med.
Club soda	
Fruit sorbet	1 scoop

SNACK:

Graham crackers	5 items
Skim milk	1 cup

DAY 2

BREAKFAST:

Oatmeal	1 cup
with raisins	*1/4 cup*
dried dates	*1/4 cup*
Milk, 1% or skim	1 cup
Coffee or tea	1 cup

LUNCH:

Tuna salad sandwich	
rye bread	*2 slices*
tuna fish in water	*3 oz.*
shredded carrot	*1/4 cup*
diced celery	*1/4 cup*
fat-free mayonnaise	*1 Tbs.*
lettuce	*1 leaf*
tomato	*1/4 med.*
Coleslaw, with fat-free mayonnaise	1/2 cup
Ginger ale	12 fl. oz.

DINNER:

Spinach pasta	4 oz.
Steamed eggplant	1/2 cup
Tomato sauce, meatless	1/4 cup
with mushrooms	*2.5 oz.*
onions	*1/4 cup*
olive oil	*1 1/2 Tbs.*
Grated parmesan cheese	2 Tbs.
Three-bean salad	1/2 cup
with low-calorie Italian dressing	1 Tbs.
Whole-wheat rolls	2 med.
Angelfood cake	1 slice
with strawberries and sauce	*3 Tbs.*
Herbal tea	1 cup

SNACK:

Fresh fruit salad	1/2 cup
Skim milk	1 cup

DAY 3

BREAKFAST:

Raisin bran cereal	1 cup
with fresh berries	1/4 *cup*
banana	1/2 *med.*
Skim milk	1 cup
Rye bread	2 slices
Fat-free cream cheese	2 tsp.
Coffee or tea	1 cup

LUNCH:

Chilled tomato juice	1 cup
Turkey sandwich	
whole-wheat bread	2 *slices*
skinless roast turkey, white meat	2 *oz.*
low-fat Swiss cheese	1 1/2 *oz.*
lettuce	1 *leaf*
tomato	1/4 *med.*
mustard	1 *Tbs.*
Waldorf salad:	
with shredded carrot	1 *whole*
diced apple	1 *med.*
raisins	2 *Tbs.*
fat-free mayonnaise	1 *Tbs.*
Iced tea, with lemon	

DINNER:

Poached salmon	3 oz.
Lima beans and corn	1 cup
Shredded broccoli slaw	1/2 cup
with nonfat vinaigrette	1 *Tbs.*
Raspberry gelatin	1 cup
Mineral water	

SNACK:

Low-fat frozen yogurt	1 cup

DAY 4

BREAKFAST:

Chilled fresh orange juice	1/2 cup
Buckwheat pancakes	3 med.
maple syrup	1 *Tbs.*
raspberry puree	1/2 *cup*
Coffee or tea	1 cup

LUNCH:

Vegetable juice cocktail	1 cup
Celery stalks	2 med.
Grilled chicken sandwich	
cracked wheat bread	*1 med.*
chicken breast, roasted without fat	*3 oz.*
low-fat Swiss cheese	*1½ oz.*
lettuce	*1 leaf*
tomato	*¼ med.*
mustard	*1 Tbs.*
Fresh peach	1 med.
Club soda	

DINNER:

Black bean soup	1 cup
Broiled swordfish, brushed with	
white wine and lemon juice	4 oz.
Brown rice	¾ cup
Steamed carrots and cauliflower	1 cup
Low-fat frozen yogurt	½ cup
with dried dates	*5 items*
apricots	*¼ cup*
Herbal tea	

SNACK:

Fig cookies	5 items
Skim milk	1 cup

DAY 5

BREAKFAST:

Chilled orange juice	½ cup
Whole-wheat bagel	1 med.
with fat-free cream cheese	*2 Tbs.*
Skim milk	1 cup
Coffee or tea	1 cup

LUNCH:

Low-fat cottage cheese	¾ cup
Fresh berries	¾ cup
Rye crackers	2 items
Mineral water with lemon wedge	

DINNER:

Chili	1 serving
with kidney beans	*½ cup*
meatless tomato sauce	*½ cup*
olive oil	*1 tsp.*
sweet peppers	*½ item*
mushrooms	*½ cup*
low-fat cheddar cheese	*1½ oz.*
Whole-wheat flour tortillas	2 med.
Brown rice	¾ cup
Cantaloupe	¼ cup
Vanilla ice milk	1 scoop
Club soda	

SNACK:

Dutch pretzels	3 items

DAY 6

BREAKFAST:

Chilled grapefruit juice	6 fl. oz.
Oat bran waffles	2 items
with powdered sugar	*1 tsp.*
fresh berries	*¼ cup*
fruit preserve	*2 Tbs.*
Coffee or tea	1 cup
Skim milk	1 cup

LUNCH:

Split-pea soup, meatless	1 cup
Pumpernickel bread	2 slices
Tossed salad	
romaine lettuce	*½ cup*
tomato	*½ med.*
shredded carrot	*¼ cup*
celery	*¼ cup*
garbanzo beans	*2 oz.*
cucumber	*¼ cup*
balsamic vinegar	*2 fl. oz.*
Fresh apple	1 item
Mint tea	

DINNER:

Sautée of turkey breast and vegetables	
skinless turkey breast	3 oz.
sweet peppers	$1/2$ *item*
carrots	$1/4$ *cup*
mushrooms	$1/2$ *cup*
peapods	$1/4$ *cup*
shredded Chinese cabbage	$1/2$ *cup*
corn	$1/4$ *cup*
vegetable oil	$1 1/2$ *Tbs.*
soy sauce	2 *Tbs.*
ground fresh ginger	2 *tsp.*
Pearled barley	$3/4$ cup
Red table wine	6 fl. oz.

SNACK:

Gingersnap cookies	2 items
Skim milk	1 cup

DAY 7

BREAKFAST:

Fresh pink grapefruit	$1/2$ med.
Egg-white vegetable omelet	
egg whites	3 *med.*
butter or margarine	$1/2$ *Tbs.*
chopped onions	2 *Tbs.*
chopped mushrooms	$1/4$ *cup*
low-fat Swiss cheese	1 *oz.*
Whole-wheat bread	2 slices
Coffee or tea	1 cup
Skim milk	1 cup

LUNCH:

Cheese pizza, reduced-fat cheese	2 slices
Tossed salad	
romaine lettuce	$1/2$ *cup*
sweet pepper	$1/2$ *item*
tomato	$1/2$ *med.*
cucumber	$1/4$ *cup*
lemon juice or nonfat dressing	1 *Tbs.*
Club soda	

DINNER:

Lentil soup, nonfat, meatless	³/₄ cup
Baked fillet of sole	4 oz.
Couscous	³/₄ cup
with olive oil	*1 Tbs.*
Ratatouille with tomato sauce, no oil	1 cup
Fruit compote	
dried, cooked apricots	*¹/₄ cup*
dried, cooked peaches	*¹/₄ cup*
cooked rhubarb	*¹/₄ cup*
dried, cooked prunes	*¹/₄ cup*
Flavored mineral water	

SNACK:

Nonfat yogurt	1 cup
Fresh berries	¹/₂ cup

CHAPTER

6

Lifestyle

Tobacco and Alcohol Use ·
The Importance of Exercise ·
How to Give Up Smoking

What's your idea of the "good life"? Not too long ago, before our society developed a greater appreciation of how personal behavior and habits influence our risk of developing cancer and other diseases, most people might have described a scene that took place around a dinner table following a sumptuous (undoubtedly fatty) meal. The players: all well tanned, sitting casually in their chairs with a glass of fine wine in one hand, a cigar or cigarette in the other and not a worry in the world.

The problem was, that kind of life could kill you.

Today the "good life" is no longer synonymous with excess. Taking care of our bodies in order to preserve our health, vitality and zest for living—*that's* the good life.

As Chapter 5 stressed, modifying your diet constitutes a major step in warding off cancer. Another is to eliminate harmful habits such as smoking, excessive alcohol use, sedentary living, risky sexual behavior and hazardous exposure to the sun, which combined account for nearly half of all cancer mortalities.

The purpose of this chapter is to show you how. We begin with tobacco use, the source of 3 in 10 cancer deaths.

FORM OF CANCER	PERCENTAGE OF CANCER DEATHS ATTRIBUTED TO TOBACCO
Lung	85 percent
Laryngeal	50 to 70 percent
Oral	50 to 70 percent
Esophageal	50 percent
Urinary bladder	30 to 40 percent
Kidney	30 to 40 percent
Pancreatic	30 percent
Cervical	Unknown

SOURCE: United States Public Health Service

TOBACCO

"Memorial Sloan-Kettering is a twelve-story hospital," remarks Dr. Michael Moore, codirector of our Evelyn H. Lauder Breast Center. "If it weren't for cigarettes, we'd probably need only four or five."

What will it take for the 46 million Americans who smoke to get the message that tobacco kills? Thirty years after the Surgeon General's historic 1964 report pronouncing smoking a health hazard, and nearly a quarter century since cigarette commercials were banned from television, one in four Americans still smokes.

The public is generally aware of the association between smoking and lung cancer, but did you know it also causes high rates of carcinomas of the larynx, oral cavity, esophagus, urinary bladder, kidneys, pancreas and cervix?

Other facts to consider:

- 435,000 men and women die annually of a smoking-related illness; that's one in five U.S. fatalities.
- According to the Centers for Disease Control and Prevention, each cigarette whittles seven minutes off a smoker's life.
- Using tobacco boosts the odds of dying not only from cancer but from emphysema, chronic bronchitis, heart disease and heart attack. What's more, it promotes dental and gum disease, peptic ulcers and wrinkles skin prematurely.

- Though pipe and cigar smokers generally don't inhale, they too up their odds of getting cancer.

For those who would reply. "It's *my* business and nobody else's if I choose to smoke," think again:

- Smokers endanger the people around them, for the sidestream smoke emitted by cigarettes contains significantly *higher* concentrations of cancer-causing compounds than found in mainstream smoke.
- Nursing mothers who insist on smoking can pass along nicotine, the addictive element of tobacco, to their newborns through the breast milk, while expectant women who smoke transfer poisonous carbon monoxide gas to their fetuses by way of the bloodstream, heightening the chances of miscarriage, premature birth, stillbirth or low birthweight.
- Each year in the United States $65 billion goes up in smoke as a result of health-care costs and lost productivity from tobacco use.
- Children of people who smoke are twice as likely to pick up the habit themselves.

Need to hear more?

We could go on for pages and pages. Except that most smokers are well aware of tobacco's dangers. Many desperately want to quit, but are physically and psychologically enslaved. You can imagine, then, their irritation every time a well-meaning friend or relative implores, *"Why can't you just stop?"* It's not that simple.

"I'm an alcoholic, so I know a fair amount about addiction," says patient Brian D., whom we profiled in Chapter 1. At age 52 he quit smoking after an x-ray revealed a suspicious lesion on his lung, which turned out not to be cancerous.

"I gave up drinking after about 30 years," Brian reflects. "It was hard, but believe me, that was duck soup next to quitting tobacco. You're alcohol free in three, five days. But with cigarettes it takes anywhere from two weeks to six months, because the nicotine can store itself in the fatty tissue, release itself and create a craving."

Brian reckons that he averaged a pack and a half a day for 30 years, which would classify him as a heavy tobacco user. According to Dr. Diane Stover, his pulmonary physician at Memorial Sloan-Kettering, "We generally consider smoking one pack or more a day for 20 years a significant smoking history." However, she adds, other factors come into play.

"Some people smoke fewer cigarettes but inhale more frequently or more deeply. Or they smoke cigarettes with higher concentrations of tar and nicotine." Yet another variable: Does the person smoke cigarettes only halfway or all the way down to the butt?

The number of years spent smoking appears to be more important than the quantity of cigarettes consumed per day, so that a 40-year, pack-a-day smoker has a greater chance of getting cancer than a 20-year, two-pack-a-day smoker. We emphasize that *any* amount of tobacco use jeopardizes your health and may predispose you to a tumor.

CIGARETTES: A SMORGASBORD OF CHEMICALS

One frustration doctors sometimes face is trying to convey to patients how their behavior can impair their health later on. Most men and women begin smoking during their early teens, a stage of life characterized by feelings of invincibility and immortality. The notion that puffing a cigarette could one day leave them gasping for breath seems abstract. Until, of course, it happens to them or someone close to them. The adverse effects of tobacco typically don't emerge for 20 years. By the time many smokers come to grips with what they've done to their health, the damage is irreversible. Perhaps if they could actually visualize what takes place inside their bodies each time they inhale, the warnings on the back of cigarette packs would carry more weight.

Tobacco smoke contains more than 4,000 chemical compounds, 43 of them confirmed carcinogens. Nicotine, a toxic alkaloid, serves as a sort of carnival-sideshow barker, keeping the customers coming back for more. When you draw cigarette smoke into your lungs, the nicotine floats out through the lung tissue and into the bloodstream, which whisks it to the brain. This all takes place within just seven seconds, twice as fast as heroin injected into a vein.

The brain instructs the body's nerve endings to release adrenaline-containing substances called catecholamines, something it normally does in response to stress. Most smokers will tell you that a cigarette relaxes them. In fact, the catecholamines rev up the heartbeat and blood pressure by constricting blood vessels and reducing the flow of blood and oxygen. This is the nicotine "buzz." The "shot." The "lift." Call it what you will, the process repeats itself with each drag. Before long, smokers need to maintain a continuous dose of nicotine or else suffer physical and psychologic withdrawal symptoms.

So now they're hooked, which enables nicotine's henchmen, assorted gases and tars, ample time in which to do their dirty work. Of the gases, carbon monoxide is the most pernicious. Once absorbed into the bloodstream, it crowds out oxygen from the red blood cells. The lack of oxygen, coupled with nicotine's forcing the heart to pump harder and faster, is what leaves heavy smokers breathless after even minimal physical exertion, like climbing a flight of stairs.

Cigarettes inflict some of their worst damage on the lungs. The tars, solid chemical particles that contain carcinogens, turn into viscous resins and clog air passages with mucus. In addition, explains Dr. Daniel Nixon of the American Cancer Society, "Some of these tars and other substances denude the inner lining of the lung. They kill the cilia, the tiny hairs that reach outward and clear out the lungs.

"And once the cilia are gone, the smoking poisons are able to accumulate and turn the oncogenes into active tumor-causing genes and gene products." About 90 percent of tobacco smoke's chemical compounds stay trapped in the lungs. The buildup can rupture the tiny air sacs, or alveoli, and cause the bronchial tube walls to thicken, further impairing breathing.

"On top of that," Dr. Nixon continues, "the toxins are absorbed into the blood of the lungs. So the lungs are hit from both sides: from the external environment as well as from the bloodstream."

Many smokers want to know if "low-tar" cigarettes are risk-free. Safer, perhaps, but by no means safe—and just as dangerous to your heart. Tobacco companies introduced so-called low-tar cigarettes in the 1950s, after sales dipped in reaction to a headline-making American Cancer Society report that linked smoking to lung cancer and a host of other diseases. In 1957 the average cigarette yielded 35 milligrams of tar, as compared with about 13 milligrams today.

However, machines, not people, assess tar yields. A 1988 study conducted by the New Jersey State Department of Health noted that participants given low-tar cigarettes "compensated for reducing tar by increasing the number of cigarettes they smoked by almost half a pack per day," negating any alleged benefit. The fact remains that any level of tar may contain chemical carcinogens.

Lung cancer's ascent from a little-seen disease at the beginning of the century to the nation's most lethal cancer among men by the 1950s paralleled the growth in cigarette sales, which, like swirls of smoke, spiraled upward at 5.6 percent a year. Although tobacco use goes back centuries, commercial cigarettes didn't appear on the market until the early 1900s, when the average American smoked a mere three packs a year.

Around the time of Surgeon General Luther L. Terry's 1964 report citing cigarettes as the primary cause of cancer in men, that figure had soared to over 200 packs per person—including nonsmokers—annually. Since then, the number of adult smokers has dropped considerably, from 42 percent to 25 percent, or to about 75 packs annually per adult.

The 1990s have witnessed two disturbing trends, however. First, there's been an increase in smoking among women, for whom lung cancer has supplanted breast cancer as the leading cause of cancer death. Second, "We still have a big problem in that children are taking it up," Dr. Peter Greenwald, director of cancer prevention and control for the National Cancer Institute, notes with concern. An estimated 3 million teenagers currently smoke, a figure that has remained stable since 1980.

"There's also been some growth," he adds, "in smokeless tobacco." According to the 1992 National Household Survey on Drug Abuse, use of chewing tobacco and snuff rose among men and women age 18 and up. Both products are every bit as addictive as cigarettes and elevate the risk of cancers of the mouth, larynx, throat and esophagus. Snuff enthusiasts, who place a pinch between their cheek and gums, exhibit a 50-fold increased incidence of cancers of those areas of the mouth.

STOP-SMOKING STRATEGIES

If you're a smoker who's wanted to kick the cigarette habit but haven't out of fear that you don't have the willpower, take heart. Every year *three million* Americans stop smoking using any of several methods. We don't advocate one over another, for there is no "best" way to give up tobacco, only what works for you.

Having said that, some techniques have demonstrated higher over-all success rates than others.

COLD TURKEY

Cold turkey, which comes from the phrase "to talk cold turkey," or to speak bluntly about something unpleasant, refers to abrupt and complete withdrawal from an addictive substance. While the most effective way to escape nicotine's clutches, it generally produces more severe side effects than cutting down gradually.

PHYSICAL SYMPTOMS	SOLUTION
Drowsiness and fatigue	Don't exert yourself during this time. When possible, treat yourself to a nap.
Coughing	About 1 in 5 smokers find they cough *more* upon stopping smoking, a result of the cilia recovering and sweeping phlegm out of the lungs again. To subdue your cough, drink warm tea or suck on sugarless hard candy or cough drops.
Dry mouth	Your mouth may feel dry as your body produces less mucus. Chewing gum, sugarless sucking candy and ice-cold water or fruit juice can help.
Insomnia	Practice deep breathing, relaxation exercises, meditation. Also, refrain from drinking coffee, tea or any other caffeinated beverage after 6:00 P.M.
Constipation	See to it that you eat at least five servings of fruits and vegetables a day, as well as whole-grain cereals and breads. In addition, drink six to eight glasses of water daily.

PSYCHOLOGIC SYMPTOMS	SOLUTION
Irritability and anxiety	Get involved in a physical activity such as walking or jogging, luxuriate in a hot bath, practice deep breathing, meditation, relaxation exercises.

Within 24 hours of your last cigarette, your body begins to heal itself. Free of smoke, the heart and lungs start repairing the damage sustained over however many years, and levels of nicotine and carbon monoxide dissipate rapidly. You may experience physical and psychological reactions ranging from headaches and diarrhea to depression and an inability to concentrate. Below we've listed the most common ones, along with suggested remedies.

Bear in mind that few people endure each and every side effect of nicotine withdrawal; some suffer none at all. What's more, these symptoms are temporary, typically lasting one to two weeks. After a few days, you'll begin to notice welcome sensations such as restored senses of smell and taste, and unencumbered breathing.

GRADUAL WITHDRAWAL

Cold turkey induces such misery for some people, they lose their resolve. For others, the mere thought of quitting all at once sends them reaching for their cigarettes. These smokers may prefer to wean themselves off nicotine over time by *tapering* or *postponing*.

Annie Beigel, a trained group facilitator with the American Cancer Society's Fresh Start stop-smoking program, observes, "I've seen these two methods work extremely well." To taper down, first switch to a brand containing less nicotine. Then gradually reduce the number of cigarettes you smoke per day. After a while, try smoking only half of each cigarette. Once you get down to about seven a day, you should be ready to set a date for full withdrawal.

"I worked with one 65-year-old woman who used to smoke two and a half packs a day," says Annie, a onetime heavy smoker herself. "She decided to knock down one cigarette a day." It took three months, "but she finally did quit."

Similarly, postponing requires you to delay lighting up for one hour. So if you normally smoke your first cigarette at eight o'clock in the morning, wait until nine. When you grow used to that, tell yourself you're going to smoke only during odd or even hours of the day. And so on, until you're able to forgo tobacco altogether.

NICOTINE REPLACEMENTS

Central to many success stories is the use of a nicotine replacement to diminish withdrawal symptoms. *Nicotine gum* releases 2 to 4 milligrams of nicotine per piece, while the *nicotine patch* adheres to the skin and releases 21 milligrams to start, tapering down to 7 milligrams. Both are available by prescription only.

"They're not for everybody," cautions Dr. Marc Manley, chief of the National Cancer Institute's public health applications research branch. "They're for people who are most addicted to nicotine and who are likely to experience significant withdrawal symptoms that will make it hard for them to stop smoking."

The two methods boast comparable success rates. However, Dr. Manley points out, "A lot of people seem to find the patch easier to use." Once a day, for 10 to 12 weeks, you simply apply a new patch "anywhere on the upper body," the doctor explains. "Preferably a spot that's not very hairy, so the patch can touch the skin." Its simplicity, he adds, "is an advantage that should not be underestimated."

Learning how to use nicotine gum properly can take time. Despite its name, you don't chomp on it like chewing gum. Rather, explains Dr. Manley, "In a sense it's treated like chewing tobacco. You chew it a little, then stick it between your gum and cheek and let the lining of the mouth absorb the nicotine.

"Without careful starter instructions," he goes on to warn, "many patients use it incorrectly and actually get no nicotine into their bloodstream." The average dosage, 10 to 12 pieces daily for three to six months, costs approximately $25 per week; nicotine patches run about $4 each, or $350 for a three-month supply. (Neither figure reflects the doctor's fee.)

According to Dr. Manley, "Both the gum and the patch have been shown to be effective when used in conjunction with some sort of behavioral intervention, either counseling by a physician or nurse, or a stop-smoking group." A word of warning: Never smoke while using a nicotine patch; even minor nicotine overdoses have triggered fatal cardiac arrhythmias in some people.

ORGANIZED SUPPORT GROUPS

It took Sally S., a 58-year-old mother and grandmother from New York City, 20 years and 10 failed attempts to unshackle herself from tobacco. "Some people I know are very much into 'I can do this myself,'" she reflects. "But it was clear to me I couldn't do it on my own." She finally gave up cigarettes by wearing the patch and attending Fresh Start for the third time.

Peer support constitutes the cornerstone of virtually all addiction groups, whether they address substance abuse, overeating or chronic gambling. Walking away from tobacco can be a perilous voyage into uncharted waters, one that's difficult to complete without the encouragement of family, coworkers and friends. A smoking-cessation group provides unconditional support from others who share the same problem and the same desire to change.

"It also gives people short-term goals," points out Dr. Manley. "For instance, they may want to not smoke for another week just so at the next meeting they can stand up and say, 'I haven't smoked all week.' The person who's quitting on his own may not have those kinds of intermediate goals to make it easier." In addition, trained group leaders dispense practical strategies on how to alleviate withdrawal symptoms, resist the temptation to smoke and so on.

Costs vary. Fresh Start charges $50; Freedom From Smoking, sponsored by the American Lung Association, $60; and Smokenders, a privately run operation, $325. For free referrals to these and other quit-smoking groups in your area, call the National Cancer Institute's Cancer Information Service (800-4-CANCER), Monday through Friday, 9 A.M. to 4:30 P.M. (In Oahu, Hawaii: 524-1234; call collect from other Hawaiian islands.)

What goes on at a typical meeting? Fresh Start, for example, consists of nine hour-long group sessions over four weeks. "At the first meeting I concentrate on trying to break the ice and develop an interaction among the group members," says Annie Beigel. It's essential, she adds, "to get them actively engaged and talking to one another about quitting smoking and their struggles and their triumphs."

For Sally S., convinced she would never conquer her habit, listening to others' experiences proved both enlightening and inspiring. "There were people who'd come through cancer surgery and still smoked," she recalls, "people with pacemakers. What it told me was that smoking is a very powerful addiction, and not to be so hard on them or myself."

Most participants seek to quit in steps rather than go cold turkey. At each session Annie assigns a behavior-modification exercise designed to make smoking as inconvenient or unpleasant as possible. "The first technique is called wrapping. It involves wrapping up their cigarette in white paper and placing two rubber bands around it. Before they smoke they have to unwrap it and write down on the paper where they are, how they feel, and rank the cigarette on a scale of one to five in terms of pleasurableness.

"What that does," she explains, "is help make people aware of the habits and automatic responses of smoking; all those cigarettes they don't even think about smoking. Not everybody's going to do this," she concedes, "but it is very effective for some people."

Subsequent meetings bring additional "homework":

- Don't smoke while talking on the phone.
- Don't borrow cigarettes.
- Change your brand.
- Change the hand you smoke with.
- Don't smoke in front of the television.
- Don't smoke while driving.
- Don't smoke while walking.

"If a person were to follow the program from day one to finish day," says Annie, "he'd be a nonsmoker by the end. But what happens is, most people don't follow all the assignments to the letter. They take what works for them and go from there. I encourage that: Do what's going to work for you." It is expected, she says, that members will gradually drop off. For a group to shrink from fifteen, the average size, to five by the end is not uncommon.

However you decide to quit—through a group or on your own, cold turkey or little by little—the National Cancer Institute recommends several ways to prepare for the day you are ready to go tobaccoless:

- Throw out all ashtrays, matches, lighters and cigarettes.
- Dry-clean any clothes that reek of cigarette smoke.
- Alert your family, friends and coworkers that you're planning to quit smoking and ask for their support and assistance.
- Begin a moderate exercise program, to help alleviate anxiety as well as keep your weight down.
- On the day you quit, treat yourself to something special.
- Know what to expect in the upcoming weeks or months. Groups such as Fresh Start instruct their members on how to surmount the hurdles that trip up many would-be quitters.

WEIGHT GAIN

"So many people are concerned with gaining weight," observes Annie Beigel, "especially women." Putting on a few pounds is common after giving up cigarettes. For one thing, the body retains fluid; for another, a smoker who enjoys wrapping his hands and lips around a cigarette may substitute food in its place. Nightmares of popping buttons and bursting seams are largely unwarranted, however. *Most ex-smokers gain only 5 to 10 pounds.*

Until you are truly free of tobacco, do not try dieting. But avoid high-calorie snacks. Instead keep hunger pangs at bay by snacking on celery, carrots, air-popped popcorn or other low-calorie foods. These and other oral substitutes will also satisfy the urge to handle a cigarette.

Other dietary tips:

- Plan meals ahead of time, to ensure that you eat a well-balanced breakfast, lunch and dinner.
- Avoid sugar.
- Acidic foods and liquids stir up the body's craving for nicotine. So stay away from coffee, nonherbal teas, alcohol, citrus juices and fruits, tomatoes and vinegar.
- Drink six to eight glasses of cold water daily. In addition to helping you feel full, water flushes tobacco toxins from the system.
- Weigh yourself every day, to prevent your weight from ballooning out of control.
- Keep plenty of noncitrus fruits, vegetables and low-fat crackers on hand.
- Don't panic if you gain a few pounds. You can always diet once you're out of the danger zone.

OVERCONFIDENCE

"You're a puff away from a pack a day." So goes a Fresh Start aphorism intended to remind members not to get too cocky once they quit smoking, particularly those who had a relatively easy time doing it.

Annie Beigel has seen this happen countless times. "Six months down the line they're at a bar, and the thought comes into their head, *Why don't you have a cigarette? It'll be great. You can always quit again. It was easy for you, remember?* So they'll smoke, and before they know it they're right back where they started." Never fool yourself into believing that one cigarette won't hurt.

BOREDOM AND LONELINESS

"A lot of people think of their cigarette as a friend," says Annie. "It's been there with them through the good times and the bad times, so when they're lonely and bored, they may relapse." That's where setting up a support network of family and friends beforehand comes in. On nights when boredom or loneliness set in, pick up the phone, not a cigarette.

TEMPTING SITUATIONS

Another popular saying among smokers in the process of quitting: Until you feel capable of resisting the desire to smoke, avoid *people, places and things* that you associate with tobacco. This might include friends who smoke; the smoky bar where you and the gang from the office assemble after work every Friday; the favorite chair you relax in at night with the TV on and a cigarette in your hand.

"It's hard to do," admits Annie, "because people don't want to give up their fun and their friends. So I tell them to plan ahead." She offers an example: "You're at a party where people are smoking and drinking. All of a sudden you get this overwhelming urge to light up. What can you do? There's always the option of leaving." Another would be to mingle with the nonsmokers there, who these days are likely to outnumber the smokers anyway. Or skip that party and make alternate plans with friends who don't smoke.

STRESS

Stress, Annie Beigel has found, is the major pitfall for men and women trying to leave tobacco behind. "I've worked with people who relapsed after twenty years," she says, "and that will be it: a new job, a divorce, moving, an illness or a death in the family."

Even relatively minor crises—a flat tire, a conflict at work—can bounce smokers off the wagon. Most times stress pounces upon us without warning, but during this time do what you can to avoid potentially stressful situations. Are you the type who fidgets and fusses any time you have to wait in a line? Then do your banking on a day other than Friday, when lines are usually longest, or go grocery shopping at night instead of on weekends.

CRAVING

After six months of abstinence, your craving for nicotine will begin to subside. But there will still be days when the sight of someone else smoking triggers the thought, *I've got to have a cigarette!* At times like those, rely on what the American Cancer Society calls the "four Ds":

• *Delay.*
• *Deep breathing.* Take a deep breath, hold it, then let it out slowly.
• *Drink* a glass of cold water.
• *Do* something else. Go for a walk, take a shower, call a friend.

Some other techniques for resisting temptation:

• Instead of lighting up after meals, brush your teeth, savoring the fresh flavor.
• Keep your hands busy: Fill in a crossword puzzle, sew, knit, get out your tool kit and build a doghouse. You don't even have to own a dog.
• Teach yourself to relax: Let your limbs go limp; close your eyes and imagine a peaceful, tranquil scene, such as a beach. Feel the breeze on your face, hear the ocean waves crashing in the distance, smell the salty air.
• Limit socializing to outdoor activities or those where smoking isn't allowed.
• Alcohol can stimulate the desire to smoke. If you drink alcohol, scale back your consumption, or better yet, stop drinking completely.
• Come up with your own stop-smoking motto to repeat in your mind whenever you hear tobacco's seductive siren song. Annie Beigel recalls one group member who would envision an angel on one shoulder and a devil on the other, daring him to smoke. With a thumb and forefinger he'd point an imaginary pistol at the devil and blow him off. Annie's own technique is to sing a rock & roll oldie to herself: "I hear you knockin', but you can't come in."

WHAT HAPPENS IF YOU RELAPSE?

The last session of Fresh Start concerns preventing relapse. "I tell them that quitting smoking is really a process," Annie explains. "You start out thinking, *One day I will quit,* then you begin to act on those thoughts—maybe make some attempts at quitting, maybe enter a program—then you quit.

"After you quit, the process continues, because you have to watch out for relapse. And people *will* relapse." According to the

Centers for Disease Control, nearly 4 in 5 quitters return to smoking within 12 months. But those who make it to the one-year mark have a recidivism rate of only 25 percent over the next five years.

Sally S. relapsed at least ten times. "A hard, hard case," Annie, her facilitator three times, calls her. "She was six months away from needing an oxygen tent in her home—she was dying—and she still couldn't quit."

Like many women, Sally didn't start smoking until relatively late in life, a trend that appears to be changing some. "I never had a cigarette until I was 38," she recalls. "I was getting divorced, and it was very stressful.

"My neighbor, who was a very heavy smoker, came over for coffee and pulled out her True Blues. 'Why don't you have a cigarette? It'll calm you down. And since you never smoked, just as soon as this mess is behind you, you'll quit.'

"Twenty years later," Sally adds with a rueful laugh, "I quit."

Averaging two and a half packs a day, she developed severe emphysema, an irreversible condition that leaves patients literally gasping for air. Whereas the average person uses just 5 percent of their energy for breathing, an emphysema sufferer depletes up to 80 percent just to get enough oxygen to live. "The doctor told me I'd done tremendous damage to my lungs," Sally says.

About seven years earlier, Sally had quit "with no effort at all," she recalls. "Then, after some stress, I went back to it and was off and running again." This time she found it impossible to get unhooked. "I'd go to the American Cancer Society quitting group once or twice a year," she says. "I was hypnotized three times. I went to two spas. I went to every length imaginable. But nothing worked."

The low point came during a stay at an upstate New York spa that promised a cure within seven days.

"I paid one thousand dollars and went off to the country," she remembers. "The first night there, I woke up at four in the morning, and I was in the most agonizing physical withdrawal. My head was spinning, my arms hurt. I'm not exaggerating: I felt insane. I got dressed and went to the kitchen, thinking I would find somebody there who smoked and would give me a cigarette." As it turned out, no one on the kitchen staff smoked.

"However," she continues, "the guys told me that a gas station five miles down the road had a cigarette machine. I went back to my room, gathered together all my quarters and singles, and set out in the dead of night in the middle of the Catskill Mountains. And I'm a person who doesn't go out in New York City at night. That's how bad it was.

"And I walked and walked, and I cried. And occasionally I sat down on the side of the road. I couldn't believe I was doing this. I couldn't believe that cigarettes were so powerful." Trucks roared past as she sat there alone in the dark. "I could have been murdered or God knows what. I didn't care. I *had* to get a cigarette."

And the punchline?

"I never found the gas station," she says, laughing. "It was light out by then. I got a lift from a woman, who, amazingly enough, was a smoker! And she gave me half her pack. I checked out that morning and came back to New York."

On the trip home, she says, "the despair was tremendous. I knew then that I would never try to quit again. And I remember, when I called my husband and told him I was on my way, the despair in his voice. We just decided that I probably was one of these people that was never going to be able to quit."

Should you relapse at any point, don't berate yourself. You've suffered a temporary setback, not a defeat. Analyze what caused you to backslide and how you can handle that situation the next time it arises. Then discard your cigarettes and begin the process again. Unfortunately, says Annie, "Many people who relapse are so disappointed in themselves, they throw in the towel, and it's another three years before they try again."

Sally S. made no pretense of trying to quit for several years. But her health deteriorated to the point where she had to leave her editorial job at a prestigious Manhattan book publisher. "I just couldn't function anymore," she recalls. "I had pneumonia and bronchitis. I was sick all the time." In 1992 she decided to give the group approach yet another try.

"I was so tired of being unwell. And I have these terrific grandchildren, and I was huffing and puffing trying to keep up with them." This time the cure took. "I was very amazed," she admits. "When I had a week free, I couldn't believe it."

Within the first month Sally no longer coughed incessantly. As she approached one year without cigarettes, she said exultantly, "I haven't sneezed once, I have not had a sore throat, I have not had bronchitis or pneumonia." A pulmonary function test has dampened her elation somewhat, confirming irreversible lung damage.

Nevertheless, at 5 years Sally's risk of lung cancer will begin to diminish, until, at 15 years, it will nearly equal that of a non-smoker. As Dr. Diane Stover explains, "What's seen before lung cancer develops is a change in the tissue: first, atypia, then dysplasia, then metaplasia, and then cancer. If you stop smoking, your cells go through those stages, but backward." An ex-smoker's chances of getting coronary heart disease or cardiovascular disease drop more quickly: beginning after one year and equaling that of a nonsmoker after 10.

Sally still attends Fresh Start meetings—but as a volunteer. "She's a walking miracle, that woman," Annie Beigel says with admiration. "I can't believe she quit; I never thought she would. Some of the other people I've worked with who were like her, they're dying now."

In order to abstain for good, it's imperative that smokers get to the root of why they smoke, for tobacco use—like any addiction —often signifies an underlying problem. Annie offers an example: "If you smoke a lot when you're nervous, and you quit but never really take care of your nerves satisfactorily, you might relapse because of that. You need to make changes."

For Sally came the realization that she used cigarettes to help ease stress. "The boss yelled at me, I lit up a cigarette," she reflects. "The phone rang at work, and it was an irate author, I lit up a cigarette. The addiction convinces a person she can't deal with any of these things unless she's smoking."

After she gave up tobacco, "I had to keep reminding myself that if I'd been able to deal with life's issues for thirty-eight years without smoking, then I could do it again. The biggest thing that keeps you smoking is the fear: 'How will I live without them?' But you really can."

Why do *you* smoke? To help you find out, take the accompanying self-quiz prepared by the National Cancer Institute. Most people's reasons for using tobacco boil down to any of these basic factors:

- Stimulation
- The enjoyment of handling cigarettes
- To accentuate pleasure/for pleasurable relaxation
- To soothe negative feelings
- Craving or psychologic addiction
- Habit

SELF-QUIZ: WHY DO YOU SMOKE?

Answer the 18 questions below using the corresponding numbers:

Always = 5
Frequently = 4
Occasionally = 3
Seldom = 2
Never = 1

A. _____ I smoke cigarettes in order to keep myself from slowing down.

B. _____ Handling a cigarette is part of the enjoyment of smoking it.

C. _____ Smoking cigarettes is pleasant and relaxing.

D. _____ I light up a cigarette when I feel angry about something.

E. _____ When I run out of cigarettes, I find it almost unbearable until I can get them.

F. _____ I smoke cigarettes automatically without being aware of it.

G. _____ I smoke cigarettes to perk myself up.

H. _____ Part of the enjoyment of smoking a cigarette comes from the steps I take to light up.

I. _____ I find cigarettes pleasant.

J. _____ When I feel uncomfortable or upset about something, I light up a cigarette.

K. _____ I am very much aware of the fact when I am not smoking a cigarette.

L. _____ I light up a cigarette without realizing I still have one burning in the ashtray.

M. _____ I smoke cigarettes to give me a lift.

N. _____ When I smoke a cigarette, part of the enjoyment is watching the smoke as I exhale it.

O. _____ I want a cigarette most when I am comfortable and relaxed.

P. _____ When I feel blue or want to take my mind off cares and worries, I smoke cigarettes.

Q. _____ I get a gnawing hunger for a cigarette when I haven't smoked for a while.

R. _____ I've found a cigarette in my mouth and didn't remember putting it there.

How to Score

1. Write the number for each question in the spaces below. For example, if you answered "4" for question A, enter "4" on the line above A.

2. Then add the three scores on each line to get your total. The sum of your scores over lines A, G and M gives you your Stimulation score, and so on. Scores range from 3 to 15, with 11 or over considered high; 7 or under, low. A score of 11 or above in any category indicates that this factor is important to you and is something you need to work on by discovering other ways of attaining this satisfaction.

Totals

_____ + _____ + _____ = _____
 A   G   M   **Stimulation**

_____ + _____ + _____ = _____
 B   H   N   **Handling**

_____ + _____ + _____ = _____
 C   I   O   **Pleasurable Relaxation**

_____ + _____ + _____ = _____
 D   J   P   **Crutch:**
                               To Soothe Tension

_____ + _____ + _____ = _____
 E   K   Q   **Craving:**
                               Psychologic Addiction

_____ + _____ + _____ = _____
 F   L   R   **Habit**

If You Score High in the Following Categories

- Stimulation—You are a smoker who is stimulated by a cigarette. You believe it helps to wake you up, organize your energies and keep you going. If you try to quit, you will need to find a safe substitute such as moderate exercise whenever you feel the urge to have a cigarette.
- Handling—There are many other ways to keep your hands occupied without lighting up or toying with a cigarette. Grab a pen,

(continued)

pencil, coin or piece of jewelry instead; doodle on a piece of paper.

- To accentuate pleasure/for pleasurable relaxation—It can be difficult to determine whether you smoke to feel good or to keep from feeling bad. About two thirds of smokers score high or fairly high in this category, while about half of those also score as high or higher in the next category.
- To soothe negative feelings—Many smokers use cigarettes as a crutch in moments of stress or discomfort. But ultimately cigarettes do not help you to handle problems effectively.
- Craving or psychologic addiction—Quitting smoking is difficult for the person who scores high in this category. As soon as she stubs out one cigarette, she craves another, so tapering off is not likely to work for her.
- Habit—This smoker no longer derives satisfaction from cigarettes but lights up without even realizing it. She may find it easy to quit and stay off tobacco if she can break her old patterns. The key to success is becoming aware of each cigarette you smoke. Ask yourself, "Do I really want this cigarette?" You may be surprised at how many times the answer is no.

OTHER STOP-SMOKING METHODS

There is little hard data on whether to recommend hypnotherapy or acupuncture, although some smokers have found success with these techniques. Both should be viewed as adjuncts to support groups, individual counseling or some other form of behavior modification.

In *hypnotherapy*, approved by the American Medical Association, you are induced into a trance state during which you become susceptible to suggestion. Speaking to your subconscious, the hypnotherapist might propose alternative ways of handling stress or encourage you to adopt a new attitude toward tobacco.

Hypnotherapy appears to be most effective when conducted over several sessions, at a cost of $120 to $350 each. William Hoffman, executive vice-president of the American Society of Clinical Hypnosis, cautions smokers to beware of any practitioner promising a cure in one session, particularly the type who temporarily sets up shop in a hotel. "It's not going to stop you from smoking," he says firmly. "Then he leaves town the next day, and just try getting your money back."

Both the American Society of Clinical Hypnosis and the Society for Clinical and Experimental Hypnosis can direct you to qualified state-licensed hypnotherapists in your area. Call for a few referrals or send a self-addressed, stamped envelope requesting an extensive list.

- American Society of Clinical Hypnosis
  2200 East Devon Avenue, Suite 291
  Des Plaines, IL 60018
  (708) 297-3317
- Society for Clinical and Experimental Hypnosis
  6728 Old McLean Village Drive
  McLean, VA 22101
  (703) 556-9222

The ancient Chinese healing art of *acupuncture* involves inserting slender needles into specific parts of the body to restore balance and energy. Treatment for nicotine withdrawal typically consists of four to six half-hour sessions costing about $50 each. The acupuncturist places two needles in your outer ear, a procedure that is completely painless. In addition, he may recommend a studlike staple that you simply press whenever a nicotine craving arises.

To receive a list of certified acupuncturists in your state, send a check or money order for $3 to the National Commission for the Certification of Acupuncturists, 1424 16th Street, N.W., Suite 501, Washington, DC 20036 (202) 232-1404.

A SMOKE-FREE SOCIETY?

Probably not in our lifetime, but several generations from now, perhaps. Currently about 1 in 4 adults use tobacco, a ratio that has remained steady since the beginning of the decade. It appears we will fall short of the National Cancer Institute's goal of 15 percent by the year 2000. Experts now expect to see the adult smoking population dwindle to around 19 percent, a noteworthy improvement nonetheless.

To maintain this pace, we'll need to concentrate on two areas. First, continuing to call attention to the dangers of cigarettes. "Public education does work," says Dr. Joseph Simone, Memorial Sloan-Kettering's physician-in-chief, and a former smoker himself. "You know what made me quit?" he says. "My kids. They were watching all those TV commercials about how bad smoking is for your health."

The other is legislative, enacting laws that prohibit smoking in public places and levying higher taxes on the sale of cigarettes. "Nobody wants to see tobacco farmers go broke," says Dr. Simone. "But on the other hand," he adds, "they're not paying the bill for taking care of all these ill people."

ALCOHOL

The most widely used drug in the United States can be purchased in your local supermarket. We're referring, of course, to alcohol, implicated in 3 percent of all cancer deaths. The 18.5 million Americans who abuse alcohol predispose themselves to cancers of the mouth, larynx, pharynx, esophagus, liver, colorectum and breast.

But even moderate drinkers increase their risk of several cancers. The National Cancer Institute defines moderate use as no more than two alcoholic beverages a day. If you must drink at all, we recommend limiting your alcohol intake to *no more than four beverages* (a 6-ounce glass of wine, one ounce of spirits or 12 ounces of beer) *per week* as part of a cancer prevention program.

Alcoholic beverages contain not only ethyl alcohol but congeners, chemical compounds or contaminants that are produced during fermentation. Neither has been shown to produce cancer in laboratory animals. However, the body metabolizes alcohol to acetaldehyde, a volatile water-soluble liquid that may in fact be carcinogenic. The International Agency for Research on Cancer (IARC) concluded in 1988, "There is sufficient evidence to suggest that alcoholic beverages are carcinogens to humans."

Although debate still rages over whether alcohol can be considered a direct carcinogen, "There is no question that alcohol is a very potent *co*carcinogen," contends Dr. Charles Lieber. "It makes carcinogens much more effective." Dr. Lieber, director of the alcohol research and treatment center at the Department of Veterans Affairs Medical Center in the Bronx, New York, outlines the numerous mechanisms by which alcohol contributes to cancer.

• *Damages Cells.* "It acts very broadly on many of the factors known to pertain to cancer," he begins. "First of all, alcohol damages many cells, which stimulates cell division. And anything that stimulates cell division is a factor in promoting cancer."

• *Activates Chemical Carcinogens.* "A number of chemical carcinogens, in order to become carcinogens, have to be activated. And alcohol stimulates some of the enzymes that do that."

• *Causes Nutritional Deficiencies.* "Alcohol depletes vitamin A, which has a general protective effect against a wide range of cancers." It also shortchanges the body of the vitamin folate and the trace mineral selenium, both believed to aid in preventing certain cancers, as well as thiamine, leading to brain and nerve damage.

• *Diminishes the Body's Capacity to Fight Off Cancer.* "The body can deactivate certain reactive molecules that may favor carcinogens," such as free radicals, "but alcohol diminishes its capacity to do that. Also, we have enzymes in the body that repair damaged DNA. Alcohol impairs that capacity as well, and anything that alters DNA favors carcinogenesis."

• *Compromises the Immune System.* "Alcohol has a suppressive effect on immune response, which is also involved in the defense against carcinogenesis."

• *Irritates Organ Linings.* Alcohol irritates the delicate lining, or mucosa, of the mouth, throat and esophagus, a possible factor in the cancers of these organs.

• *Smuggles Carcinogens into the Body.* Beer contains potent carcinogens called nitrosamines, while another carcinogenic agent, urethane, has turned up in bourbon, sherry, fruit brandies and other alcoholic beverages.

NO PROOF ABOUT PROOF

Many people assume that "hard" liquor would naturally be more harmful than, say, beer. Whiskey, for example, boasts an ethyl alcohol content of 40 to 50 percent, or 80 to 100 "proof," as compared with 3 to 6 percent for beer. But because alcoholic beverages contain other chemical compounds, proof alone does not determine cocarcinogenicity. Basically, how much you drink is more important than what you drink.

In fact, researchers who studied over 7,000 elderly Japanese men concluded in a 1990 report, "An increased relative risk of rectal cancer was associated with wine and beer consumption but not with consumption of hard liquor." Yet a 1981 study of African-American men living in Washington, D.C., the esophageal cancer capital of the United States, found that those who drank hard liquor exhibited higher rates of esophageal cancer than those who consumed equivalent amounts of wine and beer.

One thing we know for sure: Alcohol and tobacco together produce a synergistic effect that greatly compounds the risk for all cancers. The 4 percent of Americans who smoke and drink heavily are 14 times more likely to develop liver cancer, for example. According to one study, however, even moderate drinkers and smokers elevate their chances of getting cancer of the head and neck region 15-fold.

Clearly the best solution is not to drink alcohol at all. The next time you're out with friends, order mineral water, club soda, fruit juice, vegetable juice, or fruit juice mixed with club soda instead. If you feel more comfortable holding a bottle or wine glass, try one of the ever-expanding brands of nonalcoholic beers and wines.

Should you plan to imbibe, the American Institute for Cancer Research suggests you follow these tips for keeping your drinking under control:

1. Eat before you drink and while you drink. Alcohol enters the bloodstream faster when the stomach is empty, enhancing its inebriating effect.
2. Order diluted drinks such as a white-wine spritzer rather than straight wine.
3. Never guzzle alcohol when you're thirsty. Quench your thirst with water or juice. Then sip your alcoholic beverage slowly.

Men and women who consume more than two alcoholic beverages a day would be classified as alcohol abusers. Some realize they have a problem and are able to curb their drinking on their own, but as with nicotine, others find themselves physically and psychologically addicted. Since 1956 the American Medical Association has recognized alcoholism as a disease.

Cancer is but one of myriad health problems suffered by alcoholics, who on the average live 12 to 15 years fewer than nondrinkers. How do you know if you or a person close to you is an alcoholic? If *any* of the following signs apply to you/he/she, a consultation with a physician or alcohol-abuse treatment specialist is in order.

- Drinking greater amounts of alcohol with greater frequency
- Feeling uncomfortable when alcohol is not available
- Making excuses for drinking to family and friends
- Drinking early in the day
- Having episodes of total memory loss, known as blackouts

• Experiencing hallucinations, "the shakes" or phobias
• Staying drunk for days at a time

Problem drinkers have access to literally thousands of treatment programs, of which there are three basic types. Incipient alcohol abusers may find all the support they need at a peer-counseling group such as Alcoholics Anonymous, the archetype for the countless kindred organizations that have sprung up since its inception in 1935.

More intractable cases, however, require professional intervention, either on an outpatient basis or at a residential facility. Only a qualified physician or alcohol-abuse counselor can determine the appropriate therapy. For information about and referrals to alcohol-abuse treatment programs, contact the Center for Substance Abuse Treatment Referral (800-662-HELP) or the National Council on Alcoholism and Drug Dependence (800-NCA-CALL).

ILLICIT DRUG USE

It goes without saying that no one should use illicit drugs of any kind. Besides the fact that they're illegal, drugs are at the root of the violence that has turned our streets into virtual war zones, feed the AIDS epidemic through addicts sharing unsterilized needles, and are responsible for ruining or ending countless lives.

To this litany of misery, we can add increased cancer risk.

Fortunately, the 1980s and 1990s have brought a steady decrease in illicit drug use, probably for many of the same reasons behind the decline in smoking: heightened public awareness of the dangers, coupled with more health-conscious lifestyles. Nineteen ninety-three, however, witnessed a disturbing upturn in the use of marijuana, LSD and prescription stimulants among high-school students. Like platform shoes and bell-bottoms, heroin, too, has made something of a comeback.

Studies have revealed a likely association between marijuana, still the most popular so-called recreational drug, and lung cancer. The conventional wisdom of the 1960s and 1970s held that marijuana wasn't as dangerous as tobacco because marijuana users smoke far less than cigarette smokers. That notion has been discarded along with lava lamps and Day-Glo posters.

Like cigarettes, marijuana releases toxins that with habitual use can irritate the respiratory tract and give rise to a disorder called chronic obstructive pulmonary disease. One in 100 COPD patients later develop lung cancer.

But marijuana, derived from the *Cannabis sativa* plant, releases five times as much carbon monoxide into the bloodstream as cigarettes, and significantly more tar into the lungs, partly because of the manner in which it is inhaled. A 1988 study conducted at the University of California at Los Angeles School of Medicine observed male subjects smoke both filter-tipped cigarettes and marijuana. Per puff, the men drew four times longer on the marijuana "joint," filling their lungs with one third more smoke and three times as much tar.

The marijuana that makes the rounds in dorm rooms today is not the same drug that some aging members of the Woodstock generation may recall fondly from their youth. Marijuana is a mosaic of more than 400 chemicals that, when smoked, convert into 2,000. Chief among these is delta-9-tetrahydrocannabinol, or THC, *Cannabis sativa*'s main psychoactive ingredient. Whereas marijuana averaged 0.2 percent THC content in the 1960s, it now contains 5 percent, making the drug far more potent.

THC is believed to compromise the immune system, without which we cannot fend off cancer. In tests performed on laboratory rats at Tufts University in Medford, Massachusetts, THC deactivated the natural killer cells, charged with the task of destroying tumor cells.

"There are many studies that show marijuana diminishes immune capacity in certain cases," says Dr. Charles Sharp of the National Institute on Drug Abuse, "especially with higher doses. And not just natural killer cell activity, but lymphocytic and macrophage activity as well." Macrophages, a type of white blood cell, constitute the immune system's front line, scouting out and consuming bacteria and viruses, while lymphocytes, one of three mature white blood cells known as leukocytes, also help defend against infection.

Animal studies do not always correlate with human studies, but another report issued by the University of California at Los Angeles School of Medicine concluded that regular marijuana use interfered with macrophage function in the lungs.

Although other drugs have not been studied as extensively as marijuana, presumably they affect the body in similar ways. Where drugs are concerned, whether it's marijuana or amphetamines, cocaine or ecstasy, any level of use is abuse and can swiftly send you down the slippery slope to addiction.

If you're an occasional user who can quit without outside intervention, we urge you to do so. If you or someone you know needs professional help, contact the Center for Substance Abuse Treatment Referral Hotline (800-662-HELP), the National Council on Alcoholism and Drug Dependence (800-NCA-CALL) or the National Drug Abuse Treatment Referral and Information Service (800-COCAINE) for information and referrals.

SEXUAL BEHAVIOR

Sex? Cancer? Few readers would probably relate the two. But a small group of sexually transmitted viruses are known to cause neoplasms of the genitals, lymphatic system and liver.

The tie between promiscuity and cancer has been suspected for some time. As far back as 1842, an Italian physician named Rigoni-Stern reported on the low rates of cervical cancer observed among cloistered nuns and unmarried women in his country. Conversely, prostitutes exhibit a higher-than-average incidence of cervical cancer, while men who have multiple sex partners increase their susceptibility to carcinoma of the penis.

Scientists linked the *hepatitis B virus* to liver cancer in 1967. Although its transmittal was originally ascribed to blood transfusions and contaminated hypodermic needles, we've since learned that the virus can also be passed by way of bodily fluids such as semen and saliva exchanged during sex. About 1 in 10 men and women infected with hepatitis B become carriers, multiplying their chances of one day incurring liver cancer 340-fold. Ten years later another discovery associated the *human papillomavirus* with cancer of the cervix. *Herpes simplex II,* also known as the genital herpes virus, has been hypothesized as promoting cervical cancer, although no conclusive evidence yet exists. What's more, the sexually transmitted diseases herpes, gonorrhea and syphilis all add to a woman's risk of cervical cancer, as does her having had sexual intercourse before the age of sixteen.

The most recently discovered cancer-causing virus, the *human immunodeficiency virus* (HIV), progresses to *acquired immune deficiency syndrome,* or AIDS. Sufferers of this incurable disease, which ravages the immune system, show a marked propensity for one of several lymphomas and a malignancy of the skin called Kaposi's sarcoma.

AIDS does not discriminate according to sexual preference. However, because it is transmitted chiefly through receptive anal intercourse, it has devastated the male-homosexual segment of society. Other groups at great risk include intravenous drug users, recipients of blood transfusions and hemophiliacs.

It is not our place nor our intention to moralize about sexual conduct. But clearly two partners in a mutually monogamous relationship greatly mitigate their chances of contracting these viruses and other sexually transmitted diseases, not to mention ease their anxiety.

For those who've evaluated the dangers but choose to have multiple sex partners—

Men: Slip on a condom before having intercourse or oral sex.

Women: Insist your male partner wear a condom during sex.

"But it ruins the spontaneity."

"It detracts from the pleasure."

Don't let *anyone* dissuade you from protecting yourself. In this day and age, the stakes are far too high.

THE IMPORTANCE OF PHYSICAL ACTIVITY AND KEEPING FIT

Judging from the ubiquitous joggers huffing and puffing up and down the block each morning, and the gyms and health clubs sprouting up like wildflowers, you would think that Americans have never been more physically fit. While the percentage of adults reporting regular physical activity rose from 35 percent to 41 percent from 1978 to 1990, according to the Centers for Disease Control and Prevention about 6 in 10 of us still lead sedentary lives.

Pioneering industrialist Henry T. Ford once opined, "Exercise is bunk. If you are healthy, you don't need it; if you are sick, you shouldn't take it." Ironically, the automobile he mass-produced at the beginning of this century helped to foster Americans' increasingly inactive lifestyles, along with factory automation, elevators and escalators, a surge in white-collar desk jobs, and technologic advances such as television and video games, which discourage physical exertion. The CDC blames inactivity for 250,000 deaths a year, from heart disease, high blood pressure and other disorders.

Ford's appreciation of the benefits of exercise was on a par with the average physician's understanding of rotary versus piston engines. Keeping active happens to be an essential component of cancer prevention, providing protection through a variety of mechanisms.

• *Helps reduce all cancers by enhancing immune system function.* Dr. I-Min Lee, a researcher at the Harvard University School of Medicine, has coauthored several studies examining exercise's role in cancer prevention.

"There has been a fair amount of research into the immune system of individuals who exercise," she says, "and it has been fairly consistently shown that after a moderate bout of exercise, these individuals have higher circulating levels of natural killer cells." What's more, she notes, "the activity of these cells also seems to be increased." One 1990 study, conducted by San Diego's University of California and Veterans Administration Medical Center, found that exercise more than tripled participants' natural killer cell count.

• *Helps reduce the risk of colorectal cancer by promoting bowel contraction.* Increased contraction speeds waste products through the intestines, narrowing the chance for carcinogens and the colo-rectum lining to come into contact.

According to Dr. Lee, studies consistently show that "physically active individuals have a 30 to 80 percent lower risk of colon cancer than sedentary individuals." She codirected a study that followed more than 17,000 male Harvard alumni. The findings: a 25 to 50 percent lower incidence of colon cancer among those subjects who exercised at moderate to high levels, as compared with the least active men.

• *Helps reduce the risk of prostate cancer, possibly by lowering testosterone levels.* More data are needed to support this theory, but several studies have concluded that physical activity reduces testosterone, and with it a man's odds of getting prostate cancer: The disease occurs as a result of the testes producing excess levels of this male hormone.

• *Helps reduce the risk of breast cancer, uterine cancer and ovarian cancer three ways.* Similarly, an overabundance of the female hormone estrogen can stimulate abnormal cell growth in each of these organs, leading to cancer. Physical activity not only favorably alters the hormone ratio but improves body-fat distribution. Studies have noted a higher incidence of uterine cancer among women heavy in the upper and mid body. Exercise further offers protection by helping to control weight. Fatty tissue releases estrogen, making obesity a risk factor for all three cancers.

Not all scientists concur on a definition of obesity. But generally, says Dr. Lee, a person 20 percent over his or her ideal weight is considered overweight; 40 percent, obese. Men weighing 40 percent above average weight are 35 percent more likely to die of cancer; women weighing 40 percent above average weight, 160 percent.

We've reprinted the Metropolitan Life Insurance Company's weight-height-frame table, which many physicians rely on to calculate a patient's ideal weight.

Take your height and weight wearing one-inch heels and no more than five pounds of clothing for men; eight for women. Next, determine your *frame size:*

- Bend your forearm upward at a 90-degree angle.
- Keeping your fingers straight, turn the inside of your wrist toward your body.
- Place the thumb and index finger of your other hand on the two prominent bones on either side of the elbow.
- Measure the distance between your fingers with a ruler, then match it to the table below for medium-frame men and women. If your measurement is less than the one listed here, consider yourself small-framed; greater than, large-framed.

Computing the obesity range for your height and frame is simple enough to do: *Multiply 1.4 times the recommended weight range.* For a medium-frame five-foot two-inch woman, 165 to 185 pounds and above would be considered obese (1.4 × 118 = 165; 1.4 × 132 = 185).

WHAT FORM OF EXERCISE IS BEST?

Here, too, says Dr. Lee, "scientists don't really agree among themselves. In the 1980s the American College of Sports Medicine advocated an exercise regimen of at least three times a week for at least 20 minutes each time, heavy enough to increase your heart rate or for you to sweat." But in 1993 the ACSM joined with the Centers for Disease Control and several other groups and modified that to 30 minutes or more of *moderate* exercise, such as brisk walking, at least *five* days a week. The earlier recommendations,

MEN		WOMEN	
HEIGHT	*ELBOW BREADTH*	*HEIGHT*	*ELBOW BREADTH*
5'2"–5'3"	$2\frac{1}{2}"–2\frac{7}{8}"$	4'10"–4'11"	$2\frac{1}{4}"–2\frac{1}{2}"$
5'4"–5'7"	$2\frac{5}{8}"–2\frac{7}{8}"$	5'0"–5'3"	$2\frac{1}{4}"–2\frac{1}{2}"$
5'8"–5'11"	$2\frac{3}{4}"–3"$	5'4"–5'7"	$2\frac{3}{8}"–2\frac{5}{8}"$
6'0"–6'3"	$2\frac{3}{4}"–3\frac{1}{8}"$	5'8"–5'11"	$2\frac{3}{8}"–2\frac{5}{8}"$
6'4"	$2\frac{7}{8}"–3\frac{1}{4}"$	6'0"	$2\frac{1}{2}"–2\frac{3}{4}"$

RECOMMENDED WEIGHT
MEN

HEIGHT (FEET/INCHES)		WEIGHT IN POUNDS		
		SMALL FRAME	MEDIUM FRAME	LARGE FRAME
5	2	128–134	131–141	138–150
5	3	130–136	133–143	140–153
5	4	132–138	135–145	142–156
5	5	134–140	137–148	144–160
5	6	136–142	139–151	146–164
5	7	138–145	142–154	149–168
5	8	140–148	145–157	152–172
5	9	142–151	148–160	155–176
5	10	144–154	151–163	158–180
5	11	146–157	154–166	161–184
6	0	149–160	157–170	164–188
6	1	152–164	160–174	168–192
6	2	155–168	164–178	172–197
6	3	158–172	167–182	176–202
6	4	162–176	171–187	181–207

RECOMMENDED WEIGHT
WOMEN

HEIGHT (FEET/INCHES)	WEIGHT IN POUNDS		
	SMALL FRAME	MEDIUM FRAME	LARGE FRAME
4 10	102–111	109–121	118–131
4 11	103–113	111–123	120–134
5 0	104–115	113–126	122–137
5 1	106–118	115–129	125–140
5 2	108–121	118–132	128–143
5 3	111–124	121–135	131–147
5 4	114–127	124–138	134–151
5 5	117–130	127–141	137–155
5 6	120–133	130–144	140–159
5 7	123–136	133–147	143–163
5 8	126–139	136–150	146–167
5 9	129–142	139–153	149–170
5 10	132–145	142–156	152–173
5 11	135–148	145–159	155–176
6 0	138–151	148–162	158–179

it was felt, may have discouraged people from discovering the advantages of physical activity.

We're not suggesting joggers, cyclists, weight lifters and aerobics enthusiasts give up their favorite forms of exercise. But if you're unable to set aside time to work out, try incorporating physical activity into your daily life: the next time you have to go to the store, leave the car at home and walk. Instead of taking elevators and escalators, climb the stairs. And so on.

According to most studies, exercising seven days a week as opposed to five does not improve physical fitness. In fact, overdoing it can actually prove harmful. As Dr. Lee notes, "exhaustive bouts of exercise—and by that I mean a marathon run, for example—depress the immune system. Some studies have shown that it is depressed for a couple of hours, while others have shown that it stays depressed for as long as two weeks." Dr. Lee, an avid walker and cyclist, also points out that "heavy amounts of exercise cause a lot of wear and tear on joints and ligaments."

One benefit of exercise can't be measured with a scale or a

body-fat caliper: the sense of pleasure, vitality and well-being it instills. Following major surgery to remove her ovaries, uterus and a third of her colon, Mary V. says she "discovered exercise as a tremendously life-affirming, stress-reducing thing to do. Now it is a top priority with me. I do low-impact aerobics and a lot of stretch-and-tone classes.

"It has made me strong, and it has made me able to face life after cancer," Mary continues. "I can't emphasize enough what it feels like mentally to be good to your body like this."

SOLAR RADIATION

Each year more than 700,000 men and women in the United States are diagnosed with skin cancer, a disease caused almost exclusively by the damaging effects of the sun's ultraviolet rays. We include this discussion here in the chapter on lifestyle because many people's idea of an idyllic weekend or vacation consists of lounging in the sun, unprotected.

Malignant melanoma, the rarest form of skin cancer, has gradually earned the public's respect; claiming nearly 7,000 lives annually will do that. But too many people fail to take seriously the more common forms of skin cancer: basal-cell carcinoma and squamous-cell carcinoma. While rarely fatal, these diseases are capable of inflicting horrible disfigurement. Try telling a patient who had to lose part of an ear or nose that he or she "only" had skin cancer.

See Chapter 16 for details on how to enjoy the sun safely.

SUGGESTED READING ABOUT HOW TO QUIT SMOKING

From the National Cancer Institute (800-4-CANCER):
• "Clearing the Air: How to Quit Smoking . . . and Quit for Keeps"

From the American Cancer Society (800-ACS-2345):
• "Smart Move! A Stop Smoking Guide"
• "How to Stay Quit over the Holidays"

KEY WORDS

Cold turkey: The abrupt and complete withdrawal from any addictive substance.

Hepatitis B virus: A virus transmitted through the blood or sexual activity and known to cause liver disease and liver cancer.

Human Immunodeficiency Virus (HIV): An incurable virus, generally transmitted through blood and blood products as well as anal sex, that progresses to *acquired immune deficiency syndrome*. AIDS has been associated with several lymphatic cancers and Kaposi's sarcoma, a malignancy of the skin.

Human papillomaviruses: A group of sexually transmitted viruses, some of which may be associated with the development of cervical cancer.

Nicotine: The addictive compound found in tobacco smoke.

Nicotine gum: A stop-smoking aid, nicotine gum releases nicotine into the body through the lining of the mouth. Available by prescription only.

Nicotine patch: Another stop-smoking aid, the patch is applied daily to the skin for about three months and releases a tapering dose of nicotine. Available by prescription only.

Postponing: A gradual method of stopping smoking.

Tapering: A gradual method of stopping smoking.

Tar: The solid chemical particles found in tobacco smoke. Tars contain carcinogens and turn into viscous resins in the lungs.

THC (delta-9-tetrahydrocannabinol): The main psychoactive ingredient in marijuana, THC is believed to suppress the immune system.

CHAPTER

7

Carcinogens in the Home, Workplace and General Environment

How to Protect Yourself and Your Family from Radon, Asbestos, Secondhand Smoke and Other Cancer-Causing Agents

Environmental (air and drinking water) pollution probably fig-ures in only 2 percent of all cancer deaths. Nevertheless, as relatively minor as the risk may be, cancer-triggering agents do dot our surroundings. The purpose of this chapter isn't to need-lessly alarm you but to show you simple steps you can take to safeguard yourself and your family at home and at work. As with diet, smoking and exercise, here we have yet another way to lower your overall cancer risk.

CARCINOGENS IN AND
AROUND THE HOME

RADON

Radon, the second leading cause of lung cancer in the United States, is a radioactive gas produced by the natural breakdown of uranium in soil, rock and water. This unwelcome intruder slips stealthily into houses through contaminated building materials such as cinder blocks and cement, cracks and holes in the foundation, and other portals of entry, such as

- Cracks in solid floors
- Cracks in walls
- Gaps in suspended floors
- Gaps around service pipes
- Cavities inside walls
- Construction joints
- The water supply

Improperly ventilated homes trap radon inside, allowing levels to build up dangerously. As the gas decays, it releases radioactive alpha particles that, when inhaled, can damage cells in the lung, initiating cancer. The federal Environmental Protection Agency in Washington, D.C., attributes as many as 20,000 cancer fatalities a year to radon and estimates that excessive levels plague millions of U.S. homes—nearly 1 in 15.

How do you know if yours is among them? The type of house you live in is no determinant, for radon infiltrates both old and new dwellings, drafty and well-insulated structures, homes with basements and those without. Because the gas is odorless, colorless and tasteless, the only way to detect its presence is to run a radon test.

The appendix lists the phone numbers of your state's radon office, which can refer you to qualified testing contractors in your area. But the test is easy enough to perform yourself.

Most hardware stores carry radon-testing kits for about $25. You'll find several devices to choose from: charcoal canisters, charcoal liquid scintillation, and alpha track. Any is suitable for the short-term test, which takes two to three days. The long-term test lasts more than 90 days, giving you a good estimate of the

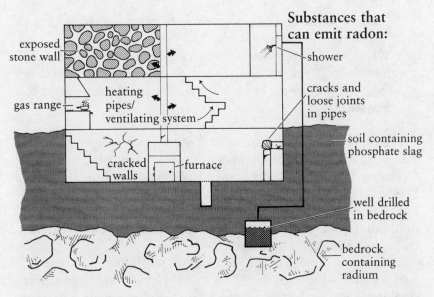

Common Sources of Radon. This odorless gas can enter your home through almost any crack, exposed brick, a sump pump, well water and contaminated building materials. Once in your home, the gas can circulate freely through heating ducts or the ventilating system.

year-long reading. For the long-term test, the EPA recommends the alpha-track detector. Whichever kind you purchase, be sure the package bears the words "Meets EPA Requirements."

How to Conduct a Radon Test

Twelve hours before beginning the short-term test, shut all windows and outside doors, and keep them closed as much as possible over the next few days. Also, do not run the short-term during extremely stormy or windy weather. Those two conditions aside, the same instructions apply for both tests:

- Place the test kit in the lowest *lived-in* level of the home. For one family, that may be the basement; for another, the first floor.
- Keep the unit in a room you use regularly—the living room or den, for example—but not a kitchen, bathroom or laundry room.
- The kit should sit at least 20 inches above the floor, where it

can't be disturbed. Keep it away from drafts, high heat or humidity, and exterior walls.

- When the testing period ends *as specified by the manufacturer,* reseal the kit and mail it promptly to the laboratory indicated on the package. Your results should arrive within a few weeks.

Radon is typically measured in *picocuries of radon per liter of air,* or pCi/L, although you may also see it expressed as *working levels,* or WL. The average level in homes is about 1.5 pCi/L. Below 4 pCi/L (0.02 WL), no corrective measures are necessary. But as Dave Rowson, deputy director of the EPA's office of radiation, points out, "Because radon is radioactive and a carcinogen, there is no absolutely safe level."

To give you an idea of the hazard involved, living in a home that tests 4 pCi/L—the minimum EPA "action level"—is equivalent to smoking half a pack of cigarettes a day; breathing in air containing 10 pCi/L would be akin to undergoing 500 chest x-rays annually. Homes have tested as high as 3,500 pCi/L.

Should a short-term test reveal a concentration of 4 pCi/L or greater, the EPA suggests following up with either a second short-term test or a yearlong test to calculate the annual level, for short-term tests taken during cooler months often greatly overestimate levels. If you decide on a second short-term test, average the results. Consider fixing your home if the average comes to 4 pCi/L or higher.

Reducing Radon Levels

"The first step," says the EPA's Rowson, "is to call your state radon office, which will have a list of radon-mitigation companies approved by the state or by the EPA. Contractors that have been through the EPA's Radon Contractor Proficiency Program are well trained in determining what will be the best mitigation system for a house. It will depend somewhat on the type of house, the magnitude of the radon problem and the way the radon is getting into the home."

For houses that have a basement or slab-on-grade foundation (concrete poured at ground level), the most common radon-reduction strategy is called active subslab suction. "What we do," Rowson explains, "is put a plastic pipe through the foundation and down into the soil. The pipe gets run up out the roof, and we put a fan on the end." The fan operates continuously and should never be shut off.

"This sucks the radon out from beneath the foundation and blows it out the top of the roof, where it disperses into insignificant concentrations. Subslab suction is usually done in combination with sealing any cracks or openings in the house." The job costs approximately $800 to $2,500 and can usually be completed in a day. Homeowners should expect to incur additional operating costs of $75 to $175 a year in higher utility bills, as most radon-reduction systems cause some heat or cool-air loss, while systems that use fans nudge up electricity consumption.

The following table, prepared by the EPA, outlines other radon-mitigation methods, including the approximate expense and efficiency of each.

METHODS OF RADON REDUCTION

TECHNIQUE	TYPICAL RADON REDUCTION	APPROXIMATE COST	COMMENTS
Passive Subslab Suction	30% to 70%	$550 to $2,250 plus some energy penalties	May be more effective in cold climates; not as effective as active subslab suction
Draintile Suction	90% to 99%	$800 to $1,700 plus $75 to $175 in annual operating costs	Works best if draintiles form complete loop around house
Blackwall Suction	50% to 99%	$1,500 to $3,000 plus $150 to $300 in annual operating costs	Only in house with hollow blackwalls; requires sealing major openings
Sump Hole Suction	90% to 99%	$800 to $2,500 plus $100 to $225 in annual operating costs	Works best if air moves easily to sump under slab, or if draintiles form complete loop

(continued)

TECHNIQUE	TYPICAL RADON REDUCTION	APPROXIMATE COST	COMMENTS
Submembrane Depressurization in a Crawl Space	80% to 99%	$1,000 to $2,500 plus $70 to $175 in annual operating costs	Less heat loss than natural ventilation in cold winter climates
Natural Ventilation in a Crawl Space	0% to 50%	$0; $200 to $500 if additional vents installed; plus there may be some energy penalties	Costs variable
Sealing Radon Entry Routes	0% to 50%	$100 to $2,000; no operating costs	Normally used with other techniques; proper materials and installation required
House (Basement) Pressurization	50% to 99%	$500 to $1,500 plus $150 to $500 in annual operating costs	Works best with tight basement isolated from outdoors and upper floors
Natural Ventilation	Variable	$0; $200 to $500 if additional vents installed; $100 to $700 typical annual operating cost range for fan electricity and heated/cooled air loss	Significant heated/cooled air loss; operating costs depend on utility rates and amount of ventilation

| Heat Recovery Ventilation | 25% to 50% if used for full house; 25% to 75% if used for basement | $1,200 to $2,500 plus $75 to $500 for continuous operation in annual operating costs | Limited use: best in tight house; for full house, use with levels no higher than 8 pCi/L; no higher than 16 pCi/L for use in basement; less conditioned air loss than natural ventilation |

NOTE: The fan electricity and house heating/cooling loss range is based on certain assumptions regarding climate, your house size and the cost of electricity and fuel. Your costs may vary. These numbers are based upon 1991 data.

In finding a radon-reduction contractor, use the same discretion as you would when hiring anyone to work on your home. To properly evaluate and compare companies, the EPA recommends asking the following questions:

1. Do you have proof that you are bonded, licensed and insured for liability? *The latter protects you in the event of injury to persons or property damage while the work is being done.*
2. Do you have proof that you are state-certified and/or listed in the EPA's National Radon Contractor Proficiency Report? *RCP contractors should carry current photo ID cards.*
3. Will you conduct any diagnostic tests on my home before recommending a radon-reduction system? And if so, is there an additional charge? *Sometimes a visual inspection is sufficient, but other times the contractor may need to use a "smoke gun" or another type of diagnostic test to help locate the source and direction of air movement in the house or under the foundation.*
4. After you've installed the system, will you test it to ensure it functions properly? *RCP contractors must see to it that a test is conducted within 30 days of installing the system, preferably within 2 to 7 days.*
5. Do you guarantee to reduce radon levels to 4 pCi/L or below, and for how long?

6. What is the total cost of the job, including taxes and permit fees? How much of a deposit is required, if any, and when must I pay the balance?
7. How long will the work take to complete?
8. Will you obtain any necessary licenses and meet all local building codes?
9. Do you clean up after the job?
10. Do you guarantee that you are responsible for any damage to my home or property?
11. Are any warranties or guarantees on parts and labor transferable if I remodel or sell my home?
12. What am I expected to do to make the work area accessible before you begin?

Once you settle on a contractor, be sure these points are included in the contract. Read the document carefully before signing. After the work is done, inspect the system yourself to ensure it meets RCP standards, using the following checklist:

_____ The system is clearly labeled.
_____ Exhaust pipes of soil-suction systems vent 10 feet or more above ground, and away from windows, doors or other openings that could allow radon to reenter the home.
_____ Exhaust fans are located in an unlivable area of the house, such as an unoccupied attic, not in a basement.
_____ The system includes a warning device to alert of a malfunction: a liquid gauge, a sound alarm, a light indicator or a needle-display gauge.
_____ The warning device is accessible, so that it can be readily seen or heard. *If a monitor indicates the system is not working properly, contact your contractor at once.*
_____ The outside exhaust fan and all electrical connections meet local codes.

Also:

• Ask for written operating and maintenance instructions and copies of any warranties.
• Retest your home for radon or have an *independent* tester take the measurement.

Selling, Buying or Renovating a Home?

With radon's dangers having been widely publicized in recent years, more and more buyers and renters now inquire about levels.

If you're thinking of selling your home, it would be a good idea to test for radon—and, if necessary, correct any problems—before you put it on the market, since a buyer's discovery of elevated radon levels could conceivably delay or scuttle a sale. (The protocols for real-estate transactions differ somewhat. They are spelled out in the booklet "Home Buyer's and Seller's Guide to Radon," available for free from the EPA Information Access Branch, Public Information Center; see Appendix for address and phone number.) Without question, being able to produce a safe test result or point to a radon-reduction system in place is a desirable selling point.

Similar foresight can benefit you when remodeling or building a home. Let's say you're planning on converting an attic into a living space. Test for radon first. That way, should your result indicate an elevated concentration of gas, the contractor could inexpensively incorporate radon-resistant building features into the construction. (After any major home renovation, be sure to test again.) Likewise, you will incur less cost by building radon-resistant features into a new home than trying to fix a problem later.

Given the health hazard radon poses, the peace of mind a mere $25 test can buy has to be considered a bargain. As Dave Rowson of the EPA points out, "Often, when the public faces environmental risks, they have to trust somebody else to take care of the problem. Radon is an issue that people can do something about to protect their health in a simple and straightforward way."

ASBESTOS

Asbestos, another undesirable tenant in the home, was a popular, versatile building material for years, used in everything from floor tiles to pipe insulation to roofing. Since its commercial introduction in 1880, more than 5,000 patents have been issued for products containing asbestos, which is both heat- and fire-resistant.

Asbestos actually refers to a group of naturally occurring mineral fibers that can be separated into thin threads and woven or compressed into blocks and tiles. These fibers crumble easily into microscopic particles that waft through the air and stick to clothing, hair and skin. When swallowed or inhaled, they lodge in the lungs and damage cells. Prolonged, heavy exposure drives up a person's risk of lung cancer and mesothelioma, a rare cancer of the thin membranes that line the chest and abdomen.

Public awareness of asbestos hazards has snowballed to a point that sometimes seems to border on hysteria. Only when the material becomes damaged is it dangerous. Asbestos that appears to be in good condition *should be left alone*.

Unless it is marked, as now required by law, you may not be able to identify all the asbestos in your home. Nevertheless, it's certainly wise to casually inspect each room. From the basement on up, here are the common household asbestos hazards to look for, according to the American Lung Association and Consumer Protection Safety Commission:

- In older homes, hot-water pipes, steam pipes, boilers and furnace ducts insulated with asbestos blankets or asbestos paper tape.
- Oil and coal furnaces insulated with asbestos; check door gaskets too.
- Wood-stove or coal-stove door gaskets containing asbestos.
- Vinyl asbestos floor tiles; the backing on vinyl sheet flooring; and adhesives used to install floor tiles.
- Walls and floors around wood-burning stoves protected with asbestos paper, millboard or cement sheets.
- Soundproofing or decorative material sprayed on walls and ceilings.
- Patching and joint compounds used on walls and ceilings.
- Textured paints.
- Artificial ashes and embers sold for use in gas-fired fireplaces.
- Insulation, particularly in homes built between 1930 and 1950.
- Roofing and siding shingles made of asbestos cement.

Should you come across material that appears worn, cut, loose, crumbly or in any way damaged, *do not touch it*. There are methods for cutting and sending asbestos samples to a laboratory for analysis, but we strongly discourage anyone from doing this themselves. Improper handling can send fibers cascading into the air or onto yourself, creating a hazard where none existed.

Sometimes, if asbestos is only slightly damaged and occupies an area where there's relatively little traffic or air flow, the best thing to do is to limit access to that section of the house and leave the asbestos undisturbed. The American Lung Association and U.S. Consumer Product Safety Commission warn homeowners *never* to:

- dust, sweep or vacuum debris that may contain asbestos.
- saw, sand, scrape or drill holes in asbestos materials.
- use abrasive pads or brushes to power-strip wax from asbestos flooring. Never use a power stripper at all on a dry floor.
- sand or try leveling asbestos flooring or its backing. When asbestos flooring needs replacing, install a new floor covering over it, if possible.
- track material that could contain asbestos through the house. If you cannot avoid walking through the area, clean it first with a wet mop. If the material is from a damaged area, or if a large area must be cleaned, call an asbestos professional.

More extensively damaged asbestos should be repaired or removed. For either job, says Vanessa Vu, deputy director of the EPA's health and environmental review division, "seek professionals trained to handle asbestos properly." The EPA-funded Toxic Hotline in Washington, D.C. (202-554-1404), can put you in touch with the agency in your state that maintains lists of approved asbestos-abatement contractors.

Have one company assess the problem and recommend a corrective measure, and another carry out the work, to avoid a conflict of interest. Asbestos repair entails treating the material with a sealant or wrapping it in a protective jacket. While less costly than removal, should future removal be necessary, it complicates the process and adds to the expense.

As with hiring a radon-removal contractor, this is not a decision to be made lightly. When interviewing prospective companies, ask to see their certification and references. Call these customers. Were they satisfied with the way the job was handled? Also, check with the state Better Business Bureau. Has the firm committed any safety violations? Have any legal actions been filed against it? To obtain the bureau's number, dial information for your state capital city.

See to it your contract specifies the work plan, including cleanup and disposal, and guarantees adherence to federal, state and local codes. (Afterward, have the contractor sign off that all procedures were followed.) While the work is under way, the American Lung Association and U.S. Consumer Product Safety Commission recommend keeping an eye out that the crew meets the following conditions:

- The work area should be clearly marked as a hazard zone. Keep people and pets away until the work is finished.

- Workers must wear approved respirators, gloves and other protective clothing.
- To prevent asbestos dust from getting tracked or blown into other rooms, the work area should be sealed off with plastic sheets and duct tape, and heating or air conditioning should be turned off.
- Before removing asbestos, the contractor should wet it with a hand sprayer, which helps prevent fibers from flaking off into the air.
- Material should not be broken down into smaller pieces but kept whole.

Once removal is completed, the work zone should be cleaned thoroughly with wet mops, rags, sponges or a high-efficiency particulate air (HEPA) vacuum cleaner—*never* a conventional vacuum—and all asbestos and disposable equipment and clothing must be deposited in sealed, leakproof, labeled plastic bags. In inspecting the area, you should see no dust or debris, but to be extra safe, we recommend having an independent firm remonitor the air for fibers.

ENVIRONMENTAL TOBACCO SMOKE

Until the 1986 Surgeon General's report on the dangers of environmental tobacco smoke (also referred to as secondhand, passive, involuntary or ambient smoke), family members who urged a tobacco user to quit did so out of concern for that person's health, unaware their own welfare was at stake. But Dr. C. Everett Koop's "The Health Consequences of Involuntary Smoking" shattered smokers' illusions that they weren't harming anyone but themselves, by verifying what had been suspected for years: Secondhand smoke causes lung cancer.

If any doubt remained, in 1993 the EPA classified environmental tobacco smoke as a class A carcinogen, putting it in the company of asbestos, radon and other substances known to trigger cancer in humans. Passive smoke kills an estimated 53,000 men and women annually, about two thirds from heart disease and 3,800 from lung cancer. Just living with a smoker increases your risk of lung cancer 30 percent, higher still if that person uses tobacco heavily.

The *mainstream* smoke that a smoker inhales and the cloud of residual smoke that envelops smokers and nonsmokers alike "are very similar," explains Dr. David Schottenfeld, for many years a colleague of ours at Memorial Sloan-Kettering, and now a professor of epidemiology and internal medicine at the University of Michigan School of Public Health.

"Tobacco is a very complex substance, with many thousands of chemicals, a number of which have been identified as having carcinogenic properties," he continues. "Several of these are at higher concentrations in sidestream tobacco smoke than in mainstream smoke." For example, the *sidestream* smoke that curls into the air contains 2 to 15 times the amount of oxygen-depleting carbon monoxide as does the smoke inhaled by the smoker.

Most sobering of all is environmental tobacco smoke's effect on children. One 1990 study reported that boys and girls whose mothers and fathers smoked had twice the risk of lung cancer later in adult life as those whose parents did not. Furthermore, Action on Smoking and Health (ASH), a Washington-based national non-smokers-rights organization, notes that each year hundreds of thousands of susceptible youngsters contract respiratory conditions that are aggravated by secondhand smoke:

- 300,000 cases of lower respiratory infection
- 1 million asthma attacks
- 26,000 new asthma cases
- 1,000 infant fatalities from sudden infant death syndrome, or SIDS.

ASH and like-minded citizens' groups have lobbied for legislation limiting or eliminating smoking in public places, with increasing success. But unless tobacco is one day declared illegal or regulated as any other pharmaceutical agent, the choice of whether or not to smoke in the privacy of their homes will rest with smokers' consciences. If the knowledge that their habit jeopardizes the health of loved ones isn't enough to persuade them to give up tobacco, it's up to family members to insist that indoor smoking not be tolerated. (See Chapter 6 for a more detailed discussion of smoking and cancer.)

PESTICIDES

For many homeowners, a lush lawn is a source of pride. However, the quest for lawn-care perfection can go too far, coming at the expense of family safety. Ever since the vast migration from the cities to the suburbs following World War II, home use of pesticides has multiplied like pokeweeds. Per acre, U.S. homeowners dust, spray and powder their property with more chemicals than do farmers: 300 million pounds a year.

Most people naturally assume that because the EPA registers and regulates these products, they present no hazard. Yet a 1986 National Cancer Institute study estimated that 2,4-D, a commonly used weed killer, significantly increased the rate of non-Hodgkin's lymphoma in farmers who used it at least 20 days per year.

Or take the insecticide dichlorvos (DDVP), used in no-pest strips, flea collars and more than 800 other consumer products. While the EPA does not consider DDVP to pose "an unreasonable risk," says Al Heier of the agency's pesticide division, "it is," he stresses, "a carcinogen." The EPA defines unreasonable risk as *greater than one additional case of cancer per one million people exposed to a given pesticide over a lifetime.* Your odds, then, of getting cancer from insecticides, herbicides and fungicides are minute, to be sure, but why take a chance?

The sensible solution is to forgo lawn and garden chemicals, which you can do without turning your yard into a jungle of weeds and vines. The EPA suggests these environmentally friendly ways of cultivating a handsome lawn:

• *Develop healthy soil.* Your grass's health hinges on the quality of the soil below. Fertilize annually to replenish nitrogen, phosphorous and potassium, and periodically test the critical balance of acidity and alkalinity. Lawns thrive in slightly acidic soil with a pH content of 6.5 to 7. A lower level indicates high acidity, which you can rectify by adding lime; sulfur produces the opposite effect.

Similarly, analyze soil texture now and then to make sure the ground isn't overly clay heavy or overly sandy, but somewhere in between. Spreading compost, grass clippings or manure can help to achieve the ideal "loamy" mix of sand, silt and a slightly lower proportion of clay. Soil that's too compacted, either from an abundance of clay or too many backyard touch-football games, prevents air and water from reaching the roots. Digging small air holes with a steel rake will loosen the earth sufficiently so that water and nutrients penetrate once again.

• *Choose a climate-compatible grass.* Just because you live in Kentucky doesn't mean you should necessarily plant Kentucky bluegrass. In choosing a type of seed or sod, take into account the grass's needs in terms of shade, moisture, wear and tear, and susceptibility to pests and disease, all of which your local nursery can advise you on.

• *Mow high and often, with sharp blades.* "That's probably the best advice," says the EPA's Heier. "If you mow high, the grass itself provides enough shade to prevent weeds from getting a foothold." The optimum length for most grasses, two and a half to three and a half inches high, can reduce weeds and disease by 50 percent to 80 percent.

• *Water slowly and deeply.* According to the EPA, no one should be watering the lawn every day. It's thoroughness, not frequency, that benefits grass. Water only when the lawn starts to wilt from dryness, losing its color and retaining footprints for more than a few seconds. Then, using a water-conserving soaker hose, slowly apply about an inch of water. Deep watering trains grass roots down, better enabling them to absorb moisture during dry spells.

• *Reduce thatch buildup.* Dead plant material that accumulates between the grass and the soil can block water and nutrients from getting to the soil and grass roots. Heavy thatch, thicker than half an inch deep, may be a sign that you're applying too much fertilizer. Two techniques for correcting the problem are to rake the lawn or sprinkle it with compost or topsoil.

• *Rely on Mother Nature's assistance.* Not all pests are pests. Earthworms, for example, help to keep thatch under control by eating it and discharging their nitrogen-rich waste into the soil. Nurseries and garden-supply mail-order firms sell beneficial parasites and predators such as ladybugs, which prey upon aphids, mites and other insects harmful to plant life.

If you do apply pesticides to your lawn, accord them the proper respect. "Remember," says Al Heier, "they are toxic, meant to kill an insect, a weed, a fungus or a rodent." First, take inventory of your garage or garden shed, for pesticides can languish on the shelf season after season, long after they've been banned. Any of the following 53 EPA-banned or severely restricted pesticides, listed alphabetically, should be discarded. *Important: Never put these dangerous chemicals out with the trash.*

"Most areas have collection days at central locations," explains Heier, "where people can bring such products." To find out how to properly dispose of hazardous pesticides, call your state pesticide agency, the number of which appears in the appendix.

Banned

1. Aldrin
2. Benzene hexachloride (BHC)
3. 2,3,4,5-Bis(2-butylene)tetrahydro-2-furaldehyde (Repellent 11)
4. Bromoxynil butyrate
5. Cadmium compounds
6. Calcium arsenate
7. Captafol
8. Carbon tetrachloride
9. Chloranil
10. Chlordimeform
11. Chlorinated camphene (Toxaphene)
12. Chlorobenzilate
13. Chloromethoxypropylmercuric acetate (CPMA)
14. Copper arsenate
15. Cyhexatin
16. DBCP
17. DDT
18. Decachlorooctahydro-1,3,4-metheno-2H-cyclobuta*(cd)*pentalen-2-one (chlordecone)
19. Dieldrin
20. Dinoseb and salts
21. Di(phenylmercury)dodecenylsuccinate (PMDS)
22. Endrin
23. EPN
24. Ethyl hexyleneglycol (6-12)
25. Hexachlorobenzene (HCB)
26. Lead arsenate
27. Leptophos
28. Mirex
29. Monocrotophos
30. Nitrofen (TOK)
31. OMPA (octamethylpyrophosphoramide)
32. Phenylmercuric oleate (PMO)
33. Potassium 2,4,5-trichlorophenate (2,4,5-TCP)
34. Pyriminil (Vacor)
35. Safrole
36. Silvex
37. Sodium arsenate
38. Sodium arsenite

39. TDE
40. Terpene polychlorinates (Strobane)
41. Thallium sulfate
42. 2,4,5-Trichlorophenoxyacetic acid (2,4,5-T)
43. Vinyl chloride

Severely Restricted (for use only by formally trained, certified pesticide applicators)

1. Arsenic trioxide
2. Carbofuran
3. Chlordane
4. Daminozide
5. EDB
6. Heptachlor
7. Mercuric chloride
8. Mercurous chloride
9. Phenylmercury acetate (PMA)
10. Tributyltin compounds

EPA GUIDELINES ON HOW TO HANDLE PESTICIDES SAFELY

Outdoors

- "Before you use a pesticide, read the label," says Al Heier, "and follow the instructions."
- Wear whatever items of protective clothing are recommended, such as long pants, long sleeves, impervious gloves, hats, goggles and shoes made of rubber, not canvas or leather. Afterward, rinse off your boots or shoes before entering the house, wash your clothes separately, and take a shower and shampoo your hair.
- Use only the amount directed.
- Do not use pesticides when the wind is above five miles per hour, to prevent drifting.
- Do not spray or dust near wells and fish ponds.
- Keep children and pets away from where you mix or apply pesticides.
- Should you spill a pesticide, don't wash it away. Promptly sprinkle it with sawdust, vermiculite or kitty litter, sweep it into a plastic trash bag and put it out with the garbage for collection.
- Never smoke while using pesticides. You could accidentally

transfer traces of pesticide from your hand to your mouth. Too, some chemicals are flammable.

- "It's prudent to wait until the pesticides have been washed off the foliage before allowing children to play on the lawn," says Heier. "The label isn't going to require that," he notes, "but it's a good practice. Because when you have pesticides on the foliage and grass, and children play in it, they're going to get an exposure that was never intended."

Indoors

- Keep children and pets away from the area.
- Remove food, dishes, and pots and pans before treating kitchen cabinets; wait until shelves dry before restocking them.
- Spray only a small area at one time, never an entire wall or ceiling.
- Keep rodent or insect baits out of children's and pets' reach.
- Allow proper ventilation. Vacate the area for *at least* as long as the label recommends.
- Once again, says the EPA's Heier, exercise extreme caution where children are concerned. "Inside the house, pesticides usually fall to the floor," he explains. "Children crawl on the floor, and because of their size, the potential danger is going to be greatest to them." According to a 1987 National Cancer Institute study, youngsters from households where indoor pesticides were used had a nearly fourfold risk of contracting childhood leukemia.

Storage

- Never transfer pesticides from their original containers.
- Make sure the contents are clearly and prominently labeled.
- Refasten all childproof closures or lids.
- Store pesticides away from youngsters and pets, preferably in a garden shed or a well-ventilated, locked utility cabinet, away from food, medical supplies and cleaning supplies.
- Keep flammable liquids outside the house and away from ignition sources.
- Don't store pesticides where flooding is possible, or in open places where they might spill or leak into the environment.
- One way to reduce storage problems is to buy only enough chemicals to last the season.

Disposal

Call your county health department (its number is in the blue pages of the White Pages phonebook) and ask if a hazardous-waste collection program is in operation for your community. If not, you may discard *up to one gallon of liquid* by tightly sealing the original container, wrapping it in several layers of newspaper, tying the package securely and placing it in a covered trash can for routine collection.

USING A LAWN-CARE SERVICE

"From all the evidence this agency has gathered," says Al Heier of the EPA, "most companies take considerable care in applying pesticides. However, people ought to be aware what products the company is applying and when. They are obligated to tell you."

Don't be satisfied with a worker telling you the chemicals being used are "safe" or "EPA approved." And let go any company whose employees do not follow the same safety guidelines regarding proper attire and protective gear that you would. Their lack of safety consciousness indicates a gross ignorance about the potential dangers of the substances they work with.

Be on the lookout for neighbors who use pesticides and keep your children, their toys and pets indoors when pesticides are being applied. Because lawn-care companies and gardening services have to follow daily appointment schedules, they may not postpone chemical treatments simply because, say, there's too much wind. Be sure unwanted chemicals are not drifting onto your property. If they are, speak to the people doing the work *and* report the offending company to the state pesticide agency immediately.

If a firm cannot adequately answer your questions about the chemicals it's using, call the National Pesticide Telecommunications Network, a toll-free information service partly funded by the EPA, at (800-858-PEST), Monday through Friday, 8 A.M. to 6 P.M. CST.

CAN YOUR DRINKING WATER CAUSE CANCER?

Probably not. Dangerous levels of known and suspected carcinogens in U.S. drinking water are "very rare," says Margaret Stasikowski, director of the health and ecological criteria division within the EPA's Office of Water.

Nevertheless, water contamination can occur, from a variety of sources. The trace metal arsenic, a proven human carcinogen, "forms naturally in the earth's crust," explains Stasikowski, "so as you take water out of the ground, you take some percentage of the arsenic with it.

"Chemicals like vinyl chloride," also a class A carcinogen, "appear in groundwater because perhaps years ago there was a manufacturing or processing plant in the area, and the chemical seeped into the groundwater." Similarly, "pesticides from fields [and lawns] may have seeped into groundwater due to improper control and overapplication."

Municipal water systems are required to test for 71 major contaminants and will send you the results upon request. The EPA sees no need for consumers to independently test municipal water themselves. However, says Stasikowski, if your water comes from a private well, "it would be a good idea to get your water tested." The American Council of Independent Laboratories in Washington, D.C. (202-887-5872), can refer you to laboratories in your area, or consult the Yellow Pages under "Water Analysis."

To interpret the results, call the EPA's Safe Drinking Water Hotline at (800-426-4791) and request a copy of its "Drinking Water Regulations and Health Advisories," which lists the permissible levels for some 300 chemicals. You will be most concerned with those classified under cancer groups A (known human carcinogens) and B (probable human carcinogens). Group C indicates possible human carcinogens; D, not classifiable due to lack of data or adequate evidence; and E, no evidence of carcinogenicity.

As an example, the maximum permissible contaminant level of milligrams per liter for benzene, an "A" carcinogen, is 0.005. In the unlikely event that your result greatly exceeded that, you would need to take corrective action, either switching to bottled water, installing a filtration system or digging a new well.

Radon, discussed earlier in this chapter, may seep into private-well water, although 95 percent of all radon that enters homes does so through the soil. The EPA estimates that indoor radon levels rise about 1 pCi/L for every 10,000 pCi/L of radon in water. To approximate how much radon in your water is elevating your indoor radon level, subtract 1 pCi/L from the indoor-air radon level for every 10,000 pCi/L detected in the water. Thus 20,000 pCi/L of radon in water would indicate that 2 pCi/L of your indoor measurement may be traceable to the water.

Unless the majority of radon appears to be coming from your

water, the EPA suggests fixing your house first, then retesting the indoor air to determine the main source of radon contamination. Should evidence point to the well, you may need to install a water-treatment system designed to remove radon.

Aeration, the most efficient process, costs roughly $3,000 to $4,500; a granular activated carbon (GAC) system, recommended for moderate levels of 5,000 pCi/L or less, $1,000 to $2,000. Devices that install on a tap or under the sink treat only a small portion of the water that enters your home and *do not effectively reduce radon*.

CLEANERS, SOLVENTS AND OTHER COMMON HOUSEHOLD PRODUCTS

Just as we advise taking stock of pesticides stored in the garage, we also suggest inventorying your utility closet or wherever you keep cleaning fluids and solvents and glues. Probably you've never given much thought to the potential hazards of these products. Many contain the known carcinogen benzene, while if you scanned the ingredients of others, you'd come across perchloroethylene or, to a lesser extent, carbon tetrachloride.

"The evidence for those isn't as clear as it is with benzene," says Dr. Aaron Blair, chief of the National Cancer Institute's occupational studies section, "but both are carcinogenic in laboratory animals. And there's enough positive evidence in the human epidemiologic data that it doesn't diminish your worry."

Another chemical to look out for is methylene chloride, found in liquid paint strippers, paints and lubricants. "It is a really potent animal carcinogen," says Dr. Blair, "causing lung, breast and brain cancers."

Dr. Blair's recommendations for using and handling such products? First, "try to avoid them where you can," he says. Second, "try to minimize exposure. If you're going to strip furniture, don't do it in your basement, like people often do. Or if you're going to do it out in the garage, make sure the door is open." In addition, wear a face mask and have a portable fan on to blow vapors away from you while you work. Then reseal the can tightly and store it outside, *never* in the house.

ELECTROMAGNETIC FIELDS (EMFs)

Short of moving to a remote cabin without electricity, it is impossible to completely avoid electromagnetic fields from overhead powerlines and household appliances. Whether you even need to is currently an intriguing, confusing question. Since 1979, several epidemiologic studies have suggested a possible connection between EMFs and certain cancers. One of the largest and most provocative of these, made public in 1992, reported on Swedish people residing near high-voltage powerlines over a 25-year period.

"The results," wrote the authors, "provide support for the hypothesis that exposure to magnetic fields increases the risk of cancer. This is most evident in childhood leukemia." But don't go evacuating your home just yet; a great deal more research needs to be conducted before any kind of consensus can be reached. At present, the EPA has issued no standards regarding EMF levels.

To explain the difference between electric fields and magnetic fields, let's look at a toaster. Merely plugging the appliance in sets up an electric field. Turning it on generates an electric current, which consequently produces a magnetic field.

Unlike electric fields, magnetic fields can penetrate any and all materials. Researchers are more concerned with the possible effects of magnetic fields associated with alternating current (AC) than with direct current (DC). AC current, the type used in North America, flows back and forth at a rate of 60 times per second, expressed as 60 hertz. On the electromagnetic spectrum, this is considered an extremely low frequency. For a point of comparison, microwaves have a frequency of about 10,000,000,000 hertz; gamma rays, at the far end of the spectrum, approximately 1,000,000,000,000,000,000,000 hertz.

One characteristic of EMFs, measured in units called *milligauss* (mG), is that their strength dissipates rapidly. Standing directly below a 230-kilovolt powerline would expose you to under 120 milligauss. Walk 100 feet away, and the level plummets to about 15 milligauss. At 300 feet, less than 2 milligauss.

The following table, adapted from one compiled by the EPA, the Electric Power Research Institute (EPRI) and the Illinois Institute of Technology Research Institute (IITRI), illustrates this correlation between magnetic-wave intensity and proximity for several everyday household appliances. Even at a difference of mere inches, milligauss levels fall sharply.

At present we're unable to apply these numbers meaningfully. Is exposure to 30 mG dangerous? 1,500 mG? No one can say. All we know for certain is that EMFs will receive close scientific scrutiny in the years ahead. In the meantime, if you believe in erring

APPLIANCE	DISTANCE FROM ELECTROMAGNETIC SOURCE			
	6"	1'	2'	4'
Can opener	1,500 mG	300 mG	30 mG	4 mG
Hair dryer	700 mG	70 mG	10 mG	1 mG
Vacuum cleaner	700 mG	200 mG	50 mG	10 mG
Electric shaver	600 mG	100 mG	10 mG	1 mG
Microwave oven	300 mG	200 mG	30 mG	20 mG
Dishwasher	100 mG	30 mG	7 mG	1 mG

on the side of caution, you might try standing at arm's length while operating an electric mixer, food processor and so on. On a more practical level, get into the habit of not watching television close up, don't sleep under electric blankets, move your electric alarm clock to the other side of the bedroom and sit at arm's length from a video display terminal.

You'll notice that running a can opener six inches away exposes you to a magnetic field more than 12 times higher (1,500 mG) than standing under an electric powerline (120 mG). However, the duration of exposure to powerlines is typically far greater than to any household appliance. What's more, neighborhood EMF levels tend to be highest around electric substations and transformers because the lines droop nearer to the ground as they pass in and out. Again, the health significance of both these factors is unknown.

The EPA neither recommends nor discourages people from measuring their homes and property for EMFs. As of now, the only benefits would be to satisfy your curiosity. Although you can rent a gauss meter for $60 to $100 per week or buy one for $75 to $650, the simplest way to go about this is to contact your local utility company.

According to Dr. William Farland, director of the EPA's office of health and environmental assessment, "These days most companies have a person who will come out and do a survey of your home, to give you an idea of what the magnetic fields are like, and probably will have some information regarding what the typical fields are for that particular location and so on. Generally that service is provided free of cost."

CARCINOGENS IN AND
AROUND THE WORKPLACE

Not that some people need another reason not to want to go to work in the morning, but occupational hazards account for at least 4 percent of cancer deaths.

Historians generally credit famed eighteenth-century British surgeon Sir Percival Pott with launching the study of industrial carcinogens. In a 1775 book, Pott noted the high incidence of cancer of the scrotum among chimney sweeps. "The disease, in these people," he wrote, "seems to derive its origin from a lodgment of soot in the rugae of the scrotum."

As the following table shows, workers in a wide range of occupations, from construction to roofing to bartending, are exposed to a plethora of known and probable carcinogens, including metals, chemical solvents, dyes, dusts, smoke and radioactive materials:

CHEMICAL/ MATERIAL	OCCUPATION	CANCER
4-Aminobiphenyl	Dye workers Chemical workers	Bladder
Arsenic	Copper refiners Sheep-dip workers Gold miners Vineyard workers Ore smelters Ceramics workers Glass-manufacturing workers	Lung Liver Skin
Asbestos	Shipyard workers Asbestos workers Insulation workers Brake liners Cigarette-filter makers Textile workers Rubber-tire manufacturing workers	Lung Mesothelioma

Auramine	Rubber workers Dye workers Paint-manufacturing workers	Bladder

Benzene	Shoemakers
	Working with glues,
	  varnishes
	Chemical workers
	Rubber-tire manufacturing
	  workers
		Leukemia

Benzidine	Chemical workers Dye workers	Pancreas Bladder
Benzo(a)pyrene	Pitch workers Roofers	Lung
Beryllium	Ceramic makers Nuclear-power workers Electronics workers	Bladder
Bis(chloromethyl)ether	Chemical workers	Lung
Cadmium	Cadmium-production workers Metal workers Electroplaters Chemical workers Nuclear workers	Lung Prostate

Chromium and
  certain chromium
  compounds
	Chromium platers
	Chromate and chromate
	  pigment manufacture
	  workers
	Metal-alloy manufacture
	Glass, brick and ceramics
	  manufacture workers
		Lung
		Nose
		Larynx

Coke-oven emissions	Coke-plant workers Steel workers	Lung Kidney
Iron oxide	Polishing compound manufacturing workers	Lung Larynx

Isopropyl oil	Isopropylene
	  manufacturing workers
	Hardwood furniture
	  makers
	Leather workers
		Nasal
		Sinuses

(continued)

CHEMICAL/ MATERIAL	OCCUPATION	CANCER
Mustard gas	Poison-gas manufacturing workers	Lung Larynx Paranasal Sinuses
2-Naphthylamine	Chemical workers Rubber-tire manufacturing workers Coal-gas manufacturing workers Dye workers Nickel refiners Copper smelters Electrolysis workers	Bladder Pancreas
Nickel	Nickel refiners	Lung Nose Sinuses
Petroleum	Petroleum workers	Skin Scrotum
Polycyclic aromatic hydrocarbons, found in soots, coal tars, paraffin waxes, creosotes, lubricating and cutting oils	Chimney sweeps Coal-gas manufacturing workers Jute processors Tool setters operating automatic lathes Wax pressmen Shale-oil workers	Skin Scrotum Lung
Radiation	Radiologists Radiographers Luminous dial painters Uranium miners	Skin Bone Pancreas Thyroid Leukemia Brain Lung Breast Stomach Multiple myeloma

Radon	Uranium, fluorspar, hematite mining	Lung
Secondhand smoke	Waiters, waitresses, bartenders and numerous other workers in offices or establishments where smoking is permitted	Lung Larynx
Ultraviolet rays	Farmers, sailors, other outdoor workers	Skin
Vinyl chloride	Polyvinyl chloride manufacturing workers Plastics workers	Liver Brain Lymphoma Lung

SOURCES: "What You Need to Know About Lung Cancer" (National Cancer Institute); "Occupational Lung Diseases" (American Lung Association); "Everything Doesn't Cause Cancer" (National Cancer Institute); Tapley et al., *The Columbia University College of Physicians and Surgeons Complete Home Medical Guide;* Stewart et al., *Understanding Your Body;* McAllister et al., *Cancer.* (See Selected Bibliography.)

ASBESTOS

Any rogues' gallery of occupational carcinogens has to begin with asbestos, "thought to be the greatest contributor to risk of cancer in the workplace," stated the National Cancer Institute's 1986 monograph *Cancer Control Objectives for the Nation: 1985–2000.*

Asbestos workers, in industries as diverse as construction, mining, and auto brake and clutch repair, face a 50 percent chance of dying from cancer—nearly three times that of the average population.

As long ago as 2500 B.C., man recognized the usefulness of asbestos, incorporating its fibers in pottery. The ancient Greeks used this fireproof mineral (*asbestos* is derived from the Greek word for *unquenchable*) to make lamp wicks and cremation cloths. Interestingly, the Roman writer Pliny "The Elder" (A.D. 23–79) observed that the slaves who wove the material contracted lung disease.

In America, industrial use of asbestos accelerated during World War II, with more than 27 million workers believed to have been exposed to asbestos dust between 1940 and 1979. Because cancer symptoms often do not arise until 20, 30, even 45 years later, both medicine and government were slow to recognize asbestos's dangers. It wasn't until the mid-1970s that regulations were implemented to reduce acceptable levels from 5 fibers per cubic milliliter of air to 2 fibers. OSHA subsequently revised the standard again, down to 0.2 fibers.

In 1989 the EPA ordered a gradual ban on most asbestos products, so that by 1997, new goods containing the mineral will have been reduced by an estimated 94 percent. Nevertheless, the material will still be found in buildings and cars built before the ban. The number of cancer deaths attributed to asbestos, 8,200 in 1982, is predicted to rise to 9,700 by the year 2000.

BENZENE

According to the U.S. Department of Labor Occupational Safety and Health Administration (OSHA), some 32 million workers are potentially exposed to one or more chemical hazards. Of the approximately 63,000 chemicals manufactured or used in American industry, up to 160 could be considered proven carcinogens, and 2,000 more, potential carcinogens. One of the most dangerous, benzene, has been linked to leukemia since the 1920s. A clear, colorless liquid that emits toxic fumes, it is widely used as a solvent and reactant in the manufacture of petrochemicals, rubber, metals, furniture and shoes. Gas-station attendants, too, are frequently exposed to benzene, which makes up 8 percent of gasoline.

CHROMIUM AND CHROMIUM COMPOUNDS

Chromium, a hard, corrosion-resistant, lustrous metallic element, and its compounds are popular in industry, used to make stainless steel and other alloys, as well as brick, glass and ceramics. Chromate-production workers, chromium platers and chromium-alloy workers have all exhibited elevated rates of lung cancer.

WOOD DUST

The bandsaws, routers, lathes and sanders used to manufacture furniture stir up a veritable duststorm of pollution. Since the 1960s, a number of studies have observed high rates of cancers of the nose and nasal passages among carpenters, furniture makers and refinishers the world over. The International Agency for Research on Cancer (IARC) associated excess risk for these cancers with exposure to dust from certain hardwoods. Therefore woodworkers should be sure to wear masks; air-suction devices mounted near saws and sanders can additionally reduce the risk of inhaling dust.

DOES YOUR JOB INCREASE YOUR RISK OF CANCER?

As the following table shows, blue-collar occupations aren't the only ones that expose employees to health hazards. In an OSHA analysis of industries with respect to worker safety, 13 exposed *at least half* their employees to dangerous chemicals:

INDUSTRY	PERCENT OF WORKERS EXPOSED TO HAZARDOUS CHEMICALS	NUMBER OF EXPOSED EMPLOYEES
Construction	70 percent	3,035,662
Agricultural production (crops and livestock)	70 percent	441,045
Oil and gas extraction	70 percent	414,200
Water transportation	70 percent	124,609
Forestry	70 percent	14,156
Health services	60 percent	3,700,745
Automotive dealers and gasoline service stations	60 percent	1,110,215
Miscellaneous repair services	60 percent	189,819
Pipelines (except natural gas)	60 percent	11,043
Business services	50 percent	2,046,410
Personal services	50 percent	534,335
Automotive repair, services and garages	50 percent	356,899
Building materials; hardware, garden-supply, mobile-home dealers	50 percent	331,026

Dr. Peter Infante is director of OSHA's Office of Standards Review. Using the construction industry as an example, he rattles off a list of carcinogenic chemicals and materials that workers in this field must contend with regularly, if not daily.

"You have quite a few exposures related to cancer in the construction industry," he says, "beginning with asbestos. Now fibrous glass is replacing asbestos, and there's some evidence that fibrous glass, ceramic fibers and mineral wool are carcinogenic.

"You've got silica from abrasive blasting," he continues, "which is related to silicosis and lung cancer; cadmium; and methylene dianiline, which is used to treat the surfaces of walls before they get painted. All of these aromatic amines—methylene dianiline, benzidine, beta-naphthylamine—are human bladder carcinogens.

"There's sufficient evidence now of painters showing, as a group, an increased incidence of cancer, probably due to the methylene chloride in paint strippers and the glycol ethers in paints. In a building that's under construction, before the plumbing and everything are put in, these workers go from floor to floor spray-painting the walls. It's a pretty hazardous operation, with regard to not only lung cancer but also lung disease."

PROTECT YOURSELF ON THE JOB

Dr. Infante raises a vital point when he says, "People have to realize that most of our permissible-exposure limits [set by OSHA] are outdated. So you shouldn't assume that something is safe just because the exposure is under the government-permissible limit.

"Even if it's a new limit," he adds, "don't assume it's safe. Presume that all kinds of chemical exposures are harmful to some degree, and take the available steps to prevent exposure."

These include, where appropriate:

- Wear protective clothing, gloves, boots and hats.
- Wear protective equipment such as masks and respirators. "Make sure what you wear fits," stresses Dr. Infante, "because everybody's face is shaped differently." Particles can slip through poor-fitting head gear and be inhaled into the lungs.
- Keep people not wearing protective clothing or devices out of your work area.
- Try not to spill chemicals or get them on your clothes. "If you

do," advises OSHA's Infante, "wash them off or change your clothes."

• At the end of the workday, clean or vacuum your work clothes, shower if you can, then change into street clothes.
• Don't smoke tobacco, which, combined with occupational exposure, greatly elevates the risk of cancer.
• Educate yourself about the materials you handle and follow all safety precautions.

"Most people don't know the risks of the chemicals they're exposed to in the workplace," comments Dr. Infante. "Employers are now required to furnish employees with material-safety data sheets, which indicate the toxicity of chemicals. Employees should ask employers for these, and see what type of toxicity is related to the chemicals they're working with.

"Then they need to follow up and ask the employer to explain the sheets to them. Because some of these data sheets are very complex, and not all people will understand what they're talking about. Employers are required to conduct a certain number of hours of training and education about safety standards and about reading and comprehending the material-safety data sheets."

OSHA is charged with enforcing workers' rights to safe, healthful conditions on the job. But as Dr. Infante readily admits, the agency doesn't have nearly enough manpower to inspect each and every work site. Therefore employees must take it upon themselves to monitor and report lapses in safety.

If you bring a violation to the attention of your supervisor, employer or union representative, and corrective action is not taken within a reasonable period of time, you can anonymously request a hazard evaluation from either OSHA (the appendix lists the phone numbers for its ten regional offices) or the National Institute for Occupational Safety and Health (NIOSH) at (800-356-4674). In order to register a confidential complaint with the latter, you need the corroboration of at least two fellow workers.

Offering a fictional scenario as an example, Dr. Infante explains, "Maybe the workers have some complaints and say, 'We don't know anything about this chemical called orthotoluidine. But somehow I don't feel good, and someone else doesn't feel good. Is there somebody that can check this place out, to see if it's safe? We don't want to lose our jobs, but we're concerned about our lives.'

"NIOSH would come out and evaluate the situation, see what

chemicals are being used, take atmospheric samples, see if the proper personal-protective equipment is being used, see if there's an appropriate respirator-fit testing program for people who have to wear them."

Section 11-C of the Occupational Safety and Health Act of 1970 guarantees workers protection against employer retaliation should their identities become known through participation in OSHA inspections, conferences, hearings or other activities. The law prohibits employers from

- Firing, demoting or laying off complainants
- Assigning complainants to undesirable jobs or shifts
- Taking away seniority
- Taking away sick leave, vacation time or any other earned benefits
- Blacklisting, threatening or intimidating complainants

"Quite often it does happen," Dr. Infante says candidly, "and it's something that needs to be improved in reform legislation. In some cases the employers won't retaliate immediately, but six months later they bring a complainant up on a charge for something else, or accuse him of sleeping on the job. They'll push him to the brink of reacting adversely, and then when he does, fire him for that." If you believe you have been discriminated against, punished or fired in retaliation, OSHA will act on your behalf to restore your job and benefits. *You or your union representative must file your complaint within 30 days of the employer's action.*

What if you are assigned a task that you believe puts you in imminent danger, and there is no time to contact OSHA or NIOSH? "You can refuse to perform that assignment," says Dr. Infante. However, you must advise your employer of the hazard and request it be corrected, and be willing to accept an alternate assignment, if offered.

One occupational health issue presently outside OSHA's jurisdiction is environmental tobacco smoke. This should concern anyone who works indoors where smoking is allowed. According to a 1993 study conducted by the Centers for Disease Control, waiters, waitresses and bartenders are 50 percent more likely to develop lung cancer due to secondhand smoke. The same study found that levels of tobacco smoke in restaurants and bars were 1.6 to 2 times higher and 3.9 to 6.1 higher, respectively, than in offices.

We believe it's everyone's right to breathe smoke-free air at work. If your place of employment still permits smoking, circulate a petition to ban it. Given the decline in tobacco use since the mid-1960s, you may be surprised at how many signatures you collect. In discussing the matter with your employer, point out that each smoker costs his or her company an additional $1,000 a year. What's more, tobacco users miss 50 percent more workdays than nonsmokers and have twice the accident rate.

A compromise solution would be to establish *separately ventilated* smoking areas. As noted in the 1986 Surgeon General's report linking secondhand tobacco smoke to cancer, merely separating smokers and nonsmokers reduces but does not eliminate nonsmokers' exposure.

X-RAYS, CHEMOTHERAPEUTIC DRUGS, RADIATION THERAPY: BAD MEDICINE?

Ironically, some medical measures, such as radiography, radiation therapy and chemotherapy, carry a slight risk of causing the very disease they are used to diagnose and treat. For example, in 1994 the Food and Drug Administration upgraded its warnings about the anticancer drug tamoxifen, which many women who've undergone surgery for breast cancer receive. Tamoxifen, two studies found, as much as triples their susceptibility to cancer of the uterus.

Does this mean those patients should discontinue the drug? Absolutely not, for tamoxifen has proved itself effective in staving off a recurrence of breast cancer. As a precaution, however, women receiving tamoxifen need to get regular gynecologic check-ups and watch out for symptoms of uterine cancer. In other words, *the benefit far outweighs the risk.* That is the standard we follow when recommending any potentially carcinogenic medical test or treatment.

Since this book concerns prevention, let's look at diagnostic x-ray procedures, used to detect cancer, hopefully in its earliest, most curable stages. Dr. Robert Heelan, a radiologist at Memorial Sloan-Kettering, emphasizes that the cancer risk from x-rays, fluoroscopies, mammographies and CT scans is so minute, "in most cases it can't even be measured."

Still, it's prudent to take steps to reduce your exposure as much as possible—to begin with, by avoiding unnecessary x-rays. Should your physician or dentist order x-rays, ask why. Or if you visit another doctor for a second opinion, ask the referring doctor to send any x-rays that were taken rather than having to undergo a second set.

Dosage is measured in units called *rads,* which stands for *radiation absorbed dose.* Over the years, dosages have been refined greatly for many routine x-ray procedures. A frontal chest x-ray, for instance, exposes a patient to 10 to 13 millirads; a lateral x-ray, 25 to 35 millirads, because the body is thicker.

Another precaution to take, then, is to make sure the radiography facility's equipment is up-to-date and that both the radiologist and the facility are certified by the American College of Radiology. You can contact the ACR at 1891 Preston White Drive, Reston, VA 22091 (800-ACR-LINE).

Radiation therapy exposes patients to doses millions of times those of diagnostic radiology. "These are doses of radiation that essentially destroy tissue as well as tumors," explains Dr. Heelan. The chest, thyroid and bone marrow tend to be particularly sensitive to the effects of ionizing radiation and are at increased risk for the development of neoplasms. "It's not a high risk, but it's certainly measurable." Once again, before recommending such treatment, the physician would weigh the benefit versus the risk.

You may be surprised to learn that you are exposed to radiation every day. Background radiation, or cosmic radiation, from gamma rays that float freely about the universe, bombard us in tiny doses of 0.1 to 0.2 rad annually. At higher elevations, where there is less atmosphere to filter out these rays, the dose increases.

SUGGESTED READING
ABOUT RADON REDUCTION AND REMOVAL

From the U.S. Environmental Protection Agency Information Access Branch, Public Information Center (202-260-2080):

• "A Citizen's Guide to Radon"
• "Home Buyer's and Seller's Guide to Radon"
• "How to Reduce Radon Levels in Your Home"

ABOUT ASBESTOS AND ITS REMOVAL

From the American Lung Association, 1740 Broadway, New York, NY 10019 (212-315–8700):

• "Asbestos in Your Home"

A plane ride from New York to Colorado exposes passengers to the equivalent of one frontal chest x-ray.

Other kinds of radiation emanate from heavy metals within the earth. According to Dr. Heelan, "There are certain areas around the globe—parts of France and the United States—where people who spend considerable amounts of time in basements and cellars are exposed to significant amounts of radiation."

KEY WORDS

Asbestos: A group of naturally occurring mineral fibers that can be separated into thin threads and woven or compressed into blocks and tiles. Because it is both fire- and heat-resistant, asbestos has been a popular building material for many years. The fibers tend to crumble easily into microscopic particles that when swallowed or inhaled lodge in the lungs, driving up the risk of lung cancer and mesothelioma, a rare cancer of the thin membranes that line the chest and abdomen.

Electromagnetic field: A field created by electric current; measured in *milligauss* (mG).

Environmental tobacco smoke: The exhaled *mainstream* smoke and residual *sidestream* smoke from a cigarette. In 1986 the Surgeon General pronounced environmental tobacco smoke a cause of lung cancer.

Radon: A carcinogenic radioactive gas produced by the natural breakdown of uranium in soil, rock and water. Radon, which is measured in *picocuries* per liter, or pCi/L, seeps into houses through the soil or the water supply.

CHAPTER 8

The Mind and Cancer

The Effects of Emotions and Stress on the Body • Stress-Reduction Techniques

Thus far we've examined physical causes of cancer and how they act upon the body. But what about the mind? What role do emotions, depression, stress, disposition or other psychologic factors play in cancer risk or survival? In an era that fervently promotes self-empowerment, the possible connections carry tremendous appeal. A spate of books, video and audio tapes and seminars assures us—in nurturing tones or exhortatory pep talks—that we have the power to mold our destinies, with regard to everything from love to longevity, and especially to control our health and illness. The fear that surrounds cancer gives these suggestions particular power.

This book is all about taking charge of one's health. But whereas we can state with reasonable certainty that a diet rich in fruits and vegetables reduces the risk of several cancers, the link between psychologic factors and cancer is far less clear. Indeed, exploring the mind-body connection is like trying to navigate a labyrinth in the dark: You turn one corner, only to encounter another. Nonetheless, the possibility of a psychogenic connection in cancer is so tantalizing that you should be aware of what we know—and don't know—about it at this point.

Psychogenic is frequently mistaken to mean a feigned or imagined illness. On the contrary, psychogenic illness produces symptoms that are quite real, even though they are ignited or made worse by emotional or mental causes. Common examples include certain types of headache and other pain syndromes and irritable bowel syndrome. In addition, many organic diseases, including asthma, hypertension, ulcers, diabetes, arthritis and numerous autoimmune diseases, are affected by psychologic factors. So it is possible that cancer may also have a psychologic component.

A BRIEF HISTORY

As with other frightening and mysterious diseases, psychological contributions to cancer have been proposed for centuries. In the second century, the Greek physician Galen noted that melancholy women developed breast cancer more often than other women, an observation that would be repeated for centuries to follow.

In a 1759 treatise on cancer, Richard Guy, a leading London surgeon, stated: "Women are more subject to cancerous Disorders than Men, especially such Women as are of a sedentary, melancholic Disposition of Mind, and meet with such Disasters in Life, as occasion much trouble and Grief." He provided two case histories as examples:

CASE 1. "Mrs. Emerson, upon the Death of her Daughter, underwent great Affliction, and perceived her Breast to swell, which soon after grew painful; at last broke out in a most inveterate Cancer, which consumed a great Part of it in a short Time. She had always enjoy'd a perfect state of Health."

CASE 2. "The Wife of a Mate of a Ship (who was taken some Time ago by the French, and put in Prison) was thereby so much affected, that her breast began to swell, and soon after broke out in a desperate Cancer which had proceeded so far that I could not undertake her case. She never before had any complaint in her breast."

One hundred years later the renowned British surgeon and pathologist Sir James Paget wrote: "The cases are frequent in which deep anxiety, deferred hope, and disappointment, are quickly followed by the growth or increase of cancer, that we can hardly doubt that mental depression is a weighty addition to the other

influences that favour the development of the cancerous constitution."

This belief was also voiced in the United States. Sixty-three-
year-old Ulysses S. Grant, the eighteenth president of the United
States, died of cancer in 1885, his reputation tarnished by a scan-
dal-ridden second administration. Not long after, a St. Louis neu-
rologist named C. H. Hughes contended that "a wounded spirit"
had brought on the Civil War hero's fatal illness.

Around the turn of the century, the notion that psychologic
factors might cause cancer was discounted. "Surgery made its big
bid," says Dr. Lawrence LeShan, a noted research psychologist
and modern-day pioneer in this field, "and then radiation. These
focused on the idea of cancer as localized disease, not as disease
of the whole person. The wisdom of one age is the foolishness of
the next, and vice versa, and the old, sophisticated psychosomatic
theories were now regarded as old wives' tales. The field dropped
out of existence, in large part, between 1900 and 1950."

Beginning in the 1950s, Dr. LeShan and others began to study
the role of personality and emotions in the genesis and development of cancer. They were particularly interested in the roles
played by depression and the repression of negative emotions.
Dr. LeShan recalls that he and his colleagues believed they were
discovering a common denominator among cancer patients who
did not respond to medical treatment. "And that is, a loss of
hope," he says. "A despair of ever achieving a really meaningful,
zestful life on one's own terms—the kind of life that really makes
you want to get up in the morning."

Dr. LeShan and colleague Richard Worthington, also a psychologist, interviewed 250 cancer patients and observed that they
shared four important characteristics:

- 77 percent had *lost a major relationship,* such as a spouse or
  children, prior to the onset of cancer. In the control group,
  consisting of 150 apparently healthy men and women, this
  was true of only 14 percent of the subjects.
- 64 percent were *unable to express hostility,* exactly double
  that of the control group.
- 79 percent admitted to *feelings of self-dislike and self-distrust,*
  as compared with 34 percent of the controls.
- 38 percent *felt tension from their relationship with one or
  both parents,* even in cases where the parent or parents had

died many years before. Only 12 percent of the healthy group claimed to feel this way.

Dr. Jimmie Holland, chief of the psychiatry service at Memorial Sloan-Kettering, notes that it is unclear how such correlations are to be interpreted when other variables, such as smoking, are taken into account. Meanwhile, research in this area continues to excite both interest and skepticism.

Scientists call the study of the interaction among the mind, the nervous system and the immune system *psychoneuroimmunology*. Perhaps psychoneuro*endocrine* immunology would be more accurate. The endocrine system's glands, organs and cells secrete *hormones,* chemical transmitters that regulate growth, reproduction and other bodily functions, including immunity. *Behavioral medicine* is the study of individuals' habits and lifestyles and their role in causing and sustaining illness.

We know quite a bit about how emotions and personality, by their *indirect* impact on behavior—smoking, sunlight exposure, diet and so on—affect cancer risk. Personality also has an indirect impact on survival because it affects a person's ability to adhere to treatment, and to come in promptly when a suspicious (and curable) symptom of cancer appears.

The data on the *direct* effects of emotions and personality on physiology, and hence upon cancer development, are less clear.

THE SOCIAL ENVIRONMENT

Considerable research shows that individuals who are poor and have less education have a higher mortality rate than those who are more affluent and better educated. While access to quality health care is an issue, it is not the whole story. One group of researchers has found evidence that in cancer patients with the same stage of disease who received the same treatment in national cooperative studies, socioeconomic status influenced survival. Other studies have found similar results. Whether nutrition or the "stress" of poverty is responsible remains undetermined, as does the influence of such factors in triggering cancer in the first place.

Epidemiological studies in various countries also show that mortality is lower from all diseases, including cancer, among men and women who have more social ties and supports. Having others who care about us may simply lead to better health habits and medical care, but there may also be a more direct physiological effect from the feeling of being loved and cared for. Two other studies, one of women with advanced breast cancer and one of patients with stage I melanoma, revealed that those who participated in weekly support groups lived longer and (in the latter group) had fewer recurrences. Again, the power of social support in *preventing* cancer remains to be investigated.

IS THERE A CANCER PERSONALITY?

Suppressing anger and a general disappointment in oneself make up part of the so-called type C personality, whose traits are said to predispose to cancer. You're no doubt familiar with the type A personality—aggressive, competitive, hostile, impatient, preoccupied with time schedules—and the opposite type B personality: patient, easygoing, noncompetitive.

The psychologic profile of the type C personality, passive and cooperative, would seem to mirror that of the type B. Only this person's calm facade conceals bottled-up anger and frustration. Dr. Paul Rosch, founder of the American Institute of Stress, takes exception to the idea of a type C personality, as do Dr. LeShan and Dr. Holland.

"I don't think that there's any good, solid scientific proof of that," says Dr. Rosch. "And I can think of nothing crueler than to add to the burden of cancer victims who are already guilt-ridden, by suggesting that their disease is of their own doing, or that their failure to improve is a result of some deficiency of character or inability to cope with stress."

Dr. Holland, who works exclusively with cancer patients, agrees. "Patients often feel victimized to have gotten cancer in the first place. They are victimized a second time when they are told their personality led to their getting cancer. The guilt becomes overwhelming for some, especially those whose families insist that they must change since their personality may affect survival as well."

Some people see a direct correlation between stress and cancer, which has been called a disease of civilization and is rarely found among primitive people. When the famed missionary Dr. Albert Schweitzer arrived in the African country of Gabon in 1913, he noted with astonishment the scarcity of cancer. But as the years passed, cases began to appear, something Schweitzer attributed to the natives living increasingly "after the manner of the whites."

The pace of life he referred to puttered along like a Model T Ford compared with today. Social, cultural and technologic changes that once unfolded over the course of a generation now seem to hurtle by before we've had a chance to adapt. Most folks would probably opine they lead more stressful lives than their grandparents did. Dr. Holland begs to differ.

"Everybody thinks his age is the worst," she remarks with a laugh. "Yes, things are changing. In the course of a day we're bombarded by many more bits of information. But while the pace and style might be different, the issues are life and death, the pursuit of happiness, and living as long and well as one can. That doesn't change.

"I have a wonderful medical textbook from 1898 that describes nervous exhaustion and says the reason for this is the pace of life. 'Do you realize there are trains going across the country at *40 miles an hour?*' "

Ask Dr. Rosch if Americans are better or less equipped to handle stress now than, say, in the 1950s, when he began practicing medicine, and he replies, without hesitation, "much less," an opinion that would seem to be borne out by rising rates of violent crime, homicide, suicide and child abuse. There's an inherent problem, however, in trying to prove that stress causes cancer. "You have to define stress," explains Dr. Rosch. "That has always been one of the drawbacks, because stress means different things to different people."

To quantify stress, Drs. Thomas Holmes and Richard Rahe of the University of Washington developed "The Social Readjustment Rating Scale," which ranked the impact of 43 major life events and assigned each a value of 1 to 100. A person who accumulated 300 or more stress points in a year, they contended, had an 80 percent chance of developing a serious illness or having an accident within two years.

Far and away the most devastating misfortune is the death of a husband or wife, awarded 100 points. Issues relating to work, from conflicts with the boss to changes in job responsibilities, also ranked throughout the scale. Interestingly, *Nature and Treatment of Cancer,* an influential medical textbook of the mid-1800s, advised men and women from families with high rates of cancer to avoid taxing, stressful occupations.

"For this reason," wrote author Walter H. Walshe, a professor of pathologic anatomy, "the professions of the Bar, Medicine, and Diplomacy should be avoided. . . . All things considered, the professions of the Army, Navy, and the Church, unless there be some special objection, offer the best chances of escape from the diseases to individuals predisposed to cancer." He added, "Females should not become governesses."

Some other sources of stress, as rated by the Holmes-Rahe scale, may surprise you:

LIFE EVENT	SCORE
Retirement	45
Pregnancy	40
Sex difficulties	39
Mortgage or loan for a major purpose (home, business, etc.)	31
Son or daughter leaving home	29
Trouble with in-laws	29
Outstanding personal achievement	28
Change in church activities	19
Change in number of family get-togethers	16
Vacation	13
Christmas	12

SOURCE: Reprinted with permission from *Journal of Psychosomatic Research,* Vol. 11, 213–18, Thomas Holmes, M.D., and Richard Rahe, M.D. "The Social Readjustment Rating Scale," 1967, Elsevier Science Ltd., Pergamon Imprint, Oxford, England.

Lacking a precise definition of stress presents one obstacle in the road to linking stress and cancer. Another is trying to isolate the effects of stress from other factors. Nuns, Mormons and Seventh-Day Adventists all have less cancer than the general population. Is it because their faith enables them to handle hardships with equanimity, or is it because they neither smoke nor drink? Most likely it's a combination of the two.

Along the same lines, personal crises may increase one's risk of cancer, but indirectly, by bringing about changes in behavior. A job dismissal can send one person reaching for a cigarette after years of not smoking. Another may be so distraught over a romantic breakup, she barely eats; or perhaps in her anguish she feels a lump in her breast but neglects to inform her physician for several crucial months.

STRESS AND CANCER: THE POSSIBLE MECHANISMS

A man is driving down a busy street, whistling along to the music on the car radio, when from out of the corner of his eye he spots a truck peeling away from the curb and directly into his path. In the space of a millisecond, his nervous system and endocrine system swing into action, a response called "fight or flight."

The pupils dilate, sharpening vision. Blood is routed to where it is most needed: the brain and the large muscles of the arms and legs. In the event of a wound or internal hemorrhaging, clots form more rapidly to stem bleeding. Nerve junctions release secretions that facilitate muscle reactions. The liver discharges glucose into the blood for quick energy. The heart and lungs work faster. Blood pressure rises. Digestive activity slows down. The nervous system secretes neurotransmitters and other substances that affect mood, emotions and behavior.

The driver hits the brake pedal and jerks the steering wheel to the left, narrowly averting an accident as the truck practically brushes his bumper.

Whether you find yourself in the above situation or bracing for upsetting news, your body prepares you to manage stress. In 1936 Dr. Hans Selye, a visionary Canadian biochemist, established the concept of stress. By exposing laboratory rats to different stressors over long periods of time, he discovered that the animals' ability to withstand stress eventually collapsed, resulting in illness or death.

The search to determine how stress might induce cancer has centered largely on its effect on the immune system, responsible for seeking out and destroying foreign invaders. Rogue cancer cells circulate through the body all the time, but under normal circumstances our natural defense mechanisms prevent them from multiplying and evolving into a tumor.

While it is generally accepted that stress impairs immunologic faculty, "There are at least 45 different parameters, or measurements, of immune system function," explains Dr. Rosch. "So we can construct an experiment where you might find that certain parameters of immune system function increase and others decrease in an individual with stress."

However, experiments have consistently shown that stress diminishes the activity of certain essential immunologic components: T lymphocytes (T cells), which inactivate or destroy foreign substances—especially a type of T cell known as natural killer cells.

Immunologist Ronald Glaser and psychologist Janice Kiecolt-Glaser, a husband-and-wife team, studied the effect of stress on Ohio State University medical students during final exams. Using a psychologic test, Kiecolt-Glaser gauged the students' stress levels; Glaser took blood samples.

Natural killer cell activity dropped noticeably in students assessed as stressed. Too, those identified as feeling lonely suffered the greatest reduction in immune function, while the reverse was true of students exhibiting the least stress and loneliness.

Emotional stress also alters the ratio of two other types of T lymphocytes, helper T cells and suppressor T cells, and suppresses interferon, a family of natural proteins that quell or destroy tumor cells and stimulate the immune system.

At the first hint of stress, the pituitary gland, located at the base of the brain, releases adrenocorticotropic hormone—ACTH, for short—which in turn stimulates a flood of cortisol from the adrenal glands atop each kidney. This hormone has been found to depress the immune system in animals.

"There certainly is evidence that these systems talk to and influence one another," says Dr. Holland, "and that there are transmitters that go in both directions. How clearly these changes in immune surveillance and function may impact upon cancer development, we don't know. But it's an area of considerable interest."

Studies of animals injected with tumor cells, she notes, have demonstrated "a relationship between helplessness, stress, the immune system's response and the rate of tumor growth." Researchers at the University of Pennsylvania subjected two groups of mice to an electric shock experiment, with the first group allowed to escape the shocks. The second group, helpless to avoid the same amount of current, developed tumors at a greater rate. Another study, conducted at the Pacific Northwest Research Foundation, revealed immune suppression and higher levels of cortisol in mice who'd been stressed. However, Dr. Holland is quick to add, it's too soon to say whether such studies are directly relevant to cancer in humans.

METHODS FOR REDUCING STRESS

Despite mounting evidence that stress affects certain immune cells, theoretically creating opportunities for cancer to take hold, it would be premature for anyone to promote stress reduction as a cancer-preventive tool per se. But since this book is about enriching life as well as prolonging it, it seems appropriate to outline the following methods, for who couldn't benefit from learning to handle stress more effectively?

RELAXATION EXERCISES

There are numerous kinds of relaxation exercises, with deep breathing, meditation, yoga and self-hypnosis among the more common. Done correctly, these techniques can reduce stress. Drs. Glaser and Kiecolt-Glaser reported that students who performed relaxation exercises heightened their levels of T helper cells, another important platoon in the body's disease-fighting force. "The whole range of relaxation therapies are very useful," says Dr. Holland.

Meditation, for example, is an age-old technique for clearing the mind of all thoughts. To aid concentration, you intone a phrase, or mantra, silently or aloud. It can be "Om," "One," whatever has personal resonance for you. Yoga, based on Hindu teachings, incorporates breathing, meditation and different physical postures to unify the mind and body and achieve inner tranquility.

Two newer variations of relaxation exercises, guided imagery and visualization, have gained considerable media attention in recent years. They can be likened to a mental vacation, one that you can embark on anytime, anywhere.

VISUALIZATION

1. In a private, quiet room, remove any constrictive clothing, dim the lights and sink into a comfortable chair, keeping your limbs outstretched and joints loose.
2. Close your eyes and take three deep breaths, releasing tension as you exhale.
3. Relax your muscles from head to toe, starting with your brow. Tense—then release. Now repeat those steps with the muscles

in your jaw, and so on. Feel the peaceful, heavy sensation traveling down your body.

4. While continuing to breathe rhythmically, "Visualize in your mind a place that's particularly restful," suggests Dr. Holland, "a place you've experienced, a place you like to be. That adds to the ability to distract yourself from every other thought."

If you're the type who finds silence deafening—you focus on the air conditioner's hum or muffled conversation from upstairs— add soothing music to your tranquil scene. Avoid anything with lyrics or rhythm, which may distract. You now have a safe haven to escape to whenever you wish.

GUIDED IMAGERY

Guided imagery is an exercise frequently suggested to cancer patients as a means of reducing stress and controlling anxiety. They may visualize a favorite place, such as a beach, and hear the waves. Or they may be instructed to set a goal and then imagine ways of achieving it. For example, the patient may set a goal of bolstering the immune system and imagine healthy white blood cells gobbling up cancer cells, perhaps like some video-game creation. Dr. Holland adds, however, "There are no data showing that creating an image of one's immune system killing cancer actually does that."

Imagery is sometimes recommended as a preventive strategy for healthy men and women as well. Dr. Holland favors visualization, which she believes is helpful to create a relaxed state. But she encourages patients who find guided imagery helpful to use it.

HYPNOTHERAPY

Approximately 15,000 health professionals currently practice hypnotherapy. This should not be confused with staged nightclub hypnosis, in which a hypnotist gets subjects to flap their arms and cluck like chickens. "The word *hypnotherapy* is rather frightening to some people," Dr. Holland acknowledges, "but it clearly has a place."

In hypnosis, subjects are guided into a trance state, during which they become susceptible to suggestions and commands. The therapist might implant ideas for reacting differently to stress. For example, a woman who complains of panic attacks during business meetings would be encouraged to take a deep breath beforehand and imagine herself as relaxed and confident in the situation about to unfold. The next step is to train her to tap into that feeling on her own.

Or hypnosis may be employed purely for relaxation purposes. "When used as we do, to make people more comfortable and to relax," explains Dr. Holland, "it's really a kind of self-suggestion for attaining a relaxed state and distracting one's thoughts to some quiet spot by the mountains or the seashore, and being able to shut out other stimuli."

You should know that some people are impervious to hypnosis and that fraudulent practitioners abound. Two national societies, the Society of Clinical Hypnosis and the Society for Clinical and Experimental Hypnosis, can refer you to qualified, state-licensed hypnotherapists in your area. For a list of names, send a self-addressed, stamped envelope; for a few names over the phone, call:

- American Society of Clinical Hypnosis
  2200 East Devon Avenue, Suite 291
  Des Plaines, IL 60018
  (708) 297–3317
- Society for Clinical and Experimental Hypnosis
  6728 Old McLean Village Drive
  McLean, VA 22101
  (703) 556-9222

BIOFEEDBACK TRAINING

Biofeedback combines Eastern mysticism with Western technology. Its basic premise is not unlike hypnotherapy's, except that patients remain conscious, hooked up to a machine that discerns electrical current and indicates involuntary functions such as a quickened pulse rate or muscle tension via an audible tone, a flashing light or some other signal. Observing the monitor enables people to regulate their responses to stress.

Dr. Holland explains, "The person may be told, 'I want you to lower your blood pressure by five points.' You relax, you look and see, and over the training period you learn to actually change these kinds of physiologic states. The degree to which people can change their actual physiology," she says, "can be quite impressive." For free referrals to biofeedback specialists in your ZIP code, call the Biofeedback Society of America, 10200 West 44 Avenue, Wheat Ridge, CO 80033 (303-422-8436).

ACUPUNCTURE

This ancient Chinese healing art is based on the theory that vital energy or life force (*chi* or *qui*) circulates through the body along *meridians,* pathways that can be likened to the blood, lymphatic and neural circuits. An imbalance in vital energy is said to cause all illnesses.

By inserting hair-thin needles into various points along certain meridians (there are over 800 known points), the acupuncturist can restore equilibrium—what Western medicine calls homeostasis, meaning "steady state." The points affecting a particular organ may sit a distance away. For example, to treat a migraine headache, the practitioner might place needles in the little toe, the back of the hand, the middle of the rib cage and the lower spine.

While frequently used to control pain and as a treatment modality, traditional acupuncture is actually intended to be administered periodically for health maintenance. "Nobody knows the mechanism," says Dr. Holland, "but some patients certainly find that acupuncture reduces their stress." The fact that we don't understand a modality doesn't diminish its apparent salubrious effects. As she advises patients, "If you find that's something you want to try, then you definitely should. You may discover that it is helpful to you; you may not. One just has to try and see." We agree, but must add a caveat: If you pursue unconventional remedies, they should be complements to—not substitutes for—traditional medicine.

To receive a list of trained acupuncturists in your state, send a check or money order for $3 to the National Commission for the Certification of Acupuncturists, 1424 16th Street, N.W., Suite 501, Washington, DC 20036 (202-232-1404).

EXERCISE

Perhaps nothing better demonstrates the principle of mind-body interaction than physical activity, which promotes a sense of well-being several ways. Besides enhancing one's body image (for some, a source of great anxiety), exercise significantly boosts natural killer cell activity and generates *endorphins,* chemical neurotransmitters that mitigate pain and produce what's been called a natural high.

We suggest 30 minutes or more of moderate exercise at least five days a week. If you can't squeeze a regular exercise session into your schedule, compensate by walking instead of driving, or by taking up a physical activity such as gardening.

Conversely, those who get winded by the mere thought of jogging or aerobics may want to concentrate on other areas of stress reduction first. It's remarkable how trimming stress from our lives encourages us to eat properly, give up tobacco and, yes, exercise.

FEELING STRESSED? TRY ZEST

In Lawrence LeShan's view, the most effective stress reducer is a satisfying, rewarding life. LeShan's form of psychotherapy was shaped in the 1950s from working with terminal cancer patients, but its principles are universal.

"For the first 10 years," he recalls, "using standard psychotherapy, 100 percent of my patients died. What we did was to devise a method deliberately designed to function on what's right with the person: what their special song to sing is, their music to beat out, and how they can move toward it. And we've found this makes a tremendous difference, statistically, in the cancer mortality rate.

"Somewhere around 50 percent of the same population go into a definite remission, which is quite a difference. If you can help the person find a way of life that gives one zest and enthusiasm, or actively work toward that, very often it's as if the immune system begins to perk up." We know of several studies showing psychotherapy or psychiatry to apparently improve immunity. According to one, published in 1989, malignant melanoma patients who received short-term group psychiatric care exhibited a marked increase in natural killer cells and large granular lymphocytes.

Any area of your life can provide the stage for singing your own song: work, family, friendships, hobbies. "It's different for everyone," says Dr. LeShan. "One person might collect fossil fish, another might go skydiving. Whatever. Once you've got the habit, try another one. What other ways can you find to enrich your life? Until you reach the problem that there are only 24 hours in the day, and you've got 36 hours of things you'd like to do.

"I had one woman who'd wanted to play the flute all her life. She started to play, and she hated it. That can happen too," he says. "But she was free for the next adventure. I never found anybody who couldn't find ways to upgrade their life so they get more out of it and put more color into it."

Dr. LeShan hastens to emphasize, "Cancer is not caused by emotions, and it isn't cured by emotions. Emotions are one factor among many others: your genetics, the environment and so forth. But one of the things we can do to help people mobilize their own self-healing resources is help them find hope in their life, and sometimes this makes a critical difference. How big a difference, I don't know. Maybe it's only 5 percent.

"But," he adds, "just think what a difference 5 percent can mean in a hard-fought election."

KEY WORDS

Acupuncture: An ancient Chinese healing art based on using thin needles to restore the normal balance of vital energy.

Biofeedback: A method of teaching subjects to regulate body functions that are normally involuntary, such as heart rate and blood pressure.

Endocrine system: Glands, organs and cells that secrete *hormones,* chemical messengers that regulate a host of body functions.

Endorphins: Chemical neurotransmitters that mitigate pain and produce a feeling of euphoria.

Hypnotherapy: A process by which subjects are guided into a hypnotic trance.

Psychoneuroimmunology: The study of the interaction among the mind, nervous system and immune system.

CHAPTER

9

Designing Your Personal Cancer Prevention Program

Guidelines for Primary and Secondary
Prevention · Common Screening
Tests · Common Diagnostic Tests

Now that you've seen the impact of heredity, diet, lifestyle, stress and exposure to environmental carcinogens on cancer, it is time to exercise your influence over the disease by combining the primary prevention guidelines below with medical surveillance, or secondary prevention:

GUIDELINES FOR PRIMARY PREVENTION: ALL MEN AND WOMEN

- Lower your dietary fat intake to no more than 20 percent of your total daily calories.
- Control your caloric intake, to prevent weight gain.
- Increase your dietary fiber intake to at least 25 grams per day.
- Eat five to nine servings of fruits and vegetables daily.
- Eat foods rich in vitamins A, C and E.
- Don't smoke cigarettes, cigars, pipes or marijuana, and avoid chewing tobacco and snuff.

- If you drink alcohol, do so in moderation: no more than four drinks per week.
- Try to maintain your ideal weight by avoiding overeating and incorporating physical activity into your daily life.
- Avoid direct exposure to the sun.
- Take steps to ensure that your home is free of cancer-causing agents such as radon, asbestos and certain pesticides.
- At work, avoid exposure to carcinogenic chemicals and materials. If necessary, report to the appropriate federal agencies any health and safety violations that may be putting you at risk.
- Try reducing the amount of stress in your life.
- Avoid promiscuous sex. If you do have multiple sex partners, use condoms, to reduce the risk of contracting a sexually transmitted virus that can lead to cancer.

GUIDELINES FOR
SECONDARY PREVENTION

Technologic breakthroughs in optical instruments and sophisticated imaging techniques enable today's physicians to view organs that previously would have been observable only through exploratory surgery. It wasn't long ago, for example, that gastroenterologists inspected a patient's lower colon for evidence of early cancer using a rigid sigmoidoscope. This solid viewing device could be inserted only into the first quarter of the rectum and colon, and the exam generally proved uncomfortable. Now we rely on a longer, narrower flexible model that not only is more comfortable for patients but detects two to three times the number of colorectal cancers.

One of the most effective cancer-screening measures, the Pap test (see following section, "Types of Screening Tests"), is performed during a routine pelvic examination. If every woman went for an annual Pap smear as prescribed by numerous cancer- and health-related organizations, we could drastically cut deaths from cervical cancer. Likewise, screening for breast cancer by mammography could reduce mortality by 30 percent, and screening for colon cancer could halve the number of deaths from that disease. With these and other forms of cancer, however, the search for reliable, cost-effective screening methods goes on.

TYPES OF SCREENING TESTS

The brief descriptions that follow are intended merely to familiarize you with the various screening procedures, which we've arranged from the simplest to the most complex. For a more thorough explanation of each, refer to the page noted at the end of the entry.

Breast self-examination: A simple four-step home exam for detecting abnormalities of the breasts, such as a change in size, color, contour or skin texture; tenderness; or nipple retraction. Women should report any of these symptoms to their physician (pages 251–54).

Skin self-examination: Everyone should conduct this home exam three or four times a year. In a well-lit room, patients examine themselves in a full-body mirror: front, sides, forearms, upper arms, underarms and palms of hands. Next they sit on the floor and inspect their legs and feet, including the soles and between the toes. Then, while standing, a hand-held mirror is used to check the back of the neck, scalp, buttocks and back. A spouse or partner can be enlisted to examine hard-to-see places (pages 368–70).

Testicular self-examination: An easy self-inspection that should be performed periodically after a warm shower or bath. With both hands, the man gently examines each testicle for hard masses, a sign of testicular cancer (pages 234–35).

Sputum cytology: A simple do-it-yourself procedure conducted at home. For three consecutive mornings the patient is asked to cough deeply and expectorate into a special jar upon waking up. The sputum samples are then either returned to the doctor's office or mailed to a laboratory, where they are studied to detect lung cancer or a precancerous condition (page 277).

Stool blood test: A test for discerning hidden blood in the stool, a possible sign of colorectal cancer. For three days in a row, the patient places a smear of fecal matter on cardboard slides specially treated with a substance that turns blue when a chemical is added. Blood in the stool can signal cancer or a noncancerous condition (pages 294–95).

Clinical breast exam: The doctor feels (palpates) the breasts with the fingers, looking for unusual lumps. In addition to manipulating the breasts and gently squeezing the nipples, he or she probes the lymph nodes above the clavicle and in the armpits (pages 254–55).

Dermatologic exam: A dermatologist, trained to visually identify skin disorders, examines the patient from head to toe, looking for potentially cancerous lesions (page 370).

Pelvic exam: A screening exam, most valuable for early detection of cervical cancer, in which the doctor inspects and feels the female genitals for abnormalities (pages 320–21).

Skin biopsy: A local anesthetic is injected into the skin. Once the area is numb, the physician cuts out a small sample of tissue using one of two instruments: a surgical knife (scalpel) or a punch. The site is either sutured closed or cauterized, and the sample sent to a *pathologist,* a doctor specializing in identifying diseases through microscopic study (page 370).

Prostate-specific antigen (PSA) test: This blood test, used to screen for prostate cancer, measures the level of a certain protein. In some prostate cancer patients, the level rises, alerting doctors to the likelihood of a tumor. However, a normal PSA level does not rule out cancer; conversely, an elevated reading can be due to a benign condition (pages 231–33).

Digital rectal exam: The physician inserts a lubricated, gloved finger into the rectum to feel for growths or abnormalities indicating cancer of either the colorectum or the prostate (pages 230–31).

Pap test: An extremely valuable office procedure used to screen for cervical cancer, in which cell scrapings are taken from the cervix and upper vagina with a spatula, cotton swabs or a tiny brush. The sample is then analyzed under a microscope by a pathologist (pages 321–22).

Chest x-ray: An x-ray of the chest used to detect early lung cancer. Although no health- or cancer-related agencies officially recommend this screening procedure on a regular basis, many doctors use it to screen men and women thought to be at high risk due to heavy smoking (pages 275–77).

Ultrasonography: An imaging procedure in which high-frequency sound waves form an image, or sonogram, of internal structures. Although primarily a diagnostic technique, it is sometimes used to screen for ovarian cancer and prostate cancer in high-risk patients (pages 223, 326).

Mammography: An x-ray of the breast. This effective technique can detect some breast tumors years before they can be felt with the fingers (pages 255–57).

Upper GI endoscopy: An examination of the esophagus and stomach, using a thin, lighted viewing instrument called an endoscope. Normally a diagnostic test, upper GI endoscopy is used to screen only patients afflicted with a condition known as Barrett's esophagus, which elevates their risk of esophageal cancer (page 348).

Sigmoidoscopy: A procedure for viewing the lower third of the colon, using a flexible lighted instrument called a sigmoidoscope. To ensure accuracy, the colon must be clear. Therefore patients need to follow a clear-liquid diet and administer themselves an enema beforehand (pages 295–96).

Colonoscopy: A screening *and* diagnostic test for viewing the entire colon, using a lighted, flexible instrument called a colonoscope. As with sigmoidoscopy, a liquid diet, laxative and enema are required before the examination (pages 296–98).

Should a screening exam reveal something questionable, the doctor may order one or more *diagnostic* tests to positively identify any disease. Several of the diagnostic tests indexed below are not exclusive to one form of cancer. To avoid repetition, we explain these in depth on the following pages:

- Upper GI series   347
- Uterine aspiration biopsy   324–25

Remember, only a biopsy can confirm a cancer diagnosis. Thus a positive result on other tests does not necessarily mean you have the disease. In many instances, a positive result merely indicates another, less-serious problem. On the other hand, incipient cancers do sometimes elude medicine's most sensitive tests. Even when results are seemingly negative, it is essential that you stay in regular contact with your doctor and be mindful of any unusual symptoms.

The early cancer detection guidelines recommended by physicians at Memorial Sloan-Kettering, contained on the following pages, adhere closely to those set by the American Cancer Society, the National Cancer Institute and the World Health Organization. At one time, no uniform standard existed, which created some confusion for the public. But in the mid-1980s a consensus emerged on most screening guidelines. "We've been very close in our recommendations ever since," says Dr. Peter Greenwald, the National Cancer Institute's director of cancer prevention and control. One point on which everyone agrees: Cancer screening saves lives.

The secondary prevention plan outlined on the following pages is designed for men and women at *average risk* for all cancers. To learn if you're at higher risk for any of the major adult cancers, take the Risk Assessment Quiz for each, found in Chapters 10 through 16. If heredity, prior health conditions, or environmental or lifestyle factors seem to place you at increased risk for one or more forms of cancer, consult your doctor about which surveillance steps are appropriate for you. A man deemed at increased risk for prostate cancer—perhaps due to a family propensity for the disease—would be urged to undergo a prostate-specific antigen (PSA) test annually beginning at age 40 rather than at age 50, the recommendation for men at average risk.

SECONDARY PREVENTION GUIDELINES

Women at Average Risk for All Cancers
Ages 20 to 34

- Monthly breast self-exam
- Periodic skin self-exam

- Annual gynecologic exam including pelvic exam and Pap smear. *(Note:* Sexually active women of any age should have an annual Pap smear. After three or more consecutive negative tests, your gynecologist may elect to perform it less frequently.)
- Clinical breast exam by a physician every three years
- General medical checkup every three years

Women at Average Risk for All Cancers
Ages 35 to 39

- Monthly breast self-exam
- Periodic skin self-exam
- Annual gynecologic exam including pelvic exam and Pap smear
- Clinical breast exam by a physician every three years
- Baseline mammogram

Women at Average Risk for All Cancers
Ages 40 to 49

- Monthly breast self-exam
- Periodic skin self-exam
- Annual gynecologic exam including pelvic exam and Pap smear
- Annual clinical breast exam by a physician
- Mammogram every one to two years
- Annual colorectal screening, consisting of digital rectal exam
- Annual dermatologic exam

Women at Average Risk for All Cancers
Ages 50 and Up

- Monthly breast self-exam
- Periodic skin self-exam
- Annual gynecologic exam including pelvic exam and Pap smear
- Annual clinical breast exam by a physician and mammogram
- Annual colorectal screening, consisting of digital rectal exam and stool blood test
- Sigmoidoscopy every three to five years
- Annual dermatologic exam

SECONDARY PREVENTION GUIDELINES

Men at Average Risk for All Cancers
Ages 20 to 39

- Monthly testicular self-exam
- Periodic skin self-exam

Men at Average Risk for All Cancers
Ages 40 to 49

- Monthly testicular self-exam
- Periodic skin self-exam
- Annual digital rectal exam for cancers of the colorectum and prostate
- Annual dermatologic exam

Men at Average Risk for All Cancers
Age 50 and Up

- Monthly testicular self-exam
- Periodic skin self-exam
- Annual digital rectal exam and stool blood test for cancer of the colorectum
- Sigmoidoscopy every three to five years
- Annual digital rectal exam and prostate-specific antigen (PSA) test for prostate cancer
- Annual dermatologic exam

DON'T LET FEAR
JEOPARDIZE YOUR HEALTH

Too often fear and embarrassment inhibit people from seeing their physician when they should. "I had that feeling," admits Henry M., the attorney whose colorectal cancer was detected at an early stage only because a friend had arranged for the two of them to participate in a screening program run by Memorial Sloan-Kettering. Henry hadn't been to a doctor for years, and so the thought that he might have some medical problem nagged at him. Yet he still wouldn't pick up the phone and schedule a physical checkup. "You're fearful of going to the doctor because of what he might tell you, so you just stay away," he says.

"But it's far, far better to find out. If you by chance have cancer, there may be an opportunity to save your life. If you ignore it, it could be a one-way ticket to death. There's no doubt in my mind," Henry adds, "that if I hadn't gone to be checked, I wouldn't be alive today."

As gastroenterologists, we see quite a few patients who admit they'd been bleeding from the rectum for some time but were afraid to make an appointment. Fear of possibly learning they have a serious illness is one source of patients' apprehension. Another is anxiety over the test itself. Will it hurt? Will I have to undress completely? Will there be a loss of dignity?

We understand that any medical procedure, comfortable or not, ranks somewhere below an IRS audit on most people's list of pleasurable activities. True, some of the more invasive exams may involve a degree of discomfort. However, a philosophical outlook can help make the experience more bearable. Remind yourself, almost as a mantra: *The discomfort is relatively minor and temporary. The potential benefits are substantial and long-term. Having this test won't harm my body and may prolong my life.*

We should point out, too, that modern instruments—such as the flexible sigmoidoscope mentioned earlier—have greatly improved the comfort level of certain procedures. One other positive development is a heightened sensitivity on the part of physicians, nurses and medical technologists to the emotional aspects of these procedures, with greater attention now paid to patients' anxieties, feelings and need for maintaining their dignity.

In our experience, a fear of the unknown can stir up patients' fears like a bellows stoking a fire. In a British survey of 600 women who received mammograms for the first time, two thirds remarked afterward that the x-ray procedure wasn't as uncomfortable as they'd anticipated.

There will always be some people for whom ignorance is bliss. But, says Dr. Michael Moore, codirector of Memorial Sloan-Kettering's Evelyn H. Lauder Breast Center, "I'd say 90 percent of patients do remarkably better if they know what's coming. Patient education is very important. I think that's true of any test." Dr. Moore hands out descriptive pamphlets outlining screening and diagnostic exams to his patients, as do many departments at Memorial Sloan-Kettering.

"I really find that to be helpful and comforting," says patient Judith K., who prepares herself mentally before screening procedures. "Just knowing what it's going to be like and what happens when you go home, so you don't have any 'surprises.' "

Educating yourself also protects you from the gusts of misinformation that tend to swirl around medical procedures. Dr. John Mendelsohn, chairman of Memorial Sloan-Kettering's department of medicine, offers mammography as a perfect example.

"Mammography used to give a fairly high dose of radiation," he says, "but now it's very low. Yet people will often hear from their friends, 'Oh, you're getting a mammography? You're subjecting your body to damage.' It's much better when the doctor explains to the patient, 'This is a special kind of low-dose x-ray; it does not emit a high dose of radiation.' "

Admittedly, not all physicians explain tests as patiently and as thoroughly as they should. *Ask questions*, such as those suggested below:

- What is the purpose of this test?
- What can it tell us? What can't it tell us?
- Where will the test be performed? In your office? A hospital outpatient clinic? On a hospital inpatient basis?
- If hospitalization is necessary, how long can I expect to remain in the hospital?
- Are any preparations necessary beforehand, such as fasting or taking an enema?
- Will I receive anesthesia? If so, what kind? Local? General?
- Will I be sedated? If so, what kind of drug will I be given, and how? Orally? Intravenously?
- Are there any health risks involved with this test?
- Can I expect any discomfort?
- Please explain the procedure from start to finish.
- How long does it take?
- Can I anticipate any side effects?
- When will the results be available, and who will inform me of them?

With so much information to digest, we suggest you carry a small notepad or journal in which to jot down the doctor's answers. If you don't understand something, ask him or her to repeat the information.

Some patients find physicians intimidating and refrain from asking questions. Either they're afraid of appearing "ignorant"—as if the average individual should be fluent in medical terminology—or they worry subconsciously that to "bother" the doctor will somehow adversely affect their quality of medical care. So they nod their head meekly even when the doctor's words have sped through one ear and out the other like a train through a tunnel. Don't hesitate to ask questions, more than once if necessary. Addressing your concerns is part of our job.

One other factor that can discourage patients from seeking preventive cancer care is cost. In a 1993 study of nearly 5,000 New Jersey women, breast cancer patients with commercial insurance survived longer than those with state-funded Medicaid or no coverage at all: Because the privately insured women enjoyed easier access to mammograms and other early-detection tests, their disease was diagnosed at earlier, more curable stages.

At the time of the study, New Jersey did not offer mammograms for women on Medicaid, a policy it has since amended. In the opinion of Dr. Joseph Simone, Memorial Sloan-Kettering's physician-in-chief, steps like that need to be taken if we are to lower the rate of cancer through screening. "People really pay attention when you hit them in the pocketbook," he says bluntly. "If you reimburse for preventive care, it will get done."

The trend appears to be moving ever so slowly in that direction. As a tertiary medical center—one that specializes in cancer—Memorial Sloan-Kettering gets referrals from all 50 states as well as from around the world and therefore works with insurers nationwide. "Over the years, I've seen the changes," says Amalia Vallance, manager of outpatient accounts. "Mammograms, for example. Most U.S. plans now cover mammography one hundred percent." That wasn't the case even just 10 years ago.

Stephen Young, New York director of the Health Insurance Association of America, which represents commercial carriers that insure over 95 million Americans, agrees. "There has been a substantial change in coverage by way of increasing preventive care," he says, adding that the majority of insurance companies reimburse for mammograms and Pap tests, and some for colorectal cancer screening. "And I think you will see more of it in the future."

He cautions, however, that while these and other preventive tests will save lives, they may not necessarily trim health-care costs, an opinion seconded by Dr. Mendelsohn of Memorial Sloan-Kettering. "It's very important to keep costs down," Mendelsohn emphasizes. "But it's unrealistic to think that we're going to build in what everybody would like, namely more preventive measures, and at the same time dramatically reduce cost."

Perhaps not, but in the long run the country might benefit economically in other ways. Cancer siphons away $104 billion annually in costs and lost productivity. Ultimately, the issue isn't "How can we afford cancer screening?" but "How can we make cancer screening affordable for everyone?"

SUGGESTED READING ABOUT SCREENING TESTS

From the National Cancer Institute (800-4-CANCER):

- "Cancer Tests You Should Know About: A Guide for People 65 and Over"

KEY WORDS

Asymptomatic: Exhibiting no symptoms of disease.

Diagnose: To confirm the existence and nature of disease.

Pathologist: A doctor specializing in identifying diseases through microscopic study.

Radiologist: A physician specially trained to interpret medical x-rays.

PART THREE

Preventing the Major Cancers

CHAPTER

10

Prostate Cancer

Digital Rectal Exam • Prostate-Specific
Antigen Test • Testicular Cancer and
Testicular Self-Exam

Though prostate cancer is exclusively a man's disease, we urge women to read this chapter, for, as many wives, daughters and mothers will attest, persuading a man to visit any doctor—much less a *urologist,* the medical specialist trained to identify and treat diseases of the genitourinary system—can be as difficult as getting him to ask directions. Taking the time to learn about this dread disease that afflicts 1 in 11 men might just save the life of a husband, father, son, brother or friend.

Men tend to speak about prostate trouble in whispers, if they broach the subject at all. For many, to acknowledge a urinary problem is to confess fears of waning virility. Thus each year thousands go silently to their graves because of prostate cancer.

Fortunately, in much the same way that First Lady Betty Ford's candor about having breast cancer inspired women to seek mammography and breast examinations in the 1970s, the past few years have seen a number of famous figures—Senator Robert Dole, Supreme Court Justice John Paul Stevens, rock musician Frank Zappa, to name a few—go public with their battle against prostate cancer, encouraging men age 40 and older to have annual rectal exams. Nevertheless, some still avoid this examination out of embarrassment or perhaps fear. If you're one of them, we hope to change your mind.

Only lung cancer takes a higher cancer toll among men than prostate cancer, which strikes almost 200,000 victims annually and kills an estimated 38,000. Many experts believe the incidence is much higher: Autopsies show that a large percentage of men who died of other diseases had undiagnosed prostate cancers.

THE PROSTATE

For a gland that looms so large in the male psyche, the prostate is surprisingly unimposing, tipping the scales at a mere half an ounce. The prostate, located under the bladder and in front of the rectum, is actually a composite of 30 to 50 smaller glands. These subglands, which produce the fluid that contributes to semen, are organized into five lobes, all held together and in place by a more or less tough covering.

Two factors give this male sex gland such a disproportionate influence in a man's life. One, it occupies a strategic position, wrapped around the neck of the bladder, where urine is stored, and the urethra, the tube through which the urine is discharged. What's more, in the sixth decade of life, the gland usually begins to enlarge. So pervasive is the process, that about a quarter of men in their early fifties, half the men in their sixties, and three quarters of those 70 and older have enlarged prostates.

Many experts attribute this growth spurt to a change in hormonal balance, in particular the male sex hormone *testosterone*. When a boy reaches puberty, a rising tide of testosterone prompts

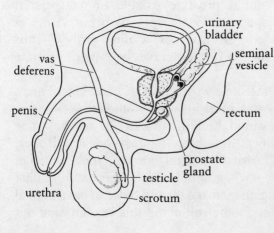

Normal Male Reproductive System. The walnut-shaped prostate gland is situated between the rectum and bladder and surrounds the male urethra.

the tiny prostate to grow to its walnutlike size. The gland remains stable until the early fifties, when hormones once again stimulate growth, by as much as 45 percent every 10 years. Given the prostate's position around the bladder and urethra, severe enlargement can trigger urinary problems.

After a man turns 50, testosterone may have a more insidious effect, spurring the growth of cancerous cells in the prostate. Just how the hormone does this is still largely a mystery, although recent years have brought glimmerings of understanding. In 1992 researchers at the University of Southern California established a possible link between prostate cancer and an enzyme known as 5-alpha-reductase. The enzyme has at least one function in the human body: to turn testosterone into a derivative called dihydrotestosterone. Among other things, dihydrotestosterone is specifically responsible for promoting development of the male sex characteristics. The scientists measured the levels of 5-alpha-reductase in three groups of men. Those with the lowest levels also had the lowest rate of prostate cancer, the implication being that the less active the enzyme, the smaller the pool of dihydrotestosterone created and the more restrained the impact on the prostate.

SIGNS AND SYMPTOMS OF PROSTATE CANCER

- Frequent urination, particularly at night
- Difficulty holding back urine or starting urination
- Weak or interrupted urine flow
- Pain or burning upon urinating
- Inability to urinate at all
- Painful ejaculation
- Bloody urine or semen
- Chronic pain or stiffness in the lower back

DIAGNOSIS AND STAGING

The signs of prostate cancer are similar to those of urethritis, benign prostate enlargement and other disorders, and their appearance should prompt an immediate visit to your doctor. In fact, *benign prostatic hypertrophy,* or enlargement of the prostate gland, is more common than cancer. Its symptoms mimic a malignancy in that the expanding gland compresses the urethra and bladder, impeding urine flow and causing it to build up in the bladder. This in turn produces many of the symptoms of cancer. Although benign enlargement and urinary obstruction require treatment, there is an important distinction: the disease does not spread to other organs, as is often the case with prostate cancer. Early prostate cancer rarely reveals itself, however, and by the time symptoms do emerge, the disease is often well advanced. And the prognosis for prostate cancer darkens once it metastasizes to adjacent tissues and/or the lymph nodes (see box on staging).

STAGING OF PROSTATE CANCER

STAGE	CHARACTERISTICS	FIVE-YEAR SURVIVAL RATE
No Stage 0		
I	Cancer has produced no palpable abnormalities in the prostate.	Greater than 90%
II	Cancer measures less than 2 centimeters in size and has not spread beyond the prostate capsule.	85%
III	Tumor has invaded nearby tissues such as the seminal vesicles, the two glands that flank the bladder and add fluid to the semen during ejaculation; and possibly the urethra.	48%
IV	Cancer has metastasized to the lymph nodes and/or the bones as well as other organs.	21%

TREATMENT OF PROSTATE CANCER

Prostate cancer is typically treated through surgery, radiation therapy, hormone therapy or a combination of these methods.

A *radical prostatectomy* entails the surgical removal of the entire prostate as well as bordering tissues. Until recently, many men found this option abhorrent, perhaps understandably. In order to reach the gland, surgeons generally made an incision through the area hosting the nerves that control erections and the opening of the bladder.

As a result, the operation left many men impotent and unable to control urination. But the technique has since been refined so that the crucial nerves may be bypassed, thus reducing the chances of incontinence and sexual dysfunction. According to Dr. Patrick Walsh of Johns Hopkins University, who developed this new operation, only 10 percent of his patients under 50 lose their ability to have erections. A man who's undergone a prostatectomy no longer produces semen, so he experiences what's referred to as a dry orgasm. But this need not interfere with sexual pleasure.

Patients with stage III tumors usually receive external or internal radiation, while the primary form of treatment for stage IV cases is hormonal therapy. This may be carried out in one of several ways:

- Patients are administered the female sex hormone estrogen to stop the testicles from producing testosterone.
- Daily or monthly injections of luteinizing hormone-releasing hormone (LHRH) agonist, a synthetic substance that also prevents testosterone production.
- *Orchiectomy,* the surgical removal of the testicles, the main source of male hormone production.

Oddly enough, sometimes the most sensible medical response to prostate cancer is to do nothing at all. By and large, the malignancy is extraordinarily *indolent,* or slow growing. Whereas breast cancer may double in size every three months, some prostate tumors can take two to four years to achieve such growth. As a result, there are instances when prostate cancer is, relatively speaking, a minor threat.

According to two 1993 studies, older men who were aggressively treated for the illness lived less than a year longer than those whose physicians merely monitored their cancer. A 60-year-old man with localized prostate cancer who'd undergone either surgery or radiation might expect to live another 15 to 17 years. Untreated, the same man would live 16 years.

Those few months of added life might seem precious, but given the potential complications from therapy, that time could well be bereft of joy or comfort. Moreover, the study revealed, the older the patient at the time of diagnosis, the lower the odds that aggressive treatment would afford him any additional time at all. The study's authors discouraged therapy for men 75 and older.

Not only age, but personal medical history and family medical history, must all be taken into account when considering treatment choices. A 71-year-old man whose brothers, father and uncles all died prematurely of heart disease or strokes may be wiser to visit his internist or cardiologist for regular checkups than to opt immediately for full prostate-cancer treatment. Based on his family history, a heart attack is more likely to kill him long before his untreated cancer does. On the other hand, a healthy, youthful 67-year-old man with a family history of longevity into the eighties and nineties might rationally decide to have the tumor rooted out immediately. Ultimately, says Dr. Willet F. Whitmore Jr., retired chief of urology at Memorial Sloan-Kettering, the decision whether or not to treat prostate cancer should rest with the patient.

WHO IS AT RISK?

- Men age 55 and older
- African-American men

Age is a major factor. As with most adult malignancies, prostate cancer afflicts mainly the elderly. More than 4 in 5 prostate tumors are found in men 65 and older, with 73 being the average age of diagnosis.

African-American men have the highest rate of prostate cancer in the world. One theory why is that they tend to produce greater levels of testosterone. Ominously, more than twice as many African-Americans die from prostate cancer as do Caucasians.

HEREDITARY RISK FACTORS

- Family history of prostate cancer

About 1 in 4 prostate cancer patients have fathers, brothers and uncles also stricken by the disease. In fact, a man whose father or brother had prostate cancer faces double the risk or more of developing the malignancy himself.

PERSONAL HEALTH HISTORY RISK FACTORS

• None identified at present

Benign prostatic hypertrophy and sexually transmitted viruses have both been suspected as possible risk factors, but there is no firm evidence of any association. Nor should you worry if you've had a vasectomy. Although data published in 1991 suggested that men who'd undergone vasectomies in the 1970s ran a slightly increased risk of prostate cancer, two subsequent studies deemed the statistical connection between vasectomy and prostate cancer insignificant. Nonetheless, the American Urological Association now recommends that men who had a vasectomy more than 20 years ago or after age 40 have a digital rectal exam and prostate-specific antigen test annually.

ARE YOU AT RISK FOR PROSTATE CANCER?

_____ Men age 55 and older

_____ African-American men

Hereditary Risk Factors

_____ Family history of prostate cancer

Personal Health History Risk Factors

_____ None identified at present

Environmental Risk Factors

_____ Occupational exposure to chemical pesticides or cadmium, the latter of which is found in the manufacture of batteries; the production of alloys, jewelry, plastics or pigments; and electroplating

Lifestyle Risk Factors

_____ Severe obesity (40 percent or more over your ideal weight; refer to height-weight-frame table in Chapter 6)

_____ Sedentary lifestyle

_____ High-fat diet (35 percent or more of daily calories)

If one or more of these risk factors applies to you, consult your physician.

ENVIRONMENTAL RISK FACTORS

Occupational exposures that appear to raise risk include the use of pesticides; cadmium, a metal used in the manufacture of batteries; the production of alloys, jewelry, plastics and pigments; and electroplating.

LIFESTYLE RISK FACTORS

- Severe obesity (40 percent or more over your ideal weight)
- Sedentary lifestyle
- High-fat diet (35 percent or more of daily calories)

HOW TO REDUCE YOUR RISK

┌───┐

GUIDELINES FOR PRIMARY PREVENTION

In addition to the general primary prevention steps recommended at the beginning of Chapter 9:

- Eat foods rich in vitamin D.

└───┘

PROSTATE CANCER AND DIET

Based on population studies, a high-fat diet appears to increase the risk of this disease. Japanese-Americans living in the United States have much higher rates of prostate cancer than do Japanese men who still reside in their homeland. A possible reason, say scientists, is that Japan's diet is significantly lower in fat than ours.

A study conducted at the Harvard University School of Public Health forged another link between prostate cancer and dietary fat in 1993. After tracking the eating habits of some 51,000 men, researchers found that subjects whose diets included up to 89 grams of fat a day exhibited nearly twice the rate of advanced prostate cancer as those who ate a more modest 53 grams of fat daily.

Interestingly, the incidence of advanced prostate cancer among men who derived most of their fat from red meat (as opposed to plant oils, fish or dairy products) was some 2.6 times higher than among participants who ate the least amount of fat. Avoiding fat didn't prevent prostate cancer but did inhibit its spread. One possible mechanism is that a fatty diet stimulates overproduction of the hormone testosterone, known to cause prostate cancer.

In addition to trimming your fat intake to 20 percent of your total calories, see to it that you eat sufficient amounts of salmon, mackerel, herring, sablefish and other cold-water fish high in omega-3 polyunsaturated oils. These may ward off prostate cancer by neutralizing the body's metabolism of testosterone. Eskimos, whose diets are laden with fish oils, have very low prostate cancer rates.

Vitamins

In preliminary animal studies, a diet rich in vitamin A seemed to reduce substantially the incidence of the disease. Given vitamin A's protective role against other cancers, that would not be surprising.

Vitamin D also has us intrigued, due to observations of especially high prostate cancer rates among African-Americans and Scandinavians. Long winters with little sun—the prime source of vitamin D—deny Nordic men and women sufficient stores of the vitamin, while an abundance of the skin pigment melanin interferes with the body's ability to produce vitamin D in dark-skinned people.

The dietary plan spelled out in Chapter 5 will provide you with adequate amounts of vitamins A and D. We do not recommend taking supplements of any kind, but this is particularly true with regard to vitamins A and D in large doses. Both are fat-soluble, which means they need to dissolve in fatty tissue for the body to use them. Whatever the body does not use is stored in the liver and, to a lesser extent, fatty tissue. When taken in megadoses, these two vitamins can build up to toxic levels.

PROSTATE CANCER AND EXERCISE

According to Dr. I-Min Lee of the Harvard University Medical School and School of Public Health, "Studies have shown that very active individuals, such as marathon runners or runners who put in a lot of mileage weekly, have lower levels of testosterone than individuals who do not exercise.

"Because testosterone is necessary for the development of prostatic cancer," she continues, "I have hypothesized that if one's testosterone levels are lower, one should have a lower risk of prostate cancer." This was borne out in a long-term health study of some 18,000 male Harvard alumni carried out by Dr. Lee and Dr. Ralph Paffenbarger Jr. Dr. Lee cautions, however, that this is not a consistent finding, and more data need to be collected before we can state authoritatively that physical activity safeguards against prostate cancer. Nevertheless, we advocate incorporating exercise into your daily life as a hedge against several cancers.

GUIDELINES FOR SECONDARY PREVENTION

For Asymptomatic Men with No Special Risk Factors

- Annual digital rectal exam, beginning at age 40
- Annual digital rectal exam and prostate-specific antigen (PSA) test, beginning at age 50

For Asymptomatic Men at Increased Risk

- Annual digital rectal exam and prostate-specific antigen (PSA) test, beginning at age 40

DIGITAL RECTAL EXAM

Albert H., a 64-year-old building contractor from New York, can testify to the benefits of this simple test. His wife, troubled by a recent spate of prostate cancer diagnoses among friends, begged her husband again and again to see her urologist. Repeatedly, he refused.

"I just saw my internist six months ago," Albert protested. "I'm perfectly healthy. I don't feel anything unusual."

"I don't feel anything in my breasts," Mrs. H. countered, "and *I* go to a doctor for a breast exam."

Her persistence eventually wore Albert down, and he reluctantly accompanied her to the urologist. By running a lubricated, gloved fingertip around the prostate, the doctor felt a suspicious mass. Diagnostic tests confirmed that his prostate was blanketed with cancer, and within days Albert began treatment. Without the digital rectal exam, he concedes, "I would have been a goner." His cancer is now in remission, and "I am a very happy camper," he says. "Everything is wonderful."

Many men are uncomfortable with the idea of having a finger inserted in their rectum, so they avoid the test. Looking back, Albert admits this was true in his case. "No one wants to go through that kind of testing," he says, "especially when you feel good."

According to at least one recent survey of physicians, many neglected to perform digital rectal examinations on male patients because of the men's embarrassment. Isn't knowing that this brief procedure can discover the earliest manifestations of a potentially fatal disease worth a few moments' embarrassment? We can tell you from experience, there is nothing more painful than seeing a patient's anguish at hearing he has an advanced cancer that could have been detected earlier.

PROSTATE SPECIFIC ANTIGEN (PSA) TEST

The idea behind *PSA testing* is simple. Prostate cells manufacture and release a substance called prostate-specific antigen. A male adult with a healthy prostate will generally have a PSA level of 4 nanograms or less per milliliter of blood, a nanogram being one billionth of a gram. But many men with prostate cancer exceed this level.

While a number of urologists consider the PSA test a valuable screening tool, others in the medical community question its routine use. They point out that some prostate malignancies are extremely aggressive and can kill quickly, while others grow so slowly as to constitute no threat to many patients. One third of all men over age 50 have microscopic traces of prostate cancer. As Dr. William Fair, chief of urology at Memorial Sloan-Kettering, notes, we have no consistent way to distinguish an aggressive tumor from an indolent one. Since even a small cancer may elevate PSA levels, the unquestioning use of the test could prompt doctor and patient to rush into an unnecessary treatment regimen, when the cancer might be the sort that would "outlive the patient."

Complicating the picture is the fact that noncancerous conditions such as prostatitis, an inflammation of the gland, and benign prostatic hypertrophy can also elevate PSA levels. With BPH, for example, the enlarging—but not malignant—prostate sheds more and more antigens, increasing the amount detectable in the blood. And given that many of the symptoms of benign prostatic hypertrophy mimic those of cancer, a so-called false-positive result may lead to needless anxiety for the patient and a battery of expensive and time-consuming tests to rule out a malignancy. All in all, 1 in 5 prostate specific antigen tests raises the specter of cancer where none in fact exists (see box).

GUIDELINES FOR FOLLOW-UP TO PSA TESTS

To reduce the odds of a false-positive, urologists adhere to the following standards:

PSA LEVEL	MEDICAL RESPONSE
4 ng to 10 ng	These levels, in conjunction with a digital rectal exam showing changes in the prostate, may raise the suspicion that cancer is present. However, a 4 ng to 10 ng level may mean you have benign prostatic hypertrophy or another noncancerous condition. Your physician will decide whether diagnostic tests are necessary.
10 ng or higher	A full diagnostic regimen for identifying a malignancy is necessary.

Conversely, the PSA test frequently fails to detect malignant disease. Up to 25 percent of prostate cancer patients may have levels well within normal range. Thus no one who has the test as part of a routine physical should rest easy, especially if he notices other symptoms of prostate trouble.

To help ensure accuracy, refrain from sexual activity, including masturbation, *one week* prior to the test. Researchers at Memorial Sloan-Kettering found that men who ejaculated beforehand had misleadingly low levels of prostate-specific antigens.

With all these reservations about the PSA test, why do we recommend it? Although it is a relatively expensive blood test, it is noninvasive and can identify patients who need further testing, even though their prostate gland may feel normal during a digital rectal exam. Furthermore, yearly tests can help to determine the *speed* at which PSA concentrations rise, which may be just as significant as the level itself. Typically, the tissue buildup from prostate cancer may be 100 times faster than the tissue growth associated with BPH. Thus the increase in PSA levels is also faster in cancer.

Furthermore, prostate cancer may produce 10 times as much prostate-specific antigen as benign disease. Thus if two tests taken within a year reveal that the pace at which the PSA levels increased has stepped up, and that the amount of the antigen has also ascended dramatically, it is likely that cancer, not benign prostate enlargement, is the problem.

TRANSRECTAL ULTRASOUND

A suspicious digital rectal exam or PSA reading opens the door to additional testing. Some prostate cancer specialists believe that *transrectal ultrasound* should be the next step. In this procedure a urologist slips a tiny ultrasound transducer, less than an inch in diameter, into the rectum and beams high-frequency sound waves toward the prostate. As the waves echo back, they are translated into an image (the *sonogram*) of the gland.

Debate rages over ultrasound's reliability for diagnosing prostate cancer. Up to one in three tumors gives off an echo indistinguishable from that of healthy tissue. Moreover, even in the hands of an experienced technologist, ultrasound does not seem able to detect some early cancers. Most researchers agree that ultrasound should be used as an adjunct to biopsy (see below).

PROSTATE BIOPSY

The final arbiter for determining the presence of prostate cancer is the *biopsy*. Many men quake at the idea of a needle being used to withdraw tissue from their prostate. But the procedure is quick and, if not completely free of discomfort, rarely painful, requiring neither general nor local anesthesia.

The morning of the biopsy you must administer yourself a Fleet enema to empty the lower bowel. You may also be asked to take antibiotics beforehand (and perhaps for 24 hours afterward) to lessen the risk of infection from the biopsy needle.

At the doctor's office, you are asked to lie on the examining table in a way that allows the physician easy access to the rectum: on your back with your knees apart; on your side with one leg straight and one bent at the knee against your chest; or on your knees and elbows.

Once you feel comfortable and relaxed, the physician inserts an ultrasound transducer into the rectum. Attached to the tiny probe is a separate plastic sheath. Once the mechanism is in place, the ultrasound machine generates pictures of the prostate. With that image before him, the urologist passes a spring-loaded needle into the sheath and up to the gland.

A gentle squeeze of a trigger, and the needle darts in and out, removing a tissue sample. The needle is carefully withdrawn; another one is passed into the sheath and guided to another area of the prostate to withdraw tissue from there. The procedure is repeated until the doctor has taken samples from half a dozen points.

Expect to spend 20 to 30 minutes on the table. "The biopsies themselves take less than a minute apiece," explains Dr. Whitmore. Because the needle can sometimes puncture the urethra, you may discover blood in your urine a day or two afterward. This is nothing to worry about. The worst side effect you are likely to experience is a mild infection, but this too is a remote possibility.

The tissue samples are sent to a pathologist for analysis. By examining the cells and looking for certain telltale signs—the shape and size of the nucleus in each cell, the number of nucleoli, among other things—the pathologist can tell if they are cancerous.

The view that early detection of prostate cancer has no bearing on the long-term mortality rate is based largely on statistics from the 1980s. Since then, medicine's approach to prostate cancer has changed a great deal, as the development and acceptance of the

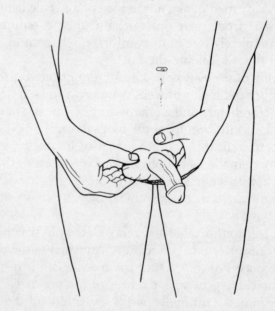

Testicular Self-examination. Use one hand to support the scrotum, and the thumb and two or three fingers of the other hand to carefully feel the testicle for any nodules or lumps.

PSA test demonstrates. Prostate cancer diagnoses are made much earlier in the disease process today, increasing the chances that the cancer will be discovered while still confined to the gland itself.

That PSA screening can find cancers earlier, when most curable,

---

PREVENTING TESTICULAR CANCER

Testicular cancer, another malignancy unique to men, is the most common form of cancer in those ages 20 to 35. But because it makes up only 1 percent of all male cancers, many men tend to ignore it. Don't! The disease seems to be on the rise, afflicting 6,800 men in 1994.

The origins of testicular cancer have yet to be pinned down, nor do we know the reasons for this increasing incidence. However, men with a history of an undescended testicle run a higher risk of developing testicular cancer than men whose testicles developed normally.

A recent study by researchers at Oxford University in England indicated that a sedentary lifestyle heightens the chance for contracting the disease. Too, evidence suggests that men whose mothers took the drug diethylstilbestrol (DES) during pregnancy may be more likely to develop testicular cancer. This drug was given to expectant mothers from the 1940s until the early 1960s to prevent miscarriage and early labor but is no longer used for that purpose.

Surgery as well as advances in chemotherapy have improved survival rates for testicular cancer, which claimed 325 lives in 1994. But the best way to defeat it is to perform a self-examination once a month. Here's how:

1. Take a warm bath or shower to relax the scrotum.
2. Afterward, examine each testicle with both hands: thumbs on top; index and middle fingers underneath. Now roll each testicle gently between the thumbs and fingers.
3. Feel for any abnormal lumps—usually the size of a pea —on the front or sides. Don't confuse a lump with the elongated, cordlike epididymis, a structure that stores and transports sperm. Also know that having one testicle larger than the other is not necessarily abnormal.
4. Report any unusual signs to your doctor immediately.

SUGGESTED READING ABOUT PROSTATE CANCER

From the National Cancer Institute (800-4-CANCER):

• "What You Need to Know About Prostate Cancer"

SUGGESTED READING ABOUT TESTICULAR CANCER

From the National Cancer Institute (800-4-CANCER):

• "Testicular Cancer Research Report"
• "What You Need to Know About Testicular Cancer"

---

was driven home recently by a study conducted at the Washington University School of Medicine in St. Louis. Of some 17,000 men, those given both a PSA test and a digital rectal exam had half the number of advanced prostate cancers as patients who underwent a digital rectal exam only.

KEY WORDS

Benign prostatic hypertrophy: A noncancerous condition marked by overgrowth or enlargement of the prostate.

Orchiectomy: Surgical removal of one or both testicles.

Prostate: A male sex gland, located under the bladder and in front of the rectum, which produces a fluid that forms much of semen.

Prostate biopsy: A spring-loaded needle withdraws approximately half a dozen tissue samples from the prostate. These are then analyzed by a pathologist for evidence of cancer.

Prostatectomy: A surgical procedure to remove the prostate.

Prostatitis: An inflammation of the prostate.

Testosterone: The most influential male sex hormone, or *androgen.*

Transrectal ultrasound: Usually the next step after a suspicious digital rectal exam or PSA test. In this procedure the urologist inserts a tiny transducer into the rectum and uses high-frequency sound waves (ultrasound) to visualize the prostate.

CHAPTER

11

Breast Cancer

Mammography · Breast Self-exam ·
Clinical Breast Exam · Breast Biopsy

The thought of developing breast cancer strikes fear in many women like no other illness. Not only is it second to lung cancer as a cause of cancer death among adult females, but for a patient who sacrifices one or both breasts as a lifesaving measure, the psychologic trauma can be devastating.

Dr. Mary Jane Massie, an attending psychiatrist at Memorial Sloan-Kettering, works extensively with breast cancer patients and women at high risk. "This is a cancer that affects a woman's sense of herself as a feminine being, as a sexual being, as a nurturing being," she explains. "So it cuts across so many different issues for women.

"I think that if you were to ask 100 women, 'What health issues do you worry about?' for the most part they'd tell you breast cancer."

Although 1,000 men get breast cancer annually, for all intents this is a women's disease. And a prolific one: Nineteen ninety-four brought 182,000 new cases and 46,000 deaths among women. Current predictions hold that 1 out of 9 women who live to age 85 will develop breast cancer, compared with 1 in 11 in 1980, and 1 in 16 in 1970. These statistics don't necessarily represent a tremendous increase in the actual incidence of breast cancer. In fact, there are some indications that at least some of the increase is due to heightened awareness of the disease and early and improved diagnosis.

The sharp upturn in diagnosed cases of breast cancer that began in the mid-1970s can be attributed largely to two factors: First, a number of prominent women went public with their fights against the disease, including First Lady Betty Ford, Happy Rockefeller, wife of the Vice President, and Shirley Temple Black, the grownup dimpled darling of cinema fame. Second, the expanding use of the imaging technique *mammography* produced more diagnoses of early-stage tumors that previously would have eluded physicians until the cancer had reached a less curable stage.

According to the American Cancer Society, timely detection of breast cancer rose significantly during the first half of the 1980s. Diagnoses of regional disease in the breast and adjacent tissues, which is 72 percent curable, increased 11 percent in women under 50 and 6 percent in those 50 and older. The detection of localized cancer, which is 93 percent curable, went up 11 percent and 39 percent, respectively, in these two age groups. And discoveries of carcinoma in situ (the earliest cancerous change in cells)—95 percent curable—soared 114 percent and 176 percent. Despite these marked increases in diagnosed breast cancers since 1970, the mortality rate has remained relatively stable and has even declined in some areas of the country.

Like all cancers, breast cancer is an insidious disease, and there is much we don't know about it. For instance, why does it seem to strike city dwellers more than rural dwellers? The exact causes of breast cancer, too, confound us at this time, though genetics, hormonal activity and dietary factors each probably share a role. We do know, however, that old wives' tales blaming the disease on blows or bruises to the breast, childbirth, nursing and sexual activity are simply untrue. And because refined screening techniques can detect breast cancer early, the outlook for large numbers of women has improved significantly.

THE BREASTS

A woman's breasts are made up almost entirely of an admixture of glandular tissue and fat that is sectioned into approximately 20 *lobes* and smaller subdivisions called *lobules*. A cluster of bulb-shaped glands produces milk, while a branchlike system of *ducts* stores milk as well as channels it to the *nipple*, which is encircled

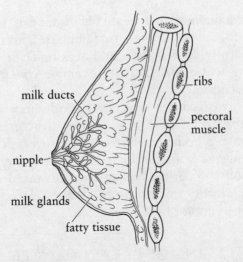

milk ducts

ribs

pectoral
muscle

nipple

milk glands

fatty tissue

Normal Breast. The typical breast is composed mostly of fatty tissue, interspersed with milk-producing glands and ducts.

by darker-pigmented skin known as the *areola*. The breasts, in addition to serving as important symbols of femininity, function as secondary sex organs as well as sources of nourishment in the months or years after childbirth.

SIGNS AND SYMPTOMS OF BREAST CANCER

Breast cancer's warning signs are rarely associated with pain and, unlike most cancers, can usually be seen or felt externally. Watch for any of the following:

- A persistent lump or thickening in the breast or armpit
- A change in the breast's size or contour
- A change in color of the breast or areola
- Dimpling, puckering, scaling or a similar change in skin texture
- An abnormal nipple discharge
- Nipple retraction or scaliness
- Noncyclical pain

Keep in mind that the breasts continually change throughout life. Sexual development, hormones, pregnancy, menopause, aging —even the monthly menstrual cycle—affect their size, shape and feel. So a patch of thickened tissue indicating a possible carcinoma in one person may be perfectly normal in another. Most breast lumps are not malignant and eventually disappear. That is why it is imperative for every woman to familiarize herself with her breasts and learn what is normal and abnormal *for her*. Later in this chapter we will explain how to examine yourself as part of secondary prevention.

Untreated, breast cancer typically spreads first to the *lymph nodes* under the arm. These bean-shaped structures, located at various sites in the body, filter bacteria, viruses, dead cells and other harmful agents from the circulatory system. Next the disease may involve nodes under the breastbone. Advanced-stage cancer, which is often deadly, metastasizes to body parts such as the bones, lungs, liver and/or brain. (See box.)

STAGING OF BREAST CANCER

STAGE	CHARACTERISTICS	FIVE-YEAR SURVIVAL RATE
0	Cancer is localized (carcinoma in situ) and affects only a few layers of cells.	Greater than 95%
I	Tumor measures 2 centimeters (approximately 1 inch) or smaller and remains localized. No lymph node involvement.	85%
II	Malignancy has grown to 2 to 5 centimeters (1 to 2 inches) and/or has invaded the lymph nodes under the arm.	66%
III	Cancer exceeds 5 centimeters (2 inches) in size and/or involves large and matted underarm lymph nodes and/or has metastasized to other regional lymph nodes or to other tissues near the breast.	41%
IV	Cancer has spread to other organs, such as the bones, liver, lungs and/or brain.	10%

TREATMENT OF BREAST CANCER

Depending on the size and location of the cancer, doctors have a number of treatments to consider. The most common surgical procedures to treat breast cancer are:

- In a *lumpectomy,* the least invasive, the localized breast cancer is removed. In addition, the *axillary* lymph nodes in the armpit are usually removed as well, and the procedure is followed by radiation and/or chemotherapy.
- In a *partial mastectomy,* the tumor is removed, as is a small rim of noninvolved healthy tissue referred to as *negative margins.* Most patients then receive radiation therapy.
- In a *total* or *simple mastectomy,* the breast is removed, and sometimes several lymph nodes as well.
- In a *modified radical mastectomy,* the most common procedure for breast cancer patients, the breast, axillary lymph nodes and the lining over the chest muscles are removed. The large chest wall muscle, the pectoralis major, is spared.
- The more extensive *radical mastectomy,* previously the standard for all breast cancer patients, is relatively rare today. In this procedure the surgeon removes the breast, chest muscles (specifically the pectoralis major), all axillary lymph nodes, and additional fat and skin.

Naturally each patient's case is unique, but generally stages I and II breast cancers have an equal choice between mastectomy and breast conservation, while women with stage III breast cancer typically undergo a combination of mastectomy and/or radiation *and* chemotherapy or hormone therapy. Stage IV, or metastatic, carcinoma affects other organs and calls for (1) chemotherapy and/or hormone therapy; (2) limited surgery to control the malignancy in the breast; and sometimes (3) radiation to distant cancers.

The effects of breast surgery vary considerably from woman to woman. Some breeze through a mastectomy and follow-up treatment with few adverse effects, but most experience at least temporary consequences. For example, cutaneous nerves that must be sacrificed during the operation may produce numbness or tingling in the chest, underarm, shoulder and upper arm. Though usually temporary, some patients experience permanent numbness.

It is not uncommon for women who lose a breast to feel weak and stiff in the arm and shoulder, from shrunken, or atrophied, muscles. But this is usually fleeting and can be ameliorated through exercise, unless it is allowed to progress to what's called a frozen shoulder, which would require long-term physical therapy. What's more, the absence of lymph nodes and their connecting vessels may bring about *lymphedema,* in which lymph fluid builds up and causes the arm and hand to swell. Though this happens to only a small percentage of patients, the effects can be profound—and permanent.

The psychosocial/psychosexual adjustments from breast surgery can be more trying than the physical effects. Fortunately, today's mastectomy patients have the choice of undergoing reconstructive plastic surgery. This may either be done at the time of mastectomy or be delayed until after treatment has been completed. The breast can be molded from fatty tissue taken from the abdomen or other areas of the body, or a soft prosthesis can be implanted.

Since breast implants were introduced in the 1960s, approximately one million women have had the operation, 80 percent for breast augmentation. Nine of ten opted for silicone-gel-filled implants; the others chose devices filled with saline, or salt water.

Implants are not without risks, particularly the silicone type. In some cases, they were found to shrink the scar tissue around the implant, resulting in a painful hardening of the breasts; cause calcium deposits in neighboring breast tissue; and change breast and nipple sensation. Although questions still remain as to whether leaking silicone gel or some devices' polyurethane envelope can increase a woman's cancer risk, the mere presence of an implant may interfere with mammography readings.

Manufacturers have claimed that ruptures occurred in only 0.2 percent to 1.1 percent of women. However, medical literature places the figure somewhere between 0 percent and 25 percent, with some doctors citing implant failure in one out of every three patients. Saline implants can leak, rupture or deflate, too, but this would merely release salt water into the body.

For these reasons, in 1992 the FDA severely restricted the use of silicone implants, except in the cases of women who want breast reconstruction for medical reasons, such as cancer, traumatic injuries, to correct severe congenital deformities, or to replace ruptured implants.

The FDA further concluded that all implants "bleed" silicone gel through their protective covering, and that patients should not expect implants of any kind to last a lifetime. A woman considering this surgery should discuss it at length with her doctor. We also suggest calling the FDA's toll-free breast-implant consumer line (800-532-4440), for up-to-date information about implants.

Women who turn down reconstructive surgery can wear a breast prosthesis (an artificial breast form) inside their brassieres. Either option allows a woman to wear her usual clothes. Still, breast cancer patients face a host of complex issues. These women have a wealth of support services available to them, not only for their physical health but also for their emotional well-being.

"Breast cancer is the one most studied in terms of its psychologic aspects," says Dr. Massie. "Over the years, major cancer centers like ours have developed highly trained staffs of related professionals. The individuals who work with the cancer patients are all highly knowledgeable: the nurses, the nurse-practitioners, the social workers and the volunteers—women who themselves have been treated for breast cancer and come back to donate their time. There is a tremendous amount of emotional support for every patient."

WHO IS AT RISK?

WOMEN AGE 40 AND OLDER

The odds of getting breast cancer increase with age. A 30-year-old woman has a 1 in 2,500 chance of developing the disease; her 50-year-old mother, 1 in 50; and her 75-year-old grandmother, 1 in 11.

Roughly three of four breast malignancies occur in women over 50. Among other reasons, the passage of time affords more opportunities for cancerous changes to infiltrate the DNA of the breast's cells as they reproduce. These genetic changes may trigger the uncontrolled cell growth that eventually causes cancer.

HEREDITARY RISK FACTORS

- Family history of breast cancer
- Family history of breast-ovarian cancer syndrome

Up to 30 percent of breast cancer patients have a family history of the disease. In a 1993 study at the Harvard University School of Public Health, nearly 118,000 women were followed for 12 years. Their findings: a 1.8 greater risk for women whose mothers had breast cancer, and a 2.5 greater risk for those who had a mother *and* a sister with the disease.

Two other factors nudge the odds higher still: a familial incidence of *bilateral* cancer (cancer of both breasts) and/or a history of early-onset disease. Both the Harvard study and an earlier one of breast cancer patients at the Creighton University School of Medicine Oncology Clinic in Omaha, Nebraska, found that women from families burdened with the latter pattern were more likely to develop breast cancer themselves.

In families beset by the extremely rare hereditary disorder *breast-ovarian cancer syndrome,* which accounts for just 1 percent of all breast cancers, women may exhibit malignancies of both the ovaries and the breast at an unusually early age, and with a high rate of bilateral tumors.

Dr. Michael Moore, a physician in the breast service at Memorial Sloan-Kettering, and codirector of the Evelyn H. Lauder Breast Center, stresses that an absence of a family history of breast cancer should not lull anyone into thinking she is immune from this disease. "Seventy percent of breast cancer patients have no known first-degree relatives with breast cancer," he points out. Yet all too often he's heard patients lament, "I thought I was safe because there was none of this in my family."

PERSONAL HEALTH HISTORY RISK FACTORS

- Personal history of breast cancer
- Personal history of ovarian cancer
- Any medical condition that required large doses of radiation to the chest
- Early menarche (beginning menstruation before age 12)
- Late menopause (ending menstruation after age 50)
- No children, or first child after age 30
- Taking hormone replacement therapy
- Using oral contraceptives (only for women at increased risk due to other factors)
- Personal history of one or more of the following conditions, confirmed by biopsy:

1. Moderate hyperplasia
2. Papilloma with a fibrovascular core
3. Atypical hyperplasia

A number of medical conditions increase the risk of breast cancer. For example, 15 percent of women with cancer in one breast eventually develop a malignancy in the other. Two less serious conditions double the propensity for breast cancer: *papilloma,* a benign tumor that arises in the skin or the ducts and in this instance has a core composed of both fibrous tissue and blood vessels, and *moderate hyperplasia,* an abnormal increase in cell-growth volume. *Atypical hyperplasia,* a borderline lesion in either the ducts or lobes of the breast, also boosts risk.

In the past, doctors believed fibrocystic breasts, in which women develop lumpy breasts with numerous cysts, predisposed them to cancer. More recent studies discount any association between cystic breasts and cancer, but there is an indirect danger in that the lumpiness may make detecting breast cancer more difficult.

HORMONES AND BREAST CANCER

Hormones have long been suspected of playing a role in breast cancer, and recent studies appear to bolster the association. Specifically, *estrogen* and *progesterone,* the major female sex hormones produced primarily by the ovaries, may promote breast cancer by stimulating cellular growth in the mammary tissue. Although the precise mechanism is unknown, researchers theorize that the rise in hormonal levels that occur during a woman's monthly ovulation cycle may somehow spur the growth of cancer cells. This would explain why the longer a woman's menstrual history, the greater her risk of breast cancer. Conversely, women who enter *menarche* (the onset of menstruation) later than the U.S. average of 12.8 years and/or undergo early *menopause* have a reduced risk of the disease. In fact, for each year the onset of menstruation is delayed, breast cancer risk falls 10 percent to 20 percent, while women who cease menstruating before age 45 see their susceptibility lowered by half.

A 1990 Norwegian study profiled women considered at reduced risk for breast cancer. In addition to late menarche or early menopause, these subjects tended to bear many children beginning at an early age. A childless woman, or one who gave birth for the first time at 30, has three times the chance of getting breast cancer as someone who had a baby before age 18. Whether or not these odds apply equally to women physically unable to conceive and those who choose not to is presently unclear.

Pregnancy elevates estrogen and progesterone levels. How could it lower risk? The answer is that during gestation, the breast tissue may somehow develop resistance to estrogen's deleterious effects.

ARE YOU AT RISK FOR BREAST CANCER?

———— Women age 40 or older*

Hereditary Risk Factors

———— Family history of breast cancer
———— Family history of breast-ovarian cancer syndrome

Personal Health History Risk Factors

———— Personal history of breast cancer
Personal history of one or more of the following conditions, confirmed by biopsy:
———— Moderate hyperplasia
———— Papilloma with a fibrovascular core
———— Atypical hyperplasia
———— Any medical condition that required large doses of radiation to the chest
———— Early menarche (beginning menstruation before age 12)
———— Late menopause (ending menstruation after age 50)
———— No children
———— First child born after age 30
———— Taking hormone replacement therapy
———— Using oral contraceptives (only for women at increased risk due to other factors)

Lifestyle Risk Factors

———— Severe obesity (40 percent or more over your ideal weight; refer to height-weight-frame table in Chapter 6)
———— Excessive alcohol use (more than two drinks per day)
———— Sedentary lifestyle
———— High-fat diet (35 percent or more of daily calories)

If one or more of these risk factors applies to you, consult your physician.

* Only 1 percent of breast cancers affect men.

LIFESTYLE RISK FACTORS

- Severe obesity (40 percent or more over your ideal weight)
- Sedentary lifestyle
- Excessive alcohol use
- High-fat diet (35 percent or more of daily calories)

WAYS TO REDUCE YOUR RISK

GUIDELINES FOR PRIMARY PREVENTION

In addition to the general primary prevention steps recommended at the beginning of Chapter 9:

- Use an alternative to oral contraception if you are at high risk for breast cancer.

BREAST CANCER AND DIET

The same low-fat, high-fiber diet that we've advocated throughout this book may be effective in protecting against breast cancer. Perhaps we should try emulating the Japanese, who on the average consume one fourth the amount of fat that Americans do and exhibit one fifth the rate of breast cancer.

How is it, then, that a Harvard University School of Public Health study concluded that a low-fat diet had no effect on preventing breast cancer? Researchers there followed 90,000 nurses for eight years. Of that group, some 600 developed breast cancer. The researchers concluded that it made no difference whether the women derived as much as 44 percent or as little as 32 percent of their calories from fat, appearing to dash earlier correlations between a low-fat diet and reduced breast-cancer risk. (In laboratory studies, for instance, rats fed low-fat meals developed far fewer breast tumors than those given richer foods.)

Dr. Michael Moore wasn't surprised by the Harvard findings, because, he contends, the participants didn't trim nearly enough fat from their diets to make the study meaningful.

"We here feel that 32 percent of calories from fat is not low enough," he says. Nor is 25 percent, which a follow-up study similarly found did not provide protection. Dr. Moore's definition of a low-fat diet? One that derives no more than 20 percent of its calories from fat.

Maintaining this level, he concedes, is not easy. For most people, "it involves some changes in their lifestyle." But, stresses Kathryn Hamilton, Sloan-Kettering's breast cancer dietitian, "it is doable." She goes on to explain: "You're not going to be eating as much beef and chicken, and you'll be adding more fruits, vegetables, grains, legumes and other carbohydrates."

What fat you do consume should include monounsaturated oils, which Kathryn calls "the lesser of three evils"—not exactly ideal, but preferable to polyunsaturated and saturated fats. Foods high in omega-3 fatty acid, a polyunsaturated fat, are also recommended as part of a breast cancer prevention diet because laboratory studies indicate it may inhibit breast cancer cells. Excellent sources of omega-3 include cold-water fish such as salmon, mackerel, herring and sablefish.

"I also suggest eating 25 to 30 grams of fiber a day," Kathryn adds. Fiber appears to safeguard against breast cancer by binding estrogen in the intestines, preventing its absorption by the bloodstream.

BREAST CANCER AND ALCOHOL

Although the jury is still out on whether alcohol actually causes breast cancer, a number of studies indicate that there is a link. Once again, let's refer to the Nurses' Health Study launched in 1980. In addition to diet, researchers surveyed participants' drinking habits. They found that women who consumed 3 to 9 drinks weekly saw their odds of breast cancer increase 30 percent, while those who consumed more than 9 drinks per week faced a 60 percent higher risk. What is worrisome is that some experts consider up to 14 drinks per week moderate.

How alcohol promotes cancer is still a matter of conjecture, but one theory holds that it may affect hormonal levels. According to a 1991 study, women who consumed two drinks daily for three months exhibited elevated levels of estrogen in their blood. And as we've seen, excessive amounts of this female sex hormone can promote breast cancer. Another hypothesis, based on animal studies, is that alcohol causes a proliferation of certain mammary-gland cells, perhaps increasing their vulnerability to carcinogens.

Significantly, nurses who said they downed fewer than three

drinks per week showed no added risk. We recommend keeping your alcohol intake to similar levels, if you must drink at all.

BREAST CANCER AND EXERCISE

Obesity increases risk for the disease, especially after menopause, probably because body fat produces extra estrogen. Regular exercise reduces body fat and may protect against breast cancer. This was emphasized in a Harvard University School of Public Health study that tracked nearly 5,400 female college alumnae. Its findings, published in 1993: Former college athletes had half the risk of breast cancer as their sedentary counterparts. Harvard researcher I-Min Lee explains, "If we believe that exercise has an influence on the hormonal milieu, then you'd expect that it would affect the risk of a hormonally mediated cancer such as breast cancer."

She cautions, however, that more data are needed before we can state conclusively that physical activity mitigates breast cancer risk. But considering its potential benefits against breast cancer, and its acknowledged salubrious effects on health in general, we recommend you incorporate physical activity into your daily routine.

BREAST CANCER AND ORAL CONTRACEPTIVES AND HORMONE REPLACEMENT THERAPY

Birth-control pills, which suppress ovulation, contain the hormones estrogen and progesterone. The increased risk of breast cancer from using the pill has been put as high as 50 percent, but only while a woman is taking it. As for long-term effects, a 1991 Columbia University School of Public Health study determined that "some evidence suggests that use of oral contraceptives for several years at an early age modestly increases the risk for breast cancer diagnosed before age 35 and perhaps age 45."

However, Dr. Moore points out that studies seeking to ascertain whether birth-control pills instigate breast cancer have produced conflicting results. In his opinion, no guidelines concerning birth-control methods are necessary for those at average risk. But, he adds, "I do recommend that women with an inordinate risk of breast cancer use other forms of contraception."

Hormone replacement therapy is used to control hot flashes and other menopausal symptoms due to decreased estrogen levels, as well as to prevent osteoporosis, the thinning of bones that commonly accelerates after menopause. Recent research additionally indicates estrogen replacement also lowers the risk of cardiovascular disease, the number-one cause of death in women after age 65.

Until recently, postmenopausal hormone therapy entailed replacing estrogen. But estrogen replacement therapy, commonly referred to as ERT, has been associated with an elevated risk of uterine cancer. In recent years, doctors have switched to a regimen of estrogen and progesterone, which appears to eliminate any increased risk of uterine cancer. As for breast cancer, estrogen replacement seems to raise the risk slightly. Therefore women going through menopause should discuss the advantages and disadvantages of hormone replacement therapy with their physicians. Experts note that the risk of premature death from a heart attack

GUIDELINES FOR SECONDARY PREVENTION

Four out of five breast cancer patients have none of the established risk factors for the disease. Therefore observing the secondary-prevention steps below assumes added importance.

For Asymptomatic Women with No Special Risk Factors
For those ages 20 to 39:
- Monthly breast self-exam
- Clinical breast exam, every three years
- Baseline mammography, used for future comparisons, between ages 35 and 39

For those ages 40 to 49:
- Monthly breast self-exam
- Annual clinical breast exam
- Mammography, every one to two years

For those age 50 and older:
- Monthly breast self-exam
- Annual clinical breast exam
- Annual mammography

For Asymptomatic Women at Increased Risk
- Monthly breast self-exam
- Annual clinical breast exam
- Annual mammography, beginning 10 years earlier than the age of a first-degree relative at the time of diagnosis of breast cancer

outstrips any risk of breast cancer, and that this fact tilts the scale in favor of hormone replacement. But ultimately the decision whether to take postmenopausal hormone therapy is a personal one.

Mary V., the patient with the extraordinary family history of cancer described in Chapter 4, thought long and hard before deciding that for her the benefits of hormone replacement outweighed its drawbacks. You'll remember that Mary's risk of gynecologic cancer was so great, she had to have a prophylactic hysterectomy, as did two of her sisters. To compound matters, she is genetically predisposed to breast cancer. "Some doctors don't recommend ERT if you've had cancer," the 44-year-old woman explains, "but to give up estrogen at a young age is very difficult. A lot of things happen to you as a woman; you rapidly age in several different ways. I was worried about my bones falling apart. I thought, *I don't want to live to age 70 and be crippled. I'm not going to go without that kind of help at this point in my life.*" Aware that ERT may raise her already increased risk of breast cancer, she says philosophically, "there are pros and cons to everything. You just have to balance them."

For Mary V. and other women at great hereditary risk for breast cancer, more intensive surveillance than the above guidelines may be necessary—as much to benefit these patients' state of mind as their physical health. "Because of my family history," she says, "I do monthly breast self-exam, I have doctors conduct breast exams on me every six months and I get annual mammograms. I'm very careful."

Because fewer than 7 percent of breast cancers afflict patients under 40, full surveillance for women of average risk isn't recommended until they reach 40. But every woman over age 20 should practice monthly breast self-examination.

BREAST SELF-EXAMINATION

Inspecting your breasts for possible warning signs of cancer does not replace a clinical exam conducted by a trained physician. Still, it can be an effective screening technique. About 80 to 90 percent of breast lumps or tumors are discovered by women themselves, and, understandably, the rate of such discoveries is highest among women who practice regular breast self-examination. At the outset, it should be stressed that the large majority of breast lumps— 70 percent or more—turn out to be benign. But all new breast

HOW TO DO BREAST SELF-EXAMINATION

All women should perform this simple self-examination each month; younger women in the week following a menstrual period when breasts are least apt to be swollen and tender, and older, postmenopausal women on the first of the month or another easy-to-remember day.

Step 1:   Stand in front of a mirror and inspect both breasts. Make sure the contour of the skin is normal, that there's no dimpling or puckering, and that both nipples point in the same direction. Change the tension on the breast tissue by placing your arms over your head, once again noting if this elicits any change in the contour, symmetry or the nipples.

Step 2:   With hands on hips, bow slightly toward the mirror while arching your shoulders and elbows and look for the same signs.

Step 3:   Now examine your breasts while showering or bathing. Wet the breasts and apply soap or a bath gel; your fingers glide more easily over wet, soapy skin, making it easier for you to feel any small lumps or changes. With your right hand, rotate your three middle fingers clockwise around the left breast. Start around the nipple at 12 o'clock, then move around the clock face in ever-increasing concentric circles outward. Alternatively, move from top to bottom, and side to side, carefully feeling every part of the breast. Then repeat this step on the opposite breast.

Step 4:   Lie flat on your back, a pillow placed under your left shoulder and your left arm raised over your head. This flattens the breast and permits easier examination. Repeat step 4 on your left breast, then change position and do the same on your right breast.

lumps that persist through two menstrual cycles must be assumed to be cancer unless proved otherwise.

Self-examination takes no more than 10 minutes, and anyone can learn how to do it. Yet only about 1 in 4 women performs this valuable procedure on a monthly basis. One encouraging sign is that women under 40 appear to be more conscientious about BSE than the older generation. For many women, including Mary V., it's a way to feel in control of their bodies.

"The breasts are one of the parts of the anatomy women have

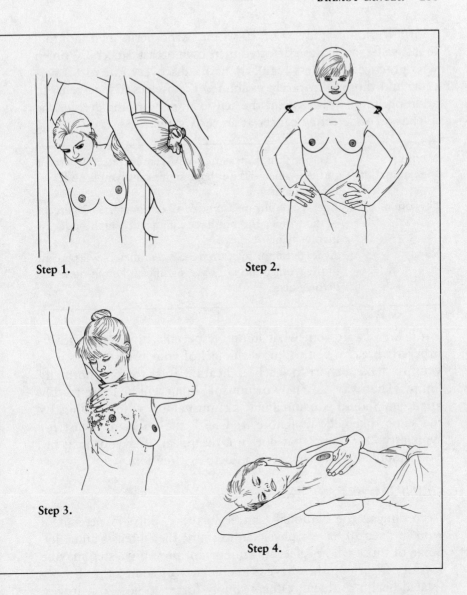

Step 1.

Step 2.

Step 3.

Step 4.

access to," she says, adding pointedly, "Why wait for the freight train to run you down, when you can step off the track now?"

Because breasts often feel lumpy, swollen and tender right before and during menstruation, the best time to examine yourself is several days to one week after your period ends. If you've already reached menopause, pick a day of the month and stick to it. (See box for illustrated step-by-step guide.) To be sure you're doing it correctly, at your next doctor's office visit, ask your physician to check your technique.

254 **PREVENTING THE MAJOR CANCERS**

In a Vermont study, 9 of 10 women who performed monthly breast self-examination detected their own breast cancers. Women who practiced BSE less regularly had a discovery rate of 82 percent, and those who rarely examined themselves, 54 percent. In addition, the more frequent the self-examination, the greater the likelihood of detecting cancer at an early stage:

Monthly examination	Average tumor measured 1.97 centimeters; 91 percent of the women did not have significant lymph-node involvement.
Less often	Average tumor measured 2.47 centimeters; 83 percent of the women did not have significant lymph-node involvement.
Rarely	Average tumor measured 3.59 centimeters; 73 percent of the women did not have significant lymph-node involvement.

All breasts are somewhat lumpy, especially in women with fibrocystic breasts. Get to know the feel of your breasts. You may want to make a chart for each, indicating areas that are normally lumpy. That way, any new or unusual lump will be more readily apparent. Should you find a new or unusual lump, don't panic. By the same token, don't ignore it: Check the opposite breast for symmetry. Any lump that does not disappear after your next period should also be brought to a doctor's attention.

CLINICAL BREAST EXAM

According to the National Cancer Institute, only 45 percent of women over 50 have a physician examine their breasts annually. Some of those who neglect this important preventive step may be fearful of learning they have a malignancy or some other breast-related health problem. Others simply forget to go. To help you remember, do what patient Mary V. does, and schedule your appointment around your birthday. The American Cancer Society recommends having a clinical breast exam performed seven to ten days after menstrual flow begins, so that the breasts will be less lumpy and tender.

First your physician inquires about any changes you've noticed in the shape, contour and feel of your breasts. "Very often," notes Dr. Moore, "the patient will tell you if there's something wrong."

Next you slip on a gown and lie on the examining table so that the doctor can inspect for changes in the skin or nipple and then *palpate* each breast, that is, touch with the fingers. Each physician has her or his own technique, but generally the exam is not unlike the one you perform yourself. You will be asked to raise your arms, hang them loosely at your sides, then press them tightly against your hips, to change the tension as the doctor evaluates the tissue and the lymph nodes above the clavicle and in the armpits. Should he or she discover a lump, it is palpated for size, texture and movability.

Two percent of all breast cancers are diagnosed during pregnancy. However, the milk glands naturally swell during gestation, making it more difficult for you and your doctor to discern potentially cancerous lumps. The American College of Obstetricians and Gynecologists therefore advises that breast exams be conducted as part of all prenatal exams.

MAMMOGRAPHY

Following the clinical breast exam, women of the appropriate age and/or risk group are sent for an x-ray of the breast called a mammogram. As noted earlier, this test can identify many breast tumors *up to two years* before they can be felt with the fingers. However, it does fail to detect growths 10 to 15 percent of the time. That is why it should be performed in combination with clinical and breast self-examinations.

Early diagnosis of cancer through mammography can reduce the mortality rate from carcinoma of the breast by nearly one third. The procedure's benefits have been clear for some time. A landmark study initiated in 1963 tracked some 62,000 women belonging to the Health Insurance Plan of Greater New York (HIP). The study group of slightly more than 30,000 subjects underwent both clinical examination and mammography, while the control group received their usual level of health care.

After five years, deaths from breast cancer were 50 percent lower among women ages 50 to 59 in the study group, and 30 percent lower after ten years. Those ages 40 to 49 showed only a 5 percent reduction in mortality after five years, but a 24 percent drop after ten. It's important to point out that mammographies weren't nearly as accurate in the 1960s and 1970s as they are today.

Medical professionals who strongly support mammography's benefits were disappointed by the results of the Canadian National Breast Screening Study, published in 1992. Researchers there ran two randomized trials for breast screening: one for females ages 40 to 49, the other for females ages 50 to 59. A total of 90,000 women entered the study. In each age group, half the participants received annual mammograms plus physical examinations; the other half, only clinical breast exams. Mammography, the authors wrote, "had no effect on the rate of death from breast cancer for up to seven years of follow-up," not even for patients over 50.

The controversial report has generated much criticism. Dr. Moore calls the researchers' methods "terribly flawed. Their mammograms were suboptimal; they were making 1992 conclusions based on mammograms that were performed mostly on obsolete equipment."

"It's too bad," comments Dr. Joseph Simone, Memorial Sloan-Kettering's physician-in-chief, "because it's an inconclusive study, and yet now anybody who's looking for an excuse not to have a mammogram has one." In 1993 the National Cancer Institute dropped its recommendation of regular mammograms for women between 40 and 50. Nevertheless, we hold firm to the earlier guideline, as do the American Cancer Society and the American College of Radiology.

State-of-the-art mammography centers use precise machines operated in a friendly, pleasant atmosphere. When the technologist is ready, you go inside, undress from the waist up and put on a gown.

The technologist places the breast between two plastic plates— one an x-ray tube, the other an x-ray cassette. Each is adjusted until the breast is properly positioned. You're asked to hold your breath—the machine takes the x-ray—now breathe. Two exposures per breast are usually required, says Dr. Moore, "one top-to-bottom view and another from the side." The entire procedure takes ten minutes.

Then, says Dr. Robert Heelan, a radiologist, "The patient waits five, ten minutes while we check the film and decide if additional shots are needed." Some women complain that the plates feel cold, and according to patient Judith K., "it's a little uncomfortable when they try to flatten out your breast" for a sharper image. But overall, she says, there's no pain involved.

Many patients express concern about radiation exposure from

mammograms. "It was probably an issue with the machines of 1973 but not today," says Dr. Moore, who offers a point of comparison: "Almost an entire lifetime's worth of recommended mammograms would equal several chest x-rays."

Because accuracy is essential, you must be sure that your mammogram will be performed by a properly trained x-ray technologist on high-quality, low-dose equipment. Ideally, the facility should be accredited by the American College of Radiology. To learn of approved mammography centers near you, call either the ACR at (800-ACR-LINE) or the National Cancer Institute's Cancer Information Service at (800-4-CANCER).

However, the ACR's program is voluntary, and not all facilities request accreditation. In that case, Dr. Moore suggests calling the center directly. Ask these questions prepared by the National Cancer Institute. If the person you speak to does not answer yes to all five, *choose another facility*.

1. *Does your facility use dedicated mammography machines?* This is equipment specifically designed for mammography and for no other purpose.
2. *Is the person who takes the mammograms a registered technologist?* Technologists should be certified by the American Registry of Radiologic Technologists or be state licensed.
3. *Is the radiologist who reads the mammograms specifically trained to do so?* The radiologist should be board certified and a graduate of special courses in mammography. Some experts recommend that two radiologists review the films, because one might see a suspicious area that the other has overlooked.
4. *Does the facility conduct mammograms as part of its regular practice?* The American College of Radiology recommends that you go only to a facility that performs at least 10 mammograms a week.
5. *Is the mammography machine calibrated at least once a year?* All equipment should be checked annually so that measurements and doses are accurate.

BREAST BIOPSY

If palpation or mammography reveals a suspicious mass, your surgeon may perform a *biopsy,* the definitive method of diagnosing a malignancy. *Fine-needle aspiration* uses a syringe-type needle to remove cells for analysis by a pathologist. When Drs. Hayes E. Martin and Edward B. Ellis introduced the technique at Memorial

Hospital in 1926, they used an 18-gauge needle. Today's much finer instruments, usually 21 or 22 gauge, make needle aspiration virtually pain free. (The higher the gauge, the thinner the needle.) A doctor's office or outpatient clinic provides the usual setting for this simple procedure.

"It takes 15 seconds," says Dr. Moore. The skin is cleansed and numbed, then a small needle is inserted into the questionable lump. "The needle is moved around, and cells are withdrawn by applying negative pressure on the piston of the syringe. They are placed on a slide and are read within hours by the pathologist," says Dr. Moore, who praises aspiration biopsy as "quite useful for giving quick diagnoses." If the growth is a benign cyst, aspirating the tissue fluid usually collapses the cyst, and no further treatment is necessary. If the cells are found to be abnormal, other methods will be used to confirm a cancer diagnosis. In a *core-needle biopsy,* the doctor extracts tissue using a special instrument with a cutting edge.

Larger masses may call for a surgical biopsy, typically performed on an outpatient basis in a hospital. Several tests may be conducted beforehand, such as blood and urine tests, a chest x-ray and an electrocardiogram (EKG), which graphically records the heart's rhythm and other actions.

In an *incisional biopsy* a portion of the mass is removed. If no cancer is discovered, it may be repeated to ensure that the entire lump is nonmalignant. Another technique is *excisional biopsy.* Here the whole growth is cut out along with a margin of normal surrounding tissue. Both can leave a small, faint scar.

Women undergoing surgical biopsies usually receive local or general anesthesia and are ready to go home within a few hours. Should your doctor recommend a biopsy requiring hospitalization, ask the reasons for this approach.

Biopsies may help pinpoint a change in breast tissue that is visible on a mammogram but cannot be felt. A physician performing a *mammographic localization with biopsy* uses the mammogram as a reference while either inserting small needles or injecting dye into the suspicious tissue, which can then be removed for analysis. A new alternative to this technique, *stereotactic biopsy,* uses mammography to aim the needle. It is so new, in fact, that many health-care centers do not offer it as of yet.

After receiving an injection of a local anesthetic, you lie face down on a padded table designed with a round opening to accommodate the breast. To precisely locate the suspicious spot seen on an earlier mammogram, a special grid is applied to the breast. We then confirm its position by taking another mammogram, this one performed as the patient continues lying on her stomach. The digital equipment differs from a conventional mammography machine in that the image appears on a computer screen instead of x-ray film.

A 14-gauge needle gun then takes five samples from the biopsy site. While somewhat uncomfortable, you should not feel any pain. Once the specimens are taken, a Band-Aid is placed over the area, and you may go about your normal activities. In all, the procedure typically lasts half an hour, and results are ready within two days.

An important final point regarding biopsies: Years ago, some patients mistakenly feared that cutting a growth or inserting a needle into it would "scatter" the cancer cells, hastening the disease's spread. There is not a shred of truth to this myth.

BEFORE A BIOPSY, ASK YOUR DOCTOR:

- How long the biopsy will take.
- Whether or not you may eat or drink beforehand.
- How soon will you be informed of the results.
- Should you have a tumor, any additional tests that will be needed.
- Whether you will have a needle aspiration, needle biopsy or a surgical biopsy.

Numerous studies have shown that physical examinations coupled with mammography beginning at age 40 can save lives. And the NCI determined that for women over 50 the two techniques decreased breast-cancer mortality by 30 percent over 10 years.

Today mammography and clinical breast exam "are a routine part of any gynecologic exam," notes Dr. William Hoskins, chief of gynecology service at Memorial Sloan-Kettering. He goes on to explain that "the vast majority of women do not routinely see a breast surgeon or someone who takes care primarily of breast disease; for most of them their obstetrician/gynecologist is the only doctor they see. So it's important that we recommend to these patients screening for breast cancer. If they do not do breast self-examinations, one of the nurses will show them how. We also explain to them the recommended frequency for physician exams and mammograms."

The National Cancer Institute hopes that by the year 2000, its effort to educate the public about the advantages of screening procedures will have influenced 4 in 5 women over 50 to go for mammography and a clinical breast exam annually. We urge all women to join this movement toward good health and to follow the screening recommendations appropriate to their particular age and level of risk.

SUGGESTED READING ABOUT BREAST CANCER

From the National Cancer Institute (800-4-CANCER):

- "Breast Exams: What You Should Know"
- "Questions and Answers About Breast Lumps"
- "What You Need to Know About Breast Cancer"

From the American Institute for Cancer Research (800-843-8114):

- "Questions and Answers About Breast Lumps and Breast Cancer"

KEY WORDS

Bilateral: Refers to both breasts; *unilateral* refers to one.

Breast biopsy: Types include *fine-needle aspiration, core needle, incisional, excisional, mammographic localization with biopsy* and *stereotactic biopsy.*

Cyst: A saclike growth filled with excess fluid or fibrous tissue.

Estrogen: A female hormone instrumental in reproduction, and a possible promoter of breast cancer.

Lumpectomy: A means of breast conservation in which only the localized breast cancer and axillary lymph nodes in the armpit are surgically removed.

Lymphedema: A condition in which lymph fluid builds up and causes swelling.

Mastectomy: Surgery to remove the breast. Classifications include *partial mastectomy, total* or *simple mastectomy, modified radical mastectomy* and *radical mastectomy.*

Menarche: The onset of menstrual periods during puberty.

Menopause: The cessation of menstrual periods and a woman's reproductive years.

Palpation: Feeling the breast with the fingers for signs of lumps or any other abnormalities indicating disease.

Progesterone: A female hormone instrumental in preparing the uterus for pregnancy.

CHAPTER

12

Lung Cancer

Chest X-Ray · Sputum Cytology · Tobacco's Effect on the Lungs

Why do they smoke? After nearly 20 years of practicing medicine at Memorial Sloan-Kettering, Dr. Diane Stover still shakes her head and ponders that question every time she prepares to tell a patient he or she has lung cancer.

"I sometimes ask them, 'Why do you do it, when you know it's been directly related to a very high risk of lung cancer?'" reflects Dr. Stover, chief of pulmonary service and head of the division of general medicine. "And there are a few blanket answers. One is: 'Well, you have to die of something.' The second is: 'I never expected that *I* would get cancer.' And the third is: 'People who don't smoke get lung cancer too.'"

True, nonsmokers sometimes do develop the disease, but smokers constitute 85 percent of lung cancer patients. Tragically, it is an ever-increasing group. From 1950 to 1988, a period in which the toll from 11 cancers fell, the death rate from carcinoma of the lung more than doubled for men and jumped nearly fivefold for women, a trend directly related to the increase in female smokers. Long the number-one killer of men among cancers, since 1985 lung cancer has held the same dubious distinction among women. In the United States, 1994 saw 172,000 new cases and 153,000 deaths, making it second only to heart disease as a cause of death.

At the dawn of the 1900s, the disease that would become the scourge of the century barely drew attention; the era's medical literature listed fewer than 80 cases. In 1912 Dr. Isaac Adler, a New York City physician and teacher, asserted in a landmark paper that lung cancer was actually more prevalent than previously thought. Physicians, he wrote, had long misdiagnosed it as tuberculosis and other pulmonary disorders. Even so, lung cancer was still relatively rare. A few years later, Dr. Alton Ochsner, founder of the famed Ochsner Clinic in New Orleans and an outspoken foe of smoking, linked cigarette smoking and lung cancer—an association that was ignored for decades.

The incidence rate among smokers is 10 times that of nonsmokers, and up to 25 times higher for heavy smokers. Fortunately, the 1964 Surgeon General's report associating smoking and lung cancer prompted many people to quit. But because lung cancer takes 20 or more years to develop, it is unlikely that we'll see any decline in lung cancer in the near future. In fact, experts predict that the disease will remain the leading cause of cancer death until at least the year 2010.

THE LUNGS

The *lungs,* the primary component of the respiratory system, occupy most of the chest cavity and flank the *mediastinum,* the chamber that houses the heart. A thin two-ply membrane, the *pleura,* envelops each lung—an organ made up of millions of tiny air sacs (alveoli), giving it the appearance of spongy, pinkish-gray tissue laced with an intricate network of blood vessels. The left lung is divided into two sections *(lobes);* the slightly larger right lung, into three.

When you inhale, air travels through the nasal and oral passages into the throat, through the larynx and the trachea, or windpipe, and into the lungs by way of two tubes called the *bronchi.* These in turn feed the *bronchioles,* smaller tubes that fan out like branches and culminate in the alveoli. The *diaphragm,* a dome-shaped muscle bordering the underside of both lungs, contracts rhythmically and enables them to expand. During exhalation the diaphragm shifts back into place, deflating the lungs and forcing air outward.

In the lungs, oxygen is exchanged for carbon dioxide and other waste gases through the thin walls of the capillaries and the alve-

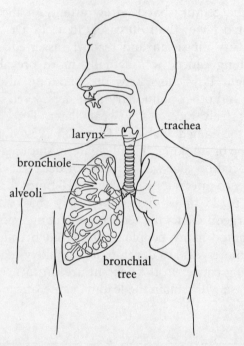

Normal Respiratory System. The respiratory tract is likened to an inverted tree, with the trachea, or windpipe, forming the trunk, the bronchial tubes making up the branches, and the alveoli, or air sacks, the leaves.

oli. Like most other functions of the human body, respiration is a remarkably complex, finely balanced process.

Lung cancer develops when a carcinogen, be it asbestos, radon, cigarette smoke or some other initiator, damages a cell's DNA. Half of all lung tumors contain a defective tumor suppressor gene —called p53 by molecular biologists—that permits uninhibited cell growth. The defective p53 gene has also been implicated in cancers of the colon, breast, liver and other organs.

Another pathogenic mechanism, this one involving a genetic mutation of proto-oncogenes in the *ras* family (H-*ras*, K-*ras* and N-*ras*), is believed to account for *adenocarcinoma,* one of four types of *nonsmall-cell* lung cancer. Adenocarcinomas tend to arise as glandular tumors along the outer perimeter of the lungs and beneath the bronchial tissue lining.

Each type of lung cancer exhibits unique cell characteristics. The other nonsmall-cell cancers include squamous-cell carcinoma, large-cell undifferentiated carcinoma and bronchoalveolar carcinoma.

Squamous-cell typically surfaces in the central portion of the lung. It is the only subtype to go through precancerous stages. As the scale-shaped cells progress from normal to *atypia* to *dysplasia* to *hyperplasia,* their size and shape grow increasingly irregular.

Large-cell undifferentiated carcinoma, so-named for its cells' size, makes up less than 20 percent of lung cancers. It usually takes hold in the smaller bronchi. The least-common form of nonsmall-cell lung cancer, *bronchoalveolar carcinoma,* manifests in the lining of the alveoli, with tumors frequently involving both lungs.

Small-cell lung cancer, found in approximately 25 percent of lung cancer cases, is also referred to as oat-cell lung cancer, an apt description of the cells' small, oval or round appearance under a microscope. An especially aggressive cancer, it spreads rapidly to other organs.

SYMPTOMS OF LUNG CANCER

SIGNS AND SYMPTOMS OF PRIMARY LUNG CANCER

- Fatigue
- A deep, wheezing cough
- Chronic chest pain
- Increased *sputum,* a mucous secretion from the lungs that is expelled through the mouth; not to be confused with the saliva produced by the salivary glands
- Bloody sputum
- Belabored breathing
- Difficulty swallowing, from pressure on the esophagus
- Hoarseness, from pressure on a nerve
- Recurring pneumonia or bronchitis
- Swelling of the face, neck or upper extremities, due to pressure on blood vessels
- *Pancoast's* syndrome, a condition in which the malignancy compresses nerves of the shoulder, arm or hand, creating pain and weakness in the affected areas

Lung cancer rarely produces symptoms (see box) until it is well entrenched in the lung. By that time it may have metastasized to other parts of the body. Fatigue, the most frequently seen sign, is often shrugged off and not considered a serious problem. The same is true of another common warning, coughing, which is caused by an irritation of the bronchial lining or a tumor blocking an air passage. Many smokers are so used to hacking and wheezing, they dismiss this as "smoker's cough" and neglect to see a doctor at this stage.

Because the brain, bones and liver are among the most frequent sites of metastasis, advanced lung cancer may produce seemingly unrelated symptoms: headaches, weakness, memory loss, impaired speech, if the brain is affected; bone pain and fractures; and jaundice, a yellowing of the skin and mucous membranes, if the liver is involved.

Lung cancer can also bring about *paraneoplastic syndromes,* tumor-related disorders of the nervous system, blood, kidneys, skin or endocrine system. The cancerous cells sometimes emit hormones, creating a hormonal imbalance that sets off a variety of symptoms: appetite loss, nausea, drowsiness, constipation, mental confusion, diabetes, weight gain and sudden hair growth.

Should any of the aforementioned consequences occur, consult a doctor. Swift medical intervention is essential for all cancers, but especially for lung tumors. As you can see from the accompanying staging classifications, the earlier the diagnosis, the greater the chance for a cure:

STAGING OF LUNG CANCER

STAGE	CHARACTERISTICS	FIVE-YEAR SURVIVAL RATE
Nonsmall-Cell Lung Cancer		
0	Carcinoma in situ: Cancer is found only in a local area and only in a few layers of cells. It has not grown through the surface lining of the lung.	70%–80%
I	Cancer is confined to the lung and surrounded by normal tissue.	50%

II	Cancer has infiltrated nearby lymph nodes.	30%
III	Cancer has spread to the chest wall, the diaphragm or other organs or blood vessels near the lung; or has spread to lymph nodes in the mediastinum or on the other side of the chest or in the neck.	Less than 5%–15%
IV	Cancer has spread to distant sites in the body.	Less than 2%

Small-Cell Lung Cancer

| Limited stage | Cancer is confined to one lung, the mediastinum and nearby lymph nodes. | 15%–30% * |
| Extensive stage | Cancer has spread to other tissues in the chest or other parts of the body. | 0%–2% * |

* 2-year disease-free survival rate

TREATMENT OF LUNG CANCER

Because fewer than one in five lung cancers are detected early, the disease frequently runs a deadly course. Complicating matters, notes Dr. Stover, "Most of these patients have underlying chronic obstructive pulmonary disease from smoking," which limits therapy options.

One new technique for treating some nonsmall-cell lung cancers, *photodynamic therapy,* allows patients to avoid surgery, radiation and chemotherapy. A photosensitizing agent is injected into the body and absorbed by the cancer cells. Using a tubular scope, the physician then beams a laser light at the agent-permeated cells, causing a chemical reaction that destroys them while sparing healthy ones nearby. Close follow-up care is essential.

For a tumor that stays confined to one lung, surgery emerges as the primary treatment. *Wedge resection* removes a small portion of a lung. In *lobectomy,* doctors excise a single lobe. And *pneumonectomy* entails taking out the entire lung. Nonsmall-cell cancers that have metastasized to neighboring lymph nodes or tissue call for a combination of surgery, radiation and/or chemotherapy.

One half of all pulmonary malignancies are inoperable, having invaded other organs by the time of discovery. In such instances, physicians utilize radiation therapy to control the tumor in the lung and combination chemotherapy to reach metastases elsewhere in the body. Fast-growing small-cell lung cancer must typically be treated in this fashion.

Although inroads have been made in improving the efficacy of treatment, the overall prognosis remains poor. Only 13 percent of all lung cancer patients survive five years, compared with 7 percent in 1963. Nonsmokers have little to fear from this sinister disease. If you are a smoker, we hope these forbidding figures convince you to take the most important step toward reducing your risk of lung cancer: Quit.

WHO IS AT RISK?

HEREDITARY RISK FACTORS

• Family history of lung cancer

The fact that nonsmoking men and women can contract lung cancer raises the possibility of an inherited tendency for cells in the lungs to activate carcinogens. No specific gene has been identified to date, yet some studies show that a family history of lung cancer elevates a nonsmoker's risk two- to threefold.

Because scientists believe it takes two independent events to spark cancer, one explanation for this pattern may be a combination of genetic susceptibility and hazardous exposure to passive, or secondhand, smoke, now recognized as a promoter of lung cancer.

PERSONAL HEALTH HISTORY RISK FACTORS

• Chronic obstructive pulmonary disease
• Personal history of lung scarring
• Any disease that required large doses of radiation to the chest
• Personal history of lung cancer

Emphysema and chronic bronchitis are forms of *chronic obstructive pulmonary disease* (COPD), which is second only to heart disease as a cause of disability among men over age 40. Dr. Curtis Harris, head of the National Cancer Institute's laboratory of human carcinogenesis, explains how COPD, caused mainly by smoking, affects the lung.

"A number of changes occur," he says. "The lungs produce more mucus, and the airways constrict, so it's more difficult for oxygen to enter the bloodstream. There's also an increased risk of infection." In addition, smoking depletes the lung tissue of elastin, a protein essential for maintaining its resiliency. About 1 in 100 COPD patients eventually develop lung cancer.

Lung scarring, a potential harbinger of adenocarcinoma, usually arises as a side effect of tuberculosis, once the leading cause of death in the U.S. The discovery of antibiotics capable of killing the tuberculosis bacterium and our improved nutrition and standards of living all but eliminated TB as a public health hazard. But worldwide, the disease remains one of the leading causes of death; in the late 1980s a new epidemic of TB erupted in New York City and other urban areas, largely as a consequence of poverty, homelessness and AIDS.

Any medical condition that requires radiation to the chest heightens a person's odds of getting lung cancer. "The risk is small," emphasizes Dr. Harris, "but significant." Survivors of Hodgkin's disease, a form of lymphoma, exhibit a higher-than-average propensity for developing lung cancer 10 to 30 years later. According to Dr. Bruce Johnson, chief of the lung cancer biology section at the National Cancer Institute, two factors appear responsible. "Our assumption," he says, "is that it's a combination of chest radiation and an underlying immunologic defect, since Hodgkin's is a disease of the lymph glands." These glands, or nodes, filter foreign substances from the lymph, a yellowish fluid that carries disease-fighting white blood cells called lymphocytes throughout the body's circulatory system. Impairment of the lymph system compromises your ability to ward off infection and possibly cancer.

ENVIRONMENTAL RISK FACTORS

Approximately 15 percent of lung cancer deaths can be linked to prolonged, unprotected exposure to the carcinogens listed in the accompanying box. The major three—secondhand smoke, radon and asbestos—are widespread in both homes and the workplace, claiming around 5,000 lives each per year.

Inhaled asbestos particles, in addition to inducing lung cancer, can also bring about *mesothelioma,* a rare malignancy that usually develops on the pleura covering the lungs, although it can also affect the protective membranes surrounding the heart, the intestinal tract or the reproductive organs. Overall, this cancer affects 1,000 to 1,500 people a year, killing 1,200.

In several surveys of mesothelioma patients, up to 80 percent could verify past occupational exposure to asbestos. Until the mid-1970s, when new regulations reducing acceptable levels went into effect, the material was as ubiquitous in U.S. industry as the punch clock. That we are now seeing a rise of the disease in white males age 55 and older can be attributed to the 30 to 40 years that mesothelioma takes to develop.

There are numerous other occupational carcinogens, with workers in metal refining and chemical manufacturing at especially high risk. Anyone who works with known carcinogens should follow recommended safety procedures. Above all, they should not smoke, which compounds the danger of both the tobacco and the chemical or metal carcinogen. In white males, asbestos exposure in conjunction with tobacco use boosts the chances of getting lung cancer *90-fold* over someone who has never smoked or worked with asbestos.

ENVIRONMENTAL CAUSES OF LUNG CANCER

- Asbestos
- Radon
- Secondhand smoke
- Arsenic
- Benzo(a)pyrene
- Bis(chloromethyl) ether
- Bis(chloromethyl) sulfide
- Cadmium
- Chromium and certain chromium compounds
- Coal gas
- Coal tars
- Coke-oven emissions
- Iron oxide
- Mustard gas
- Nickel
- Petroleum
- Polycyclic aromatic hydrocarbons, found in soots, tars, mineral oils
- Radiation
- Rock wool
- Slag wool
- Vinyl chloride

ARE YOU AT RISK FOR LUNG CANCER?

Hereditary Risk Factors

_____ Family history of lung cancer

Personal Health History Risk Factors

_____ Chronic obstructive pulmonary disease, such as emphysema or chronic bronchitis

_____ Personal history of lung scarring

_____ Any medical condition that required large doses of radiation to the chest

_____ Personal history of lung cancer

Environmental Risk Factors

Prolonged, unprotected exposure to:

_____ Asbestos

_____ Radon

_____ Secondhand smoke

Also:

_____ Arsenic

_____ Benzo(a)pyrene

_____ Bis(chloromethyl) ether

_____ Bis(chloromethyl) sulfide

_____ Cadmium

_____ Chromium and certain chromium compounds

_____ Coal gas

_____ Coal tars

_____ Coke-oven emissions

_____ Iron oxide

_____ Mustard gas

_____ Nickel

_____ Petroleum

_____ Polycyclic aromatic hydrocarbons, found in soots, tars, mineral oils

_____ Radiation

_____ Rock wool

_____ Slag wool

_____ Vinyl chloride

Lifestyle Risk Factors

_____ Tobacco use (highest risk)

If one or more of these risk factors applies to you, consult your physician.

LIFESTYLE RISK FACTORS

• Heavy tobacco use

"The risk of lung cancer increases with the number of cigarettes smoked and the duration," Dr. Stover explains, "but it also depends on the person's age, the degree of inhalation, the levels of tar and nicotine, and whether the cigarettes are filtered or unfiltered."

Although heavy smokers—defined as smoking a pack or more a day for 20 years—have the highest risk, *no* amount of smoking is safe, with regard not only to cancer but also to numerous other diseases, including emphysema, chronic bronchitis and heart disease.

HOW TO REDUCE YOUR RISK
GUIDELINES FOR PRIMARY PREVENTION

In addition to the general primary prevention steps recommended at the beginning of Chapter 9:

• *Avoid all forms of tobacco!*
• Eat foods rich in folic acid.

At the top of the list, and italicized for emphasis: *Do not use tobacco in any form.* If you are currently a smoker, stop, through the methods discussed in Chapter 6. We say this well aware that quitting is a difficult challenge. Nicotine may be legal, but it is no less pernicious than the most addictive illicit narcotic. Pulmonary doctors tell countless stories of terminally ill lung cancer patients who can no longer breathe without the aid of an oxygen tank yet still crave the nicotine responsible for putting them on their death bed. They sneak cigarettes or light up defiantly, and continue to do so until the end of their shortened lives.

A serious health scare frightened one of Dr. Stover's patients into finally giving up cigarettes after more than 30 years. In 1992 Brian D., a 52-year-old divorced father of two grown children, went to his primary-care physician complaining of poor health.

This partner in a successful New York City investment firm normally smoked a pack and a half a day. "But if I was under great stress," he says, "I'd go up to three packs." When a CT scan revealed a suspicious lesion on one lung, his doctor feared the worst. Even after a battery of tests and several consultations, the exact nature of the white spot on the x-ray remained uncertain. So Brian underwent a surgical biopsy at Memorial Sloan-Kettering, aware that should the pathologist's verdict come back "cancer," the surgeon would proceed at once with a wedge resection or lobectomy. He awoke in his hospital room, surrounded by two children anxious to impart wonderful news: The growth turned out to be benign scar tissue, probably from two earlier bouts of pneumonia.

He resolved right then to stop smoking. Compared with many smokers, Brian did so with relative ease, through a combination of cold turkey and wearing a nicotine patch that eases withdrawal symptoms. He has not touched a cigarette in a year. The longer he shuns tobacco, the more his lungs will heal themselves. Eventually his risk of pulmonary cancer will approach that of a nonsmoker.

"Already I feel better, sleep better and have more energy," says Brian, who adds that he'd feel better still if his children, "both smokers, sad to report," followed their father's example. If Dr. Stover has any say in the matter, they will.

The last time Brian visited her office for a routine checkup, the first in nine months, "She came into the waiting room," he recalls, "hugged me and asked, 'Now, have you gotten your children to quit smoking yet?'"

LUNG CANCER AND DIET

A number of human studies have examined fruits' and vegetables' possible protective effect against lung cancer in smokers and non-smokers. More research is needed, though, to pinpoint just which of their many vitamins and nutrients could possibly lower risk. Thus far, candidates include vitamins A, C, E, the trace mineral selenium and many other compounds.

According to Dr. Susan Pilch, a health scientist/administrator with the diet and cancer branch of the National Cancer Institute, "Most of the studies are showing a stronger association with beta-carotene." Another form of vitamin A, retinol, also appears to boast potential protective properties. Both are currently being administered in pill form to high-risk patients as part of several research projects intended to determine their effectiveness and safety. (A 1994 Finnish study that followed patients at high risk of lung cancer found no preventive benefits from beta-carotene.)

How may fruits and vegetables reduce the risk of lung cancer?

One theory holds that vitamins C, E and beta-carotene—all anti-oxidants—demobilize and eliminate the free-radical molecules that can impair lung-cell DNA and thus promote tumor growth. In a second scenario, Dr. Pilch explains, "compounds in these foods increase the activity of certain enzymes in the lungs that could detoxify carcinogens."

Yet other foot soldiers in the fight against lung cancer may be the many beneficial compounds found in cruciferous vegetables such as broccoli, cauliflower and cabbage, and folic acid, which has demonstrated promise in diminishing metaplasia, the transitional step from dysplasia to full-fledged squamous-cell carcinoma. Spinach, turnip greens and other leafy vegetables, asparagus, brussels sprouts and parsnips are just some of the foods that contain folic acid, a B-complex vitamin. (For extensive lists of excellent dietary vitamin sources, refer to Chapter 5 on nutrition.) We must emphasize that no clear proof exists that altering your diet will safeguard you from lung cancer *if you continue to smoke.*

GUIDELINES FOR SECONDARY PREVENTION

For Asymptomatic Men and Women with No Special Risk Factors (nonsmokers)
• No screening recommended at present

For Asymptomatic Men and Woman at Increased Risk (smokers and others)
• Annual chest x-ray

For Those with a History of Cured Lung Cancer
• Annual chest x-ray
• Annual sputum cytology

SCREENING AND DIAGNOSIS

"The role of screening for lung cancer is a delicate issue," says Dr. Stover. Nevertheless, "many of us do recommend annual chest x-rays for high-risk patients," while a lesser number of physicians additionally depend on sputum cytology to help detect early lung cancer.

Dr. Stover came to Memorial Sloan-Kettering in 1977, the final year of a National Cancer Institute study to determine the efficacy of both procedures. Our center, Baltimore's Johns Hopkins University and the Mayo Clinic in Rochester, Minnesota, each divided more than 10,000 men age 45 and older, all heavy smokers, into two groups. The study group received annual chest x-rays and sputum cytology every four months for six years; members of the control group were advised to go for annual x-rays, with no further attempts made to ensure their compliance.

Little difference in mortality was seen between the single-screening group and the dual-screening group. However, both groups in the Memorial Sloan-Kettering Lung Project had a five-year survival rate of 35 percent—almost three times the national average —suggesting that chest x-rays and sputum cytology could save lives.

"What the study showed," contends Dr. Stover, "was that a chest x-ray was the best screening device for patients with a tumor in the lung periphery, and sputum cytology was the best screening device for those with a centrally located tumor. So it was recommended that we might alternate chest x-ray with sputum cytology every six months. But because the yield [the number of cancers diagnosed] was so low and the cost was so high, that was not implemented."

The American Cancer Society originally recommended against either test. But in 1990 it modified its position, leaving the decision up to physician and patient. Dr. Stover, while emphasizing that Memorial Sloan-Kettering has no official policy on screening for lung cancer, believes in annual chest x-rays for high-risk patients, and yearly x-rays and sputum cytology for lung cancer survivors.

"Even though the clinical trial showed these not to be cost-effective or to have a major impact on mortality," she says, "for the persons in whom you do pick up lung cancer, it *is* cost-effective and has an impact on *their* mortality."

CHEST X-RAY

Taking radiographic pictures of the chest, one of the oldest techniques in our diagnostic armament, is still the simplest and one of the most effective methods for detecting a suspicious growth or area in the lungs. (To confirm the presence of cancer, a biopsy is necessary.) Patient Brian D., a veteran of numerous chest x-rays, as well as CT scans and other imaging procedures, says, "There's nothing to be afraid of with a chest x-ray. The most unpleasant thing about it is waiting for the technician."

The procedure itself takes but minutes. First you are asked to disrobe from the waist up and put on a hospital gown. Then you stand in front of an x-ray cassette containing a piece of photographic film. An x-ray tube aims an x-ray beam at the cassette, producing an image on the film. As radiologist Dr. Robert Heelan explains, "For someone in whom we suspect lung cancer, we take two exposures: posteroanterior, which is a frontal view, and lateral, which is a side view. Those are then interpreted in conjunction. The radiologist puts up the films side by side and looks at both of them."

From these he or she can clearly identify the size and location of a peripheral tumor. Has it infiltrated the chest wall or mediastinum? Blocked the bronchial tube? Chest x-rays can sometimes answer these and other essential questions; if doubt exists, CT scans can provide more definitive data.

Because malignancies typically double in volume in 18 months to two years, annual chest x-rays of patients at high risk of lung cancer are highly useful for comparison purposes. The appearance of an abnormality where none was present a year before would alert doctors to a possible cancerous or precancerous condition and warrant further diagnostic testing.

Dr. Stover tells of how having past x-rays on file can preclude unnecessary tests. "Often a patient will exhibit a nodule on an x-ray," she says. "If they underwent an x-ray five years previously, and it was there, then most likely it is benign, and we would do nothing about it."

"Isn't the radiation emitted by x-ray machines dangerous?"

Dr. Stover says she hears that question "all the time." Her response is to tell patients that the benefits far transcend the risk. "Of all of the x-ray procedures," Dr. Heelan adds reassuringly, "chest radiography exposes patients to the least amount of ionizing radiation": a dosage of 10 millirads per exposure for a mere 1/60 to 1/20 second. That said, however, the cumulative effects of repeated chest x-rays are not yet known—one reason why they are not recommended routinely for men and women at average risk of lung cancer.

It is imperative that the facility administering the x-ray be approved by the American College of Radiology and, Dr. Stover stresses, that a radiologist analyze the film. "We've had cases," she explains, "where an x-ray taken in a doctor's office is read as normal by a nonradiologist. One year later the patient comes in with inoperable lung cancer, and it turns out the nodule was there on that x-ray." To learn of ACR-accredited imaging centers in your area, call its toll-free number (800-ACR-LINE).

SPUTUM CYTOLOGY

As long ago as the 1860s, doctors used sputum cytology to ferret out silent lung cancer. *Cytology* is the microscopic study of cell structure—in this instance, cells found in mucus coughed up from the lungs. "It has been shown to pick up centrally located tumors before the patient is symptomatic," says Dr. Stover, who prescribes annual sputum cytology for lung cancer survivors.

Cytology's ability to diagnose lung cancer isn't as high as we would like—in the cooperative study by Memorial Sloan-Kettering and two other cancer centers, alluded to earlier in this chapter, 42 percent; 77 percent when performed in conjunction with chest x-rays—but it involves zero risk or pain, costs relatively little and couldn't be easier.

Upon rising three mornings in a row, you are asked to brush your teeth and rinse your mouth before coughing deeply and expectorating phlegm into a wide-mouthed receptacle. Your doctor may require five specimens, as several studies have demonstrated a higher yield this way.

The National Cancer Cytology Center, an educational and research organization in Plainview, New York, makes cyto-sputum kits available free of charge to the public. A kit consists of a jar containing an ethyl alcohol preservative, an airtight snap-on cap, a medical history form to be filled out, and a mailing container that you send to the laboratory. There the specimens are examined under a microscope. Cancerous or precancerous cells will appear noticeably different from normal ones. Currently, sputum cytology remains our only means for identifying microinvasive malignancies and carcinoma in situ of the lung.

For a free cyto-sputum kit, write the NCCC at 88 Sunnyside Boulevard, Suite 307, Plainview, NY 11803 (516-349-0610). Be sure to include your name and address, as well as the name and address of your physician. A minimal fee is charged for laboratory processing.

BRONCHOSCOPY

Chest x-ray and sputum cytology by themselves cannot diagnose lung cancer. One frequently used technique, *bronchoscopy*, permits physicians to visually inspect the tracheobronchial tree by way of a fiber-optic viewing instrument called a *bronchoscope*, which is inserted into the nose or mouth and fed into the bronchi.

Reading about it may be more difficult than undergoing the actual procedure, which is performed on a hospital outpatient basis under systemic sedation (usually Demerol) and Novocain application to the nose and behind the mouth. "Not terribly formidable," patient Brian D. describes it.

"Bronchoscopy is uncomfortable," he adds, "because it's an intrusive test; it's strange to have something in your lung through your nose or throat. But it's not painful at all. You don't feel anything sharp. In fact, you don't feel very much at all." As often happens, Brian found it difficult to keep from gagging. "But they assure you it's not a problem," he recalls. "The nurses encourage you to take deep breaths, to relax as much as you can, and to gag when you have to.

"From beginning to end, including waiting time, with any efficiency it's over in half an hour. The actual test usually takes fifteen or twenty minutes. Afterward they sit you there to make sure that your pulse, heart rate and so forth return to normal." According to Dr. Stover, the only memento most patients take home is a mildly sore throat.

LUNG BIOPSY

Biopsying tissue, the definitive method for diagnosing any cancer, can be accomplished a number of ways. One advantage to bronchoscopy is that biopsying tools can be passed through the scope to brush or excise samples. Sometimes this is done along with a *fluoroscope*, an x-ray machine that projects a moving image on a TV-type screen rather than a photographic plate. "We use the fluoroscope to place a forceps into a lesion and biopsy it," explains Dr. Stover. "It doesn't hurt," she adds, "because the lung has no pain fibers."

Lesions outside the range of the bronchoscope, or those less than 2 centimeters in size, usually call for another form of biopsy, *transthoracic fine-needle aspiration*. After first cleansing the skin with antiseptic, the doctor gives an injection of Novocain. Then he uses a long, thin needle to gently penetrate the chest wall and the pleura, aspirating tissue and fluid from the lesion.

"When the needle is put in," says Dr. Stover, "occasionally patients will feel a sharp, momentary pain, because the pleura does have pain fibers." To guide them, physicians rely on either fluoroscopy or a CT scan, an imaging technique described in detail on pages 326–27. Fine-needle aspiration is not without potential complications. "You can collapse the lung," says Dr. Stover, "or patients can bleed during the procedure. These are not major problems, however, and they are readily treatable."

Another technique, *thoracentesis,* is reserved for patients who have pleural fluid. A thin needle is used to withdraw fluid from the space between the two layers of pleura. Evidence of cancer in the fluid would indicate advanced-stage disease. (A biopsy needle can also be inserted to sample the pleura itself for cancer.) As with fine-needle aspiration, patients receive local anesthesia and may experience a flash of pain as the needle or biopsy instrument pierces the pleura.

A different imaging procedure, ultrasound (explained on pages 233, 326), may be used to direct the doctor. "Usually before we remove fluid, we take an x-ray on the patient's side, to see if it's free-flowing," says Dr. Stover. "Free-flowing fluid will layer out on the side that's down. If the fluid is trapped in a particular area of the chest, the ultrasound is helpful for identifying where it is and where to put the needle." During the procedure, patients straddle a chair, resting their head and arms on the back.

After the doctor removes the needle, a gauze pad impregnated with petroleum is applied over the thoracentesis site, and sterile dressing covers the area. You rest in bed while a nurse observes you for signs of dizziness or changes in skin color and monitors heart and respiration rates. A chest x-ray will be taken in about an hour to ensure the lung did not collapse. If not, you will be released. Once home, watch for symptoms of complications, which include excessive coughing, blood-streaked sputum and pain or tightness in the chest.

While neither chest x-rays nor sputum cytology is presently recommended for routine screening, perhaps they will be in the future. Dr. Curtis Harris of the National Cancer Institute notes that work is under way "to make these tests more specific and more efficient."

Even in their present form, we believe these procedures can be useful and therefore advise patients at high risk of lung cancer to consult their doctors about having x-rays taken on an annual basis. But ultimately no medical procedure can safeguard you from America's number-one cancer killer as effectively as refraining from tobacco.

SUGGESTED READING ABOUT LUNG CANCER

From the National Cancer Institute (800-4-CANCER):
• "What You Need to Know About Lung Cancer"

KEY WORDS

Bronchi: The two large air passages of the lungs, which branch out into smaller tubes called the *bronchioles*. These in turn culminate in millions of tiny air sacs called *alveoli*.

Bronchoscopy: A diagnostic procedure in which a lighted tube called a *bronchoscope* is inserted through the nose or mouth and into the lungs, enabling physicians to examine the tracheobronchial tree.

Chronic obstructive pulmonary disease: A chronic condition that gradually restricts air flow in and out of the lungs. Emphysema and chronic bronchitis are common examples.

Diaphragm: The dome-shaped muscle between the chest and the abdomen.

Fluoroscope: An x-ray machine that projects a moving image of the body's deep structures on a monitor rather than on a photographic plate.

Lobectomy: Surgical removal of a single lobe of the lung.

Mediastinum: The compartment that houses the heart and other organs and is located between the lungs.

Paraneoplastic syndrome: A disorder caused by the abnormal secretion of hormones from a tumor.

Photodynamic therapy: Laser destruction of nonsmall-cell lung cancer through a bronchoscope after the injection of a photosensitizing agent.

Pneumonectomy: Surgically removing an entire lung.

Pulmonary mesothelioma: A rare cancer of the *pleural mesothelium*, the lung's two-layer protective membrane.

Thoracentesis: A method for tapping fluid from the pleural space. Cancer cells in the fluid would indicate advanced-stage lung cancer.

Trachea: The windpipe, which connects the larynx (voice box) and the bronchi.

Transthoracic fine-needle aspiration: A biopsy in which a long, thin needle is inserted into the lung to draw out fluid and tissue samples from a lesion.

Wedge resection: Surgical removal of a small portion of the lung.

CHAPTER
13

Colorectal Cancer

Digital Rectal Exam •
Stool Blood Test • Sigmoidoscopy •
Colonoscopy • Barium Enema

In 1994 about 150,000 Americans developed carcinoma of the colon or rectum, the incidence of which rose 10 percent from 1973 to 1987. Colorectal cancer claims approximately 56,000 U.S. lives a year, making it second only to lung cancer as a cause of cancer death.

Yet the overall picture is not as bleak as these figures suggest. The past decade and a half has seen tremendous advances in understanding the nature of colorectal cancer, yielding new possibilities for prevention. At the same time, a growing body of evidence indicates that diet plays a key role in preventing the disease.

Such encouraging news ought to prompt everyone to follow the low-fat, high-fiber diet described in Chapter 5 and, beginning at age 50 for those at average risk, undergo periodic examinations to detect any cancer in an early, highly curable stage. Unfortunately, many people are so terrified of colorectal cancer, or so embarrassed by any procedure involving the bowel, that they avoid medical tests and ignore symptoms that should be evaluated at once.

So before going any further, let's dispel the two most pervasive myths about this cancer: one, that it always leads to a *colostomy*, an opening made in the lower abdomen for eliminating solid waste when normal bowel movements are no longer possible, and two, that it is invariably fatal. Modern surgical techniques make it possible to avoid colostomies in 99 out of 100 cases. Even in those rare instances where the operation is necessary, the vast majority of patients lead full, active lives, as one famous example, the late Speaker of the House Tip O'Neill, certainly demonstrated.

To refute the second myth, you need only look at another figure from the political arena: former President Ronald Reagan, still very much alive and well long after surgeons removed a section of his colon due to a localized malignancy in 1985. While it is true that only half of all colorectal cancer patients survive five years after diagnosis, this reflects the late stage at which most colorectal tumors are discovered. The facts are that 89 percent of localized colorectal cancers are curable and that, since the 1950s, the death rate has dropped 30 percent for women and 7 percent for men. Increased emphasis on prevention and early detection could improve those numbers significantly. So put your fears and embarrassment aside and take an active role in understanding and reducing your risk.

THE COLON

The adult colon, also called the bowel or large intestine, consists of five main sections that lie as if draped at right angles up, across and down inside the abdominal cavity. Appropriately, these sections are referred to as *ascending, transverse, descending* and *sigmoid* colon, plus the *rectum*.

The small intestine, responsible for completing the process of digestion and absorption of nutrients into the bloodstream, empties the indigestible waste fluids and certain minerals into the pouchlike *cecum* at the beginning of the ascending colon. As muscular contractions propel it through the bowel, much of the water and mineral content is reabsorbed, until all that remains is semisolid fecal matter containing billions of bacteria, many of which normally inhabit the intestinal tract and aid in digestion. These waste products collect in the sigmoid and rectum, the final eight to ten inches of the five-foot-long colon, before being excreted through the inch-long passageway known as the anal canal.

The colon is lined with *mucosa,* a pinkish tissue made up of millions of tiny, tubular passages, or *crypts*. New mucosal cells form at the base of each crypt and work their way up the sides to

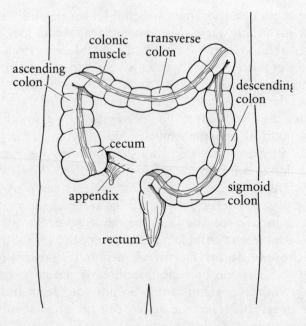

Normal Colon. In a typical adult, the colon is about 6 feet long and divided into five main segments. It curves around the abdomen, with a long muscle running its entire length. Because this muscle is somewhat shorter than the colon itself, the intestine looks as if it were drawn into a series of pouches.

the mucosa's surface. There they replace old cells that are continuously sloughed off over a period of four to five days.

POLYPS: PRECURSORS OF CANCER

Sometimes the mechanisms and controls that regulate mucosal cells go awry, so that new cells emerge faster than old ones can be discarded. In some cases this produces a buildup of cells on a small area of the lining's surface. When enough of these cells accumulate, they form a barely visible bump, or *polyp. Sessile* polyps attach directly to the mucosa, while *pedunculated* polyps resemble tiny mushrooms and affix themselves by way of stalks.

Polyps are extremely common, present in two of three people over age 65. The National Polyp Study, a 10-year multicenter study directed by researchers at Memorial Sloan-Kettering, has clarified many characteristics of polyps. One third are harmless

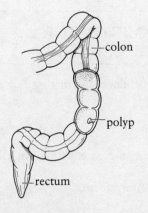

colon

polyp

rectum

Colon Polyps. A polyp may appear as a mushroom-shaped growth on a stem, as shown here, or in clusters scattered throughout the colon. Most are harmless, but because some do become cancerous, any colon polyp should be removed and analyzed.

and benign, and do not turn malignant. However, the other two thirds are *adenomas,* a type of growth that has a 1-in-20 chance of progressing into cancer. We've discovered that adenomas generally occur in clusters, so should one be found, the odds are that more exist. This discussion focuses on the latter, using the words polyp and adenoma interchangeably.

The polyp's transformation into cancer takes from five to ten years in most adults. At first the benign polyp continues to grow, but in time it develops *dysplasia,* a cellular condition characterized by abnormal size, shape and internal organization, all of which a pathologist can identify under a microscope. At the same time, the cells proliferate out of control, so that eventually the adenoma changes into a small cancer. Ninety-nine percent of all colorectal cancers evolve from polyps.

Since the only way to distinguish adenomas from harmless polyps is to examine them microscopically, all polyps are deemed suspect and need to be removed through one of two methods explained later in this chapter. Doing so cuts the chance of colorectal cancer by 90 percent. However, patients with a history of polyps tend to grow new ones over time and therefore must be monitored.

DIAGNOSIS AND TREATMENT

Early colorectal cancer and polyps rarely produce warning signs and symptoms, but the presence of any of the indicators listed in the accompanying box requires prompt medical investigation, especially if it persists for two weeks. Blood in the stool, usually the most notable sign of polyps or colorectal cancer, may be your

SIGNS AND SYMPTOMS OF COLORECTAL CANCER

Advanced colorectal cancer may produce one or more of the following:

- Cramping and gas pains
- Bloating
- A sudden change in bowel habits, such as constipation, diarrhea or unusually narrow stools
- A "full" feeling even after bowel movements
- Chronic, unexplained tiredness
- Dark-red or bright-red blood in the stool

only clue that something could be wrong. Chances are, you have a comparatively minor problem such as hemorrhoids. Nevertheless, alert your doctor at once.

Once formed, colorectal cancer progresses through several stages (see box). Doctors usually treat carcinoma of the colon or rectum surgically, sometimes in combination with radiation therapy or chemotherapy.

STAGING OF COLORECTAL CANCER

STAGE	CHARACTERISTICS	FIVE-YEAR SURVIVAL RATE
0	Cancer is found only on the top of the lining of colon or rectum.	100%
I	Cancer is localized and remains within bowel or rectum wall or lining.	75%–95%
II	Disease has spread to adjacent tissues but not lymph nodes.	50%–75%
III	Disease has spread to nearby nodes but not other body sites.	30%–50%
IV	Tumors are present in distant sites; most frequently liver, lungs and ovaries.	Less than 10%

WHO IS AT RISK?

- Men and women age 50 and older

HEREDITARY RISK FACTORS

- Family history of colorectal cancer and/or adenomatous colon polyps
- Family history of one or more of the following syndromes:

  1. Hereditary nonpolyposis colorectal cancer (HNPCC)
  2. Familial adenomatous polyposis (FAP)
  3. Gardner's syndrome

A large number of colorectal cancers may be traced to hereditary patterns. For example, having a parent, child or sibling with colorectal cancer triples a person's own lifetime risk. Nearly 2 in 10 cases afflict families where one or more first-degree relatives have the disease, but a pattern of colorectal cancer among second-degree family members increases risk as well.

Hereditary nonpolyposis colorectal cancer (HNPCC), also known as *Lynch syndromes I and II*, constitutes between 5 and 15 percent of colorectal tumors. In families beset by Lynch I, relatives develop small numbers of polyps, then carcinoma of the colorectum at an early age; Lynch syndrome II leaves family members prone not only to colorectal cancer but malignancies of the uterus, ovaries and other organs.

In about 1 percent of cases, polyps and colorectal cancer result from rare inherited disorders such as *familial adenomatous polyposis,* or FAP. This hereditary disease, first reported in a brother and sister in 1882, is present in about 1 of every 5,000 babies. While most patients with polyps grow only one or a few, those with familial adenomatous polyposis have thousands of potentially cancerous polyps, which usually arise around the time of puberty.

Another similar form of hereditary polyps, *Gardner's syndrome,* occurs in 1 of every 14,000 births. According to recent research, the process by which normal colorectal cells turn cancerous can be linked to inherited abnormalities in several genes.

PERSONAL HEALTH HISTORY RISK FACTORS

- Personal history of inflammatory bowel diseases such as ulcerative colitis or Crohn's disease
- Personal history of breast, ovarian or uterine cancer
- Personal history of polyps and/or colorectal cancer

Crohn's disease, which can affect the entire digestive tract, and *ulcerative colitis,* which is confined to the colon and perhaps the

---

ARE YOU AT RISK FOR COLORECTAL CANCER?

_____ Men and women age 50 or older

Hereditary Risk Factors

_____ Family history of colorectal cancer
_____ Family history of adenomatous polyps
Family history of any of the following hereditary syndromes:
_____ Hereditary nonpolyposis colorectal cancer (HNPCC), also known as Lynch syndromes I and II
_____ Familial adenomatous polyposis (FAP)
_____ Gardner's syndrome

Personal Health History Risk Factors

_____ Personal history of inflammatory bowel diseases (IBD) such as ulcerative colitis or Crohn's disease
_____ Personal history of breast cancer
_____ Personal history of ovarian cancer
_____ Personal history of uterine cancer
_____ Personal history of adenomatous colorectal polyps or cancer

Lifestyle Risk Factors

_____ Obesity (40 percent or more over your ideal weight; refer to height-weight-frame table in Chapter 6)
_____ Excessive alcohol use
_____ Sedentary lifestyle
_____ High-fat, low-fiber diet (35 percent or more of daily calories; less than 25 grams of fiber daily)

If one or more of these risk factors applies to you, consult your physician.

lowermost inches of the small intestine, produce acute attacks that can flare up periodically throughout life. Symptoms include bloody diarrhea that lasts days, weeks or months, fever, abdominal cramps and weight loss.

Sufferers of chronic ulcerative colitis are several times more likely to develop colorectal cancer than the general population. The chances of getting cancer are even greater for patients whose entire colon is inflamed. Therefore these men and women need to have their colons examined annually.

LIFESTYLE RISK FACTORS

- High-fat, low-fiber diet (35 percent or more of daily calories; less than 25 grams of fiber daily; low in fruits and vegetables)
- Obesity (40 percent or more over your ideal weight; refer to height-weight-frame table in Chapter 6)
- Sedentary lifestyle
- Excessive alcohol use

WAYS TO REDUCE YOUR RISK

GUIDELINES FOR PRIMARY PREVENTION

In addition to the general primary prevention steps recommended at the beginning of Chapter 9:

- Consume at least 800 milligrams of calcium daily (1,200 milligrams for children and young adults), mostly from nonfat or low-fat dairy products.

COLORECTAL CANCER AND DIET

Time and again, animal studies have found that high-fat diets enhance colorectal tumors. It's interesting to note that this malignancy barely exists in Asian and African countries where diets are typically low in fat and high in fiber, but it thrives in the West, with our fat-heavy eating habits. In fact, moving from areas with low colorectal-cancer rates to Western nations dramatically increases a person's risk, as demonstrated by studies of Japanese and Chinese who immigrated to the United States, and of Poles who relocated to Australia. After a number of years, both groups and their offspring developed colorectal cancer at high rates approaching those of longstanding Americans and Australians, a phenomenon attributed to dietary changes.

No one is certain just how dietary fat promotes colorectal cancer, although a number of biochemical mechanisms have been suggested:

- Fat increases the colonic level of bile salts, which are believed to damage the colon lining and induce the unchecked cell growth that can result in cancer.
- Products of broken-down fat present in fecal matter may likewise harm the colorectum's lining or give rise to other substances that stimulate mucosal-cell growth to spiral out of control.
- Excess fat might foster a favorable environment within the colon for the growth of cancer-promoting bacteria.

Yet another explanation holds that the problem is not fat per se, but its high caloric density that cultivates cancer. Whereas one gram of fat yields nine calories, one gram of protein or carbohydrates yields only four. And a diet high in fat is usually high in calories, which increase a person's susceptibility to cancer.

As numerous population studies have demonstrated, fiber seems to protect against colorectal cancer. A 1982 Scandinavian report revealed more cases in Denmark than in Finland, even though the latter population ate a diet high in meat, protein and fat. One likely explanation is that the Finns also consume far more fiber, through sources such as porridge and whole-grain bread. The average American eats only about 11 grams of fiber per day, less than half the optimum amount.

How does fiber help to guard against colorectal cancer? There are several theories: (1) It neutralizes cancer-promoting materials in the stool and aids the growth of bacteria that break down those substances. (2) Fiber absorbs water, producing a soft, bulky stool that moves swiftly through the colon and thus reduces exposure to cancer-causing agents. (3) Similarly, it dilutes the colon's contents, so that carcinogens and the mucosa are less likely to make contact.

Therefore we recommend you eat adequate amounts of these foods:

- All kinds of fruits
- Vegetables, especially cruciferous vegetables such as broccoli, cabbage and brussels sprouts
- Legumes (beans, peas, lentils)
- Whole-grain cereals, breads and pastas
- Low-fat, high-fiber snacks such as popcorn, and whole-grain crackers and flatbreads

The National Cancer Institute estimates that if these or equivalent dietary recommendations were widely followed, deaths from colorectal cancer *could be cut in half within ten years.* A 1992 American Cancer Society study followed more than 750,000 men and women for six years. Those who ate more vegetables and high-fiber grains had a lower risk of deadly colorectal cancer, causing researchers to conclude: "These prospective data support the hypothesis that a diet high in vegetable and grains may protect against fatal colon cancer."

Calcium

This mineral is believed to protect the colon's lining from damaging compounds in the stool, particularly free fatty acids and bile acids, and also reduce the rate of cell turnover. Finlanders' love of dairy products contributes to their low colorectal-cancer rate.

No convincing studies on calcium's value in preventing colorectal cancer yet exist. Nevertheless, considering its other health benefits, we advise all adults to consume at least 800 milligrams a day, the recommended dietary allowance established by the nutrition board of the National Research Council. If you plan to increase your intake substantially, discuss it with your doctor first, for excessive amounts can prove harmful to some people, such as those with kidney stones. Milk and milk products are especially rich in calcium (a full glass of milk contains about 250 milligrams), but *be sure to buy brands that are low in fat.*

COLORECTAL CANCER AND ALCOHOL

Since 1957 researchers have noted a definite association between alcohol consumption and elevated risk of colorectal cancer, particularly carcinoma of the rectum. One 1990 report contended that a single drink raises a person's risk of colorectal cancer by 5 percent. The evidence is not considered strong, but suffice to say, you should drink in moderation (no more than four drinks per week), if at all. This includes beer and wine, which seem to be more closely linked with rectal cancer than hard liquor.

COLORECTAL CANCER AND EXERCISE

Studies have consistently shown that obesity heightens one's risk, especially for men. According to the *Journal of the National Cancer Institute:* "In a large prospective study, the principal sites of excess cancer mortality among overweight men (but not women) were found to be in the colon and the rectum." A 1992 summary of a long-term study of nearly 18,000 Harvard alumni brought to light that obesity during young adulthood or middle age increases the chance of getting colorectal cancer later in life. To determine your ideal weight, refer to the height-weight-frame chart in Chapter 6.

Exercise appears to be particularly beneficial in guarding against colon cancer, although evidence that it helps protect against rectal cancer has yet to be confirmed. In the Harvard Alumni Health Study, the most sedentary subjects had up to twice the incidence of colon cancers as those engaged in high levels of exercise.

"Individuals who exercise have a faster rate of transit through their intestines," explains Dr. I-Min Lee, the study's codirector. "That is, food seems to pass from the mouth to the rectum faster than in those who do not exercise. If this is the case, then any potential carcinogens in the diet have less chance of contact with the colonic mucosa."

Other studies, both in the United States and in China, corroborate Dr. Lee's findings. Moreover, the Harvard study found that keeping active may lower the risk of colon cancer even in overweight men. For these and other health-related reasons we advise our patients to get involved in some form of regular physical activity.

COLORECTAL CANCER AND ASPIRIN

Aspirin? To help prevent colon cancer? Possibly. According to a 1991 American Cancer Society study of 662,424 men and women, participants who ingested as few as 16 aspirin tablets monthly had a 40 percent lower colon cancer mortality rate. But even its lead researcher cautioned that it was too early to recommend taking aspirin every other day as a hedge against colorectal cancer. More research is needed to determine whether the drugs themselves and

GUIDELINES FOR SECONDARY PREVENTION

For Asymptomatic Men and Women with No Special Risk Factors

- Annual digital rectal exam, beginning at age 40
- Annual digital rectal exam and stool blood test, beginning at age 50
- Sigmoidoscopy every three to five years, beginning at age 50

For Asymptomatic Men and Women at Increased Risk

1. Those with a family history of colorectal cancer or colorectal polyps:

- Colonoscopy every three to five years, beginning between ages 35 and 40

2. Those with a family history of hereditary nonpolyposis colorectal cancer (HNPCC, also known as Lynch syndromes I and II):

- Colonoscopy every two years, beginning at age 25
- Annual colonoscopy, beginning at age 40
- In addition, members of Lynch II families need to be carefully scrutinized for other cancers; in particular, uterine and ovarian

3. Those with a personal history of chronic ulcerative colitis lasting eight years or longer:

- Annual colonoscopy

Regular examinations of the colon and biopsies of the lining are included in the care of people with ulcerative colitis, starting about eight years after the initial diagnosis. The purpose of these examinations is to find early cancer, premalignant polyps and changes in the colon lining. The time to begin this monitoring and the intervals between examinations may vary, depending on how much of the colon is involved. People with Crohn's disease, which also carries an increased risk of colorectal cancer, also require periodic examinations.

4. Those with a personal history of colorectal polyps or colorectal cancer:

People who have had polyps removed tend to develop new ones over time. Therefore surveillance is necessary after removal. The National Polyp Study recently demonstrated the most effective follow-up program yet devised:

- Follow-up colonoscopy every three to five years; more or less often in some circumstances not some other factor aspirin users have in common is responsible for this apparent benefit. Still, it's an area that merits watching, especially when you consider that aspirin has been shown to reduce the risk of heart attacks by inhibiting clots from forming in the arteries.

DIGITAL RECTAL EXAM

About 10 percent of colorectal cancers can be detected before symptoms arise by way of a rectal examination, recommended as part of regular checkups for all adults age 40 and older. While perhaps not everyone's favorite test, it really is simple and painless and requires no enema beforehand. Your physician inserts a lubricated, gloved finger in the rectum and probes for any irregularity, nodule or mass in the inner wall of the rectum.

STOOL BLOOD TEST

Traces of blood in the stool are one of the early warning signs of colorectal cancer and polyps, as well as other, less worrisome conditions. In many instances the amount of blood is so minute, however, it cannot be detected with the naked eye. We hear from our patients all the time: "Blood in the stool? I didn't see any." That is why a stool blood test is so helpful.

During your initial office visit, you receive a set of stool blood test slides and accompanying instructions to take home with you. Each card has been impregnated with a substance called *guaiac,* which undergoes a chemical reaction with hemoglobin, the oxygen-carrying molecule in blood.

Stool samples should be collected on three successive days. You place a smear of fecal material on the slide, then close its cover. The slides can be returned to your doctor either in person or by mail. Developing liquid is then dropped onto each card. If the guaiac turns blue within 30 seconds, we have probable evidence of blood in the stool.

To ensure accuracy, we suggest you follow these dietary guidelines:

- The day before taking your first stool sample, eat plenty of fruits, cereals and vegetables, especially raw ones. A high-fiber diet will irritate any abnormalities in the colorectum, increasing the chance that they will bleed and thus reveal themselves. Continue this diet until the day of your last sample.

- From the day before the test until day three, do not eat red meat or take aspirin, vitamin C or iron pills, all of which can produce a positive result even if no stool blood is present.

SIGMOIDOSCOPY

A thorough screening program should include sigmoidoscopy. In this procedure, a physician uses a flexible lighted instrument called a *sigmoidoscope* to view the rectum, sigmoid and part of the descending colon, where up to 45 percent of colorectal cancers and polyps form.

Scopes measure 60 centimeters (25 inches) long and less than half an inch in diameter and contain computer chips that transmit images to a video screen. Accuracy is contingent upon the patient's lower colon being clear. Therefore, one day prior to your appointment it's necessary to observe a clear liquid diet consisting of:

Soups	Clear broth or bouillon, clear consomme, packaged broth
Sweets and desserts	Gelatin, popsicles, sugar, honey, sugar substitutes, sucking candy
Beverages	Apple, cranberry, white-grape juices; black coffee, tea; ginger ale, seltzer water

At noon patients drink a 10-ounce bottle of citrate of magnesia, available in most pharmacies. The morning of the procedure, following a clear liquid breakfast, you administer yourself an enema using lukewarm tap water. The enema must be repeated until the water you expel is clear, indicating an empty lower colon. An alternative preparation, the Fleet enema, stimulates the colon to empty and therefore requires neither laxatives nor a special diet.

An important point: Patients must refrain from taking aspirin or other anti-inflammatory drugs the week before their sigmoidoscopy. Other medications can be continued, but only after you've raised this matter with your physician.

A sigmoidoscopy lasts about 10 minutes. You are handed a gown and asked to lie on your left side on the examining table, knees bent. First the doctor examines your rectum with a lubricated finger. Then he or she slowly inserts the sigmoidoscope. As it advances, you may feel some mild cramping, which you can

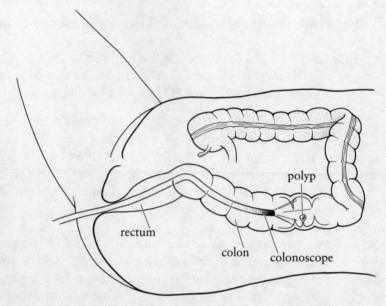

Colonoscopy. A flexible tube with magnifying and lighting devices is inserted into the colon via the anus and rectum, allowing a physician to view the entire interior of the colon. In this illustration, a polyp is clearly visible and can be removed during the examination. Samples of other suspicious tissue can also be collected for laboratory study.

relieve by breathing deeply. The physician may also biopsy a tiny sample of tissue for laboratory examination. This is not painful, since the colon lining contains no nerves.

Once the examination is completed, the scope is carefully withdrawn. A few minutes of rest, and you are ready to go about your normal activities and diet, unless your doctor instructs otherwise. Patients who needed a biopsy may experience minor rectal bleeding for about 24 hours. Should the bleeding persist, become heavy or occur between bowel movements, alert your doctor.

COLONOSCOPY

This procedure, introduced in the early 1970s, is considered the "gold standard" among gastroenterologists and colon surgeons. It dramatically enhances our ability to examine the colon and makes it possible to obtain biopsies at the same time rather than as part of a separate procedure.

A colonoscope is a flexible fiber-optic viewing instrument similar to the sigmoidoscope but approximately double the length, so that it can reach the entire colon. Because all sections of the colon must be clear, it requires slightly more extensive preparation than a sigmoidoscopy.

Patient Judith K., whom you first met in Chapter 1, makes it a point to schedule her annual colonoscopies for a Monday, giving her the weekend to prepare. That way, she explains, she doesn't have to lose extra days of work. Some preparations take one day; others, two days.

A day or two before a colonoscopy, you eat a normal breakfast, then switch to an all-liquid diet around lunchtime. At 3 P.M. the next day you drink Fleet Phospho Soda, a laxative. An alternative is to drink a salt solution and adhere to a liquid diet one day prior to the exam.

The morning of the procedure, you may brush your teeth or rinse your mouth, but *do not eat or drink anything for six hours prior to your appointment.* Some physicians have their patients take enemas at least two hours before they leave for the hospital or doctor's office.

"On the day before the procedure," says Judith, "I'm usually pretty hungry. But by the next morning I've just lost my appetite." As with a sigmoidoscopy, no aspirin, ibuprofen or other anti-inflammatory drugs should be taken a full week prior to the test, and your physician should be apprised of any medical conditions you may have, especially diabetes or heart disease, or any medications you are taking.

A colonoscopy takes approximately 20 minutes, though you should expect to spend one to two hours at the health-care facility. You will likely lose track of time, due to the sedatives, Demerol and Versed, that are introduced *intravenously* (IV) shortly beforehand.

A nurse or doctor inserts a needle into the patient's forearm, then injects the medication directly into the vein. The two sedatives relax patients and block sensations of pain or discomfort. "It usually knocks me out completely," says Judith.

Dressed in a hospital gown, you lie on an examining bed in a fetal-type position, though you may be asked to lie on your back, which helps the colonoscope to advance. As with a sigmoidoscopy, the doctor first performs a digital rectal exam, then gently inserts the flexible tube. Air is instilled through the colonoscope and into the bowel, creating a sensation of fullness, as if you're about to have a bowel movement. No need to worry: Your bowel is completely empty. You may also experience mild cramping.

Colonoscopy has another major advantage, in that if a polyp is found, we can remove it through a painless procedure known as a *polypectomy*. A wire snare is passed out the end of the scope, over the head of the polyp and around its stalk, like a lasso. Electrical current is then generated through the snare, cutting the polyp and cauterizing the area, so as to prevent bleeding.

Sometimes bleeding does occur. In rare cases where it is excessive, a transfusion may be necessary. Another complication, a perforation of the colon wall, must be repaired surgically. Keep in mind, though, that only one in a hundred patients experiences any complication from colonoscopy or polypectomy.

In a second technique, a *"hot" biopsy,* a forceps is inserted into the colonoscope and used to grasp the polyp and withdraw a portion for analysis. Electrocautery is then applied through the forceps, destroying the remaining tissue. Especially large polyps may call for surgical removal.

After the examination, you remain in the hospital or office for several hours, until the sedative has worn off and the doctor has discussed the results with you. You might think that after a day of fasting, patients would crave a seven-course meal, but Judith says, "All I wanted was something light." We recommend that you eat sparingly and absolutely abstain from alcohol for 24 hours. Also, make plans to have someone escort you home, since you may still be drowsy and should not drive until the next day.

BARIUM ENEMA

Physicians usually rely on barium enemas only if the colonoscopy hasn't performed to their satisfaction or if the patient has a medical condition that would preclude him from receiving sedation. This x-ray study is less expensive, but also less accurate.

Once again, a clean colon is essential for clarity. You lie down on the table, and an enema bag containing a chalky solution called barium sulfate is instilled into the rectum. The liquid fills the bowel, forming a silhouette on a fluoroscopic screen. From this, radiologists can spot suspicious growths. In an air-contrast enema, air is injected into the colon to improve accuracy.

During this process, you'll be asked to hold the barium in and to turn over in different positions so that various x-ray pictures can be taken. Most patients feel little discomfort other than a sensation of fullness toward the end of the study. Once the x-rays are obtained, you may go to the bathroom and evacuate the liquid. However, notes radiologist Dr. Robert Heelan, "Some people, especially those who are prone to spasms of the gastrointestinal tract, can have considerable cramping." These patients are given a medication, glucagon, to relax the GI tract.

According to the American Cancer Society, screening for colorectal cancer can boost survival rates 55 to 85 percent and decrease deaths by 60 percent. One study estimated that if 10,000 average-risk men between the ages of 50 and 75 went for annual stool blood tests and flexible sigmoidoscopies every three years, as we recommend, the result would be 153 fewer cases of colorectal cancer and 126 fewer deaths. Project those figures over the entire population, and you can see this would save a significant number of lives.

SUGGESTED READING ABOUT COLORECTAL CANCER

From the National Cancer Institute (800-4-CANCER):
• "What You Need to Know About Cancer of the Colon and Rectum"

KEY WORDS

Barium enema (lower GI [gastrointestinal] series): An x-ray examination of the colon taken after a chalky solution, barium sulfate, is introduced into the colon.

Colostomy: A temporary or permanent opening made surgically in the abdomen to allow the exit of fecal material.

Familial adenomatous polyposis: In this rare inherited condition, thousands of polyps arise in the colon and rectum, putting patients at increased risk of colorectal cancer.

Inflammatory bowel disease: Diseases such as *ulcerative colitis* and *Crohn's disease,* which increase the risk of colorectal cancer.

Polyp: A protruding growth or mass that forms in the mucous membranes that line the intestines and other organs. The most common colorectal polyps, *adenomas,* have a 5 percent chance of turning malignant. *Sessile* polyps attach directly to the mucosa; *pedunculated* polyps affix themselves by way of stalks.

Polypectomy: A painless technique for removing polyps, using a colonoscope and electrocautery.

CHAPTER

14

Gynecologic Cancers

Cervical Cancer • Uterine Cancer •
Ovarian Cancer • Pelvic Exam •
Pap Test

The umbrella term *gynecologic cancer* encompasses carcinomas of the cervix, uterus, ovaries, vulva, vagina and fallopian tubes. We will focus on the first three, which make up 95 percent of all gynecologic tumors.

Once a leading cause of death among women, mortalities from gynecologic cancers have dropped considerably over the last 40 years: from cancers of the uterus and cervix, by 70 percent and 50 percent, respectively; and from ovarian cancer, by approximately 10 percent. Credit this largely to heightened public awareness. In the late 1940s the American Cancer Society sponsored "Uterine Cancer Year," "Let No Woman Be Overlooked" and other educational campaigns aimed at encouraging women to visit their gynecologist, a physician who specializes in diagnosing and treating diseases of the female reproductive system.

Of the three major gynecologic malignancies, *cervical cancer* is the one we're able to screen most effectively, using procedures such as the Pap test and pelvic exam. What's more, the disease typically lingers in a noninvasive state for anywhere from 8 to 30 years before finally invading the cervix. In addition, 40 to 50 percent of the 15,000 cases of invasive cancer reported annually are detected in stage I, which is highly curable.

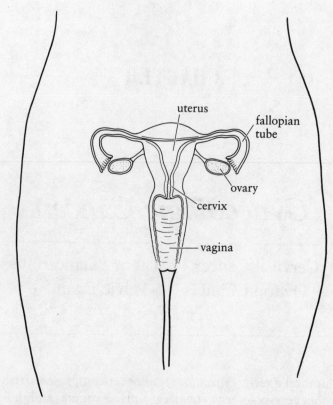

Normal Female Reproductive Tract. A woman's reproductive organs are protected within the pelvic cavity.

Uterine cancer, which was diagnosed in 31,000 women in 1994, accounts for nearly 50 percent of all gynecologic tumors. In the U.S., white women have almost twice the incidence of uterine cancer as African-American women (29.9 cases versus 14.6 cases per 100,000). In fact, American whites rank among the world's most common victims of this disease, with Jewish women and those of northern European descent appearing to be especially vulnerable.

Ovarian cancer, the most fatal gynecologic malignancy, caused 13,600 deaths in 1994, more than cervical (4,600) and uterine (5,900) cancers combined. Because early ovarian cancer does not produce symptoms, two in three cases are detected in advanced stages, by which time the disease has infiltrated the lymph nodes and/or intestine.

THE FEMALE REPRODUCTIVE ORGANS

The female reproductive organs lie hidden within the pelvic cavity. The hollow *uterus,* commonly known as the womb, resembles an upside-down pear. During pregnancy its muscular outer layer, the *myometrium,* swells 500 to 1,000 times its normal size to accommodate the growing fetus. Most uterine cancers occur in the

---

SIGNS AND SYMPTOMS OF GYNECOLOGIC CANCERS

Cervical Cancer
- Abnormal vaginal bleeding or spotting
- Abnormal vaginal discharge
- Painful intercourse
- Bleeding following intercourse

Advanced-stage cervical cancer can also send these signals:

- Persistent lower-back pain
- Urinary obstruction or sharp pain in the kidney region

Uterine Cancer
- Bleeding, especially after menopause

Because three of five women who get uterine cancer no longer menstruate, the sudden discovery of fresh, red blood or a watery, bloody discharge can be alarming indeed. According to Dr. William Hoskins, chief of Memorial Sloan-Kettering's gynecology service, "About 90 percent of early endometrial cancers will cause vaginal bleeding. If every woman who has abnormal bleeding reports it to her doctor, the vast majority of endometrial cancers would be detected when most of them are highly curable."

Ovarian Cancer
- Acid indigestion
- Appetite loss
- Gas
- Nausea
- A vague discomfort in the lower abdomen
- Abdominal swelling, which may be accompanied by constipation and frequent urination

spongy inner *endometrium,* so much so that physicians often refer to uterine cancer as endometrial cancer.

From the domelike upper portion (the *fundus*) of the uterus branch a pair of four-inch-long *fallopian tubes.* Each leads to an *ovary,* one of the two almond-shaped glands that hold and ripen the egg cells, or *ova.* Once a month one of the ovaries releases a ripened egg, which is propelled into a fallopian tube for possible fertilization by a male sperm cell. If conception takes place, the fertilized egg implants itself in the uterus to begin the approximately 40-week period of gestation. Should fertilization not occur, the uterus discharges blood, fluid and shreds of the thickened layer of endometrial tissue it had produced in preparation for pregnancy. This process is *menstruation.*

Toward its bottom, the uterus tapers into a rubbery, cylindrical section called the *cervix,* which opens into the birth canal, or *vagina.* The mucus produced by the glands that line the cervix serve a dual purpose. It protects the uterus from bacterial infection and, during ovulation, facilitates the sperm cells' perilous journey through the cervical canal and up the fallopian tubes in search of the egg. Like the uterus, the cervix is remarkably resilient, capable of stretching 50 times its normal width to accommodate the soon-to-be-born baby.

BENIGN CONDITIONS

Some of the aforementioned symptoms, particularly abnormal bleeding, may telegraph a noncancerous gynecologic disorder such as cervical polyps or endometriosis. Three related conditions, while almost always benign, can have a bearing on a woman's chance of getting gynecologic cancer and therefore merit discussion.

• Cervical polyps. Polyps, tiny protrusions of epithelial tissue, are quite common, forming in the cervical canal either singly or multiply. Large growths may reveal themselves by bleeding, but most are discovered by a gynecologist in the course of a routine pelvic exam. Polyps can be painlessly removed in the doctor's office with a forceps. They are rarely cancerous.

• *Fibroid tumors,* also referred to as *uterine leiomyomas, fibromyomas* or *myomas,* afflict 1 in 5 women over 30, although they are sometimes seen in younger patients. These firm, round lumps often develop in clusters and can range from pea size to cantaloupe size. Fewer than 5 in 1,000 are malignant.

Most fibroids are detected during pelvic exams, before symptoms appear. Barring severe side effects, women whose tumors are small or who are nearing menopause often forgo surgery, for once menstruation ceases, leiomyomas usually diminish in size or disappear altogether.

We don't want to downplay the impact uterine fibroids can have on a woman's life, especially if she wishes to have children. Other than hysterectomy, the lone surgical option is a *myomectomy*, in which only the myomas are removed. This procedure can weaken the uterine wall, however, and lead to complications during birth. Hormonal therapy appears promising: By lowering a patient's estrogen level to the equivalent of menopause, doctors can shrink the tumors to a more operable size.

• *Ovarian cysts and tumors.* In women under 30, 90 percent of ovarian growths are noncancerous cysts, fluid-filled sacs that usually recede on their own. Women under 30, who rarely grow tumors to begin with, have but a 2 percent chance that a solid growth will turn out to be cancerous. The incidence of malignancies rises with age, however. Women 50 and older have a greater chance of developing a malignant tumor.

PRECANCEROUS CONDITIONS

CERVICAL DYSPLASIA (also known as Cervical Intraepithelial Neoplasm, or CIN)

Dysplasia, which literally means "abnormal growth," can occur in the cells of the cervix. In this instance, dysplastic cells reproduce wildly, crowding out the squamous cells that normally compose the cervical wall. If not treated, approximately one third to one half of all cervical dysplasias eventually progress to cancer.

ATYPICAL UTERINE HYPERPLASIA

Similarly, hyperplastic cells multiply uncontrollably and in time dominate the epithelial lining of the uterus, causing it to thicken. *Hyperplasia* ("excessive growth") is usually benign. But a form called atypical hyperplasia does denote precancerous activity, placing a woman at higher risk for carcinoma of the uterus.

STAGING OF GYNECOLOGIC CANCERS

STAGE	CHARACTERISTICS	FIVE-YEAR SURVIVAL RATE
Cervical Cancer		
0	Carcinoma in situ: Cancerous cells have replaced normal cells in the cervix's outer layer.	100%
I	Cancer is found throughout the cervix but has not spread beyond it.	65%–90%
IA	A very small amount of carcinoma has penetrated the deeper tissues of the cervix.	65%–90%
IB	A greater amount of cancer is found in the cervix's tissues.	65%–90%
II	Cancer has spread to nearby areas but remains within the pelvic cavity.	45%–80%
IIA	Cancer has metastasized beyond the cervix and involves the upper two thirds of the vagina.	45%–80%
IIB	Cancer has spread to the tissue around the cervix.	45%–80%
III	Cancer has metastasized throughout the pelvic area. Malignant cells may have spread to the cells of the pelvic bone and/or invaded the lower part of the vagina. Metastatic cells may also block the tubes connecting the kidneys to the bladder.	Up to 61%
IV	Cancer has invaded other parts of the body, including the bladder, rectum and other nearby organs and/or distant sites such as the lungs.	Less than 15%

Uterine Cancer

No Stage 0

I	Cancer confined to the body of the uterus.	75%–100%
II	Cancer has invaded the uterine body and cervix but remains within the uterus.	Up to 60%
III	Cancer has traveled beyond the uterus and involves ovaries or tubes; surface of pelvic organs; vagina; or pelvic and/or para-aortic lymph nodes.	Up to 30%
IV	Malignancy has spread to the bladder and/or bowel or to other parts of the body.	Up to 5%

Ovarian Cancer

No Stage 0

I	Cancer is found only in one or both ovaries.	Up to 90%
II	Cancer is found in one or both ovaries and/or has spread to the uterus and/or the fallopian tubes and/or other body parts within the pelvis.	Up to 70%
III	Cancer is found in one or both ovaries and has spread to lymph nodes or to other body parts within the abdomen, such as the surface of the liver or intestine.	25%
IV	Cancer is found in one or both ovaries and has spread outside the abdomen or to the inside of the liver.	10%

TREATMENT OF GYNECOLOGIC CANCERS

Hysterectomy is a common treatment for gynecologic malignancies, sometimes in conjunction with radiation therapy and/or chemotherapy. Young patients with endometrial hyperplasia may be spared this major operation and given an oral hormone medication; young women suffering from cervical dysplasia or cervical carcinoma in situ are sometimes candidates for one of the following alternatives:

- *Cryosurgery.* A virtually painless office procedure in which intense cold is applied to the affected area.
- *LEEP,* or *Large Electro-Surgical Excision Procedure,* uses an electric current through a thin wire to excise the abnormal tissue. This can be performed in the office.
- *Laser treatment* uses a carbon-dioxide laser to evaporate a thin area of the surface tissue.
- *Cervical conization,* also called a *cone biopsy,* is performed in a hospital setting under general anesthesia. The surgeon excises a cone-shaped section of cervical tissue containing the tumor.

HYSTERECTOMY

There are two major types of hysterectomies: total and radical. The former removes the uterus and cervix, while the latter excises the cervix, uterus, parametria (tissue around the uterus and cervix) and part of the upper vagina. Both operations terminate a woman's ability to have children; with either type of hysterectomy, the ovaries and fallopian tubes may also be removed *(salpingo-oophorectomy),* resulting in surgical menopause in young women.

Every patient's case is unique, but generally hysterectomy would be justified in the following circumstances:

Cervical Cancer

- Stages I or II. In women who have yet to reach menopause, however, the ovaries may be left intact to maintain normal hormone function.

Uterine Cancer

- Stage I or II.
- Stage III. Following successful radiation therapy to reduce the tumor to a more operable size.

Ovarian Cancer

- Stage I. A young woman whose cancer is limited to one ovary and is well differentiated may undergo a salpingo-oophorectomy, in which the ovary and fallopian tube are taken out, but not the uterus, to preserve a woman's ability to have children. Most other cases, though, warrant a total abdominal hysterectomy and bilateral salpingo-oophorectomy.

Hysterectomy is so common that many people view it as inevitable, routine and minor. Make no mistake, this is major surgery that requires general anesthesia and hospitalization for approximately seven days. Moreover, the frequency with which hysterectomy is recommended has been questioned in recent years. As with any medical procedure, we recommend obtaining a second opinion whenever possible, to reassure yourself that it is indeed the proper course.

A diagnosis of gynecologic cancer often raises many of the same psychologic issues associated with breast cancer: a distorted sense of body image, femininity and sexuality. A University of Iowa study of gynecologic cancer patients and breast cancer patients reported that women in the first group had a poorer self-image of their bodies by a more than 2-to-1 margin. Although surgical treatment for advanced gynecologic cancer does not disfigure the body, it usually means an abrupt end to a woman's childbearing years, an outcome that can be emotionally devastating.

Regrettably, gynecologic cancer patients have not been afforded the same degree of study and support as survivors of mastectomy. That appears to be changing, says Lynn Gossfield, a clinical nurse specialist in the gynecology service at Memorial Sloan-Kettering.

"On a national level," she observes, "you don't see support groups like you see for breast cancer patients. But we're starting to see some networking occur now. Here at Memorial, we've just started up monthly support meetings for gynecologic cancer survivors."

WHO IS AT RISK?

CERVICAL CANCER

- Women age 18 or older
- Sexually active women of any age

Hereditary Risk Factors

- None identified at present

Personal Health History Risk Factors

- Exposure to the drug diethylstilbestrol (DES) in utero
- Personal history of a sexually transmitted disease, including the human papillomavirus (HPV), herpes, gonorrhea and syphilis
- Personal history of vulvar or vaginal dysplasia or cancer
- Personal history of cervical dysplasia or cancer

Lifestyle Risk Factors

- Tobacco use
- Multiple sexual partners
- Intercourse before age 16
- First pregnancy before age 18
- Multiple pregnancies
- Using oral contraceptives

UTERINE CANCER

- Postmenopausal women
- Women ages 55 to 70

Hereditary Risk Factors

- Family history of Lynch syndrome II, also known as hereditary nonpolyposis colorectal cancer (HNPCC)

Whereas Lynch syndrome I leaves relatives vulnerable to colorectal cancer, *Lynch II,* originally dubbed cancer family syndrome, additionally increases their risk of uterine and ovarian tumors, so that women with Lynch II need to be closely scrutinized for all three cancers.

Personal Health History Risk Factors

- Diabetes
- High blood pressure
- Estrogen replacement therapy
- Personal history of colorectal, ovarian and/or breast cancer
- Early menarche (beginning menstruation before age 12)
- Late menopause (ending menstruation after age 50)
- No children
- Personal history of atypical uterine hyperplasia

Lifestyle Risk Factors

- Severe obesity (40 percent or more over your ideal weight; refer to height-weight-frame table in Chapter 6)
- Sedentary lifestyle
- Never having taken oral contraceptives

OVARIAN CANCER

- Women over 60

Hereditary Risk Factors

- Family history of one of the following syndromes:

1. Lynch syndrome II, also known as hereditary nonpolyposis colorectal cancer (HNPCC)
2. Breast-ovarian cancer syndrome
3. Site-specific ovarian cancer syndrome

Cancer researchers have identified three major ovarian cancer syndromes. Lynch II, explained earlier, cuts across a spectrum of cancers. *Breast-ovarian cancer syndrome,* the most common, also weaves a disturbing pattern of multiple disease. Women in these families characteristically exhibit malignancies of the ovaries and breast, usually at an early age, and with a high incidence of tumors on both sides of the body.

By contrast, *site-specific ovarian cancer syndrome* heightens family members' odds of getting ovarian cancer only. "If you belong to a hereditary ovarian cancer family," Dr. Hoskins explains, "and you have two first-degree relatives with the disease, then theoretically you have a 50 percent chance of carrying the gene if you're female.

"Not everybody who has the gene expresses the disease," he emphasizes. "The actual incidence of cancer may be only 30 percent. Nevertheless, that's tremendously high compared to the normal incidence of 1.5 percent." The American Cancer Society estimates that a maternal or sororal history of ovarian cancer more than doubles a woman's risk.

Personal Health History Risk Factors

- Diabetes
- High blood pressure
- Personal history of colorectal, uterine and/or breast cancer
- First birth after age 30
- No children
- Early menarche (beginning menstruation before age 12)
- Late menopause (ending menstruation after age 50)

Lifestyle Risk Factors

- Severe obesity (40 percent or more over your ideal weight; refer to height-weight-frame table in Chapter 6)
- Sedentary lifestyle
- Never having taken oral contraceptives

HORMONES AND GYNECOLOGIC CANCERS

From the preceding lists, you can see that uterine and ovarian cancers have several risk factors in common: obesity, never having taken oral contraceptives, a prolonged menstrual history, late childbirth or no childbirth. These, in turn, share an association in that each influences the hormonal factors believed to trigger cancers of the breast, uterus and ovaries.

The ovaries are part of the endocrine system, which is made up of hormone-producing glands and tissues. Estrogen, the hormone formed in the ovaries, adrenal cortex and placenta, is essential to the development of a woman's female physical characteristics. It also aids in controlling menstruation and pregnancy.

Therefore women who enter the childbearing years early and exit late exhibit higher incidences of uterine and ovarian cancers.

Childless women, too, are more prone to these malignancies. According to the National Cancer Institute, "Childbearing is the most important known factor in preventing ovarian cancer."

The hormonal impact upon cervical cancer is not nearly as pronounced. However, daughters born to mothers who during pregnancy took the drug diethylstilbestrol, better known as DES, are considered at increased risk for both cervical and vaginal cancers. During the 1940s, 1950s and early 1960s, physicians prescribed this synthetic estrogen compound for expectant mothers to prevent miscarriages and premature labor. It wasn't until 1971 that scientists noticed a higher-than-average incidence of rare cervical and vaginal cancers in women from sections of the country where the drug had been widely used. An estimated 4 million to 6 million mothers and offspring were exposed to DES before its use during pregnancy was halted.

ARE YOU AT RISK FOR CERVICAL CANCER?

_____ Women age 18 and older
_____ Sexually active women of any age

Hereditary Risk Factors

None identified at present

Personal Health History Risk Factors

_____ Personal history of a sexually transmitted disease such as genital herpes, gonorrhea, syphilis or genital warts (human papillomavirus, or HPV)
_____ Personal history of vulvar dysplasia or cancer
_____ Personal history of vaginal dysplasia or cancer
_____ Personal history of cervical dysplasia or cancer
_____ Exposure to the drug diethylstilbestrol (DES) before birth

Lifestyle Risk Factors

_____ Tobacco use
_____ Multiple sexual partners
_____ First intercourse before age 16
_____ First pregnancy before age 18
_____ Multiple pregnancies
_____ Oral contraceptive use

If one or more of these risk factors applies to you, consult your physician.

ARE YOU AT RISK FOR UTERINE (ENDOMETRIAL) CANCER?

_____ Women ages 55 to 70
_____ Postmenopausal women

Hereditary Risk Factors

_____ Family history of Lynch syndrome II

Personal Health History Risk Factors

_____ Diabetes
_____ High blood pressure
_____ Estrogen replacement therapy
_____ Personal history of atypical uterine hyperplasia
_____ Personal history of colorectal cancer
_____ Personal history of ovarian cancer
_____ Personal history of breast cancer
_____ Early menarche (beginning menstruation before age 12)
_____ Late menopause (ending menstruation after age 50)
_____ No children

Lifestyle Risk Factors

_____ Severe obesity (40 percent or more over your ideal weight; refer to height-weight-frame table in Chapter 6).
_____ Sedentary lifestyle
_____ Never having taken oral contraceptives

If one or more of these risk factors applies to you, consult your physician.

ARE YOU AT RISK FOR OVARIAN CANCER?

_____ Women age 60 and older

Hereditary Risk Factors

_____ Family history of site-specific ovarian cancer syndrome
_____ Family history of Lynch syndrome II
_____ Family history of breast-ovarian cancer syndrome

Personal Health History Risk Factors

_____ Diabetes
_____ High blood pressure
_____ Personal history of colorectal cancer

_____ Personal history of uterine cancer
_____ Personal history of breast cancer
_____ First child born after age 30
_____ No children
_____ Early menarche (beginning menstruation before age 12)
_____ Late menopause (ending menstruation after age 50)

Lifestyle Risk Factors

_____ Severe obesity (40 percent or more over your ideal weight; refer to height-weight-frame table in Chapter 6)
_____ Sedentary lifestyle
_____ Never having taken oral contraceptives

If one or more of these risk factors applies to you, consult your physician.

HOW TO REDUCE YOUR RISK

GUIDELINES FOR PRIMARY PREVENTION

Because no reliable screening tests yet exist for uterine cancer or ovarian cancer, primary prevention is your greatest asset against these diseases. Adhere to the general primary prevention steps recommended at the beginning of Chapter 9.

GYNECOLOGIC CANCERS AND DIET

The protective element against carcinoma of the uterus mirrors that for breast cancer. Dietary fat, it is believed, causes the intestine to reabsorb estrogen. Fiber, on the other hand, has the reverse effect: It binds this hormone in the gut, preventing reabsorption.

In addition to observing a low-fat, high-fiber diet:

• Use monounsaturated oils in place of polyunsaturated or saturated.
• Include cold-water fish such as salmon, mackerel, herring and sable, which are high in omega-3 fatty acid.

Although no correlation has been demonstrated between dietary fat and ovarian cancer, a fat-heavy diet can obviously increase weight. Obesity and its hormonal consequences are most definitely factors in promoting both malignancies of the ovaries and uterus.

Vitamins

Scientists have used retinoids, a synthetic form of vitamin A, to arrest or prevent cervical dysplasia in laboratory animals. Studies also point to the benefits of whole milk, deep-yellow vegetables, deep-orange fruits and other foods containing this vitamin in helping to stave off ovarian cancer.

One such study, conducted at Roswell Park Cancer Institute in Buffalo, New York, tracked 274 women for eight years. The authors reported that among those ages 30 to 49, "increased risk [for ovarian cancer] was seen in women reporting diets low in fiber and vitamin A from fruit and vegetable sources."

The National Cancer Institute has cited both vitamin C and folic acid as useful in reducing a woman's risk of cervical dysplasia and carcinoma in situ. By now you know that oranges and other citrus fruits, green and red peppers, and a host of other fruits and vegetables are high in vitamin C, but you may not be as familiar with folic acid, or folacin, a member of the B-complex family. (See box for sources.)

FOODS HIGH IN FOLIC ACID

- Green, leafy vegetables such as kale, spinach and turnip greens
- Dried beans and peas
- Wheat germ

- Asparagus
- Corn
- Parsnips
- Beets

GYNECOLOGIC CANCERS AND EXERCISE

Fatty *(adipose)* tissue metabolizes estrogen, which stimulates cell growth in the uterus. Therefore an obese woman is twice as likely to develop endometrial cancer, and the greater her weight, the greater her danger: Being 50 pounds overweight multiplies the odds ninefold.

Interestingly, body-fat volume may be less of a factor than how it is distributed. Several studies have found that subjects with apple-shaped figures—heavy in the upper and midtorso—exhibited a higher incidence of uterine tumors than those with pear-shaped builds. One 1991 study conducted at Tampa's H. Lee Moffitt Cancer Center concluded: "Women with upper-body fat localization are at increased risk of developing endometrial cancer." It is believed that abdominal fat is more active metabolically than fat elsewhere on the body.

While evidence connecting obesity and ovarian cancer is less compelling, excess weight can lead to diabetes and hypertension, both of which elevate the risk of uterine and ovarian cancers. For an adult, blood pressure that is consistently above 140/90 is considered abnormal and potentially dangerous.

Just as exercise is an important aspect of controlling diabetes and high blood pressure, it is also recommended to help avoid gynecologic cancer. According to a 1993 Harvard University School of Public Health study, female participants who trained regularly had lower rates not only of uterine cancer, but also of ovarian, cervical and vaginal tumors. Researchers hypothesize that besides reducing body fat, exercise alters the hormone ratio as well.

GYNECOLOGIC CANCERS AND ORAL CONTRACEPTIVES AND HORMONE REPLACEMENT THERAPY

In the late 1960s a rash of uterine cancers arose among women receiving estrogen replacement therapy (ERT) to relieve the adverse effects of menopause. The longer a patient took the estrogen pills, the greater her chances of getting the disease, with seven years of therapy boosting the risk 14-fold.

Word of this uterine cancer "epidemic" sent hormone prescriptions tumbling by nearly half. But estrogen replacement therapy provides substantial benefits, helping to prevent osteoporosis, a thinning of the bones mainly in elderly females, and cardiovascular disease.

So doctors studied new approaches to hormone replacement, giving lower doses of estrogen and adding progesterone to the regimen to prevent a buildup of endometrial tissue by promoting a periodic shedding of the lining—similar to what happens during menstruation. A regimen of estrogen and progesterone decreases the risk of uterine cancer to the same level of risk as in the general population. Any woman considering hormone replacement therapy should discuss this matter at length with her doctor.

Similarly, some birth-control pills originally administered nothing but estrogen for the first half of their cycle, then a combination of estrogen and progesterone for about seven days, followed by a week off. These "sequential" oral contraceptives were found to double the risk of uterine cancer, and the U.S. Food and Drug Administration took them off the market in 1976. The "combination" oral contraceptive provides estrogen and progesterone simultaneously throughout the cycle. The results have been striking. Combination birth-control pills are believed to halve a woman's risk for both uterine and ovarian cancers. The Centers for Disease Control in Atlanta credits oral contraceptive use for preventing an estimated 4,000 cases of gynecologic cancers per year.

Dr. Hoskins explains the process by which the pills may work: "For ovarian cancer, one theory is that they stop ovulation, which adds a period of protection. The other theory is that they block the pituitary hormones that constantly stimulate the ovary." As for uterine cancer, he says, they "probably protect the endometrium simply by exerting a constant progestational effect that keeps the endometrium very inactive."

Curiously, "Women who take oral contraceptives have a slightly *increased* risk of cervical cancer," he notes, although just why is not yet clear. Recent studies point to something in the pill itself. Another reason may be oral contraception's influence on sexual mores. It was the introduction of the birth-control pill in 1960 that contributed to the so-called sexual revolution, with its permissive attitudes toward premarital and casual sex. This leads to our next topic.

CERVICAL CANCER AND SEXUAL BEHAVIOR

A well-known study compared incidences of cervical cancer among prostitutes and nuns. Women in the former group showed four times the rate of disease among the general population, while not one case was reported among 13,000 nuns. The issue, however, isn't promiscuity per se, but *unprotected* sex with multiple partners, which increases exposure to sexually transmitted diseases such as herpes, gonorrhea and syphilis, and to *human papillomaviruses*. All add to a woman's risk of cervical cancer.

Sixty human papillomaviruses, present in up to 30 percent of the population, have been identified to date. Approximately 18 of these infectious agents cause benign genital warts. But other HPVs lead to cervical dysplasia and vulvar hyperplasia, conditions that can progress into cancer. According to Dr. Hoskins, "Some people have theorized that all cervical cancer is papillomavirus related." A possible association between cervical cancer and the genital herpes virus, also referred to as herpes simplex II, is less well established.

Certainly the threat of AIDS has somewhat dampened the sexual revolution, but a frighteningly high number of men and women still practice unsafe sex. If you're in a monogamous relationship, how essential is protected sex? That is a matter of mutual trust only you can answer. A woman may be monogamous, but if her partner has multiple sexual partners, then her exposure is influenced by *that* person's multiple partners.

Cervical cancer flourishes in the disadvantaged areas of the world, where multiple partners and early intercourse (before age 16) and early childbirth (before age 18) are often part of the cultural landscape. "There's no one clear factor," says Dr. Hoskins, who goes on to explain how all three are interrelated.

"The outside of the cervix is lined with a skinlike [squamous-cell] epithelium, while the inside of the cervix is lined with a columnar epithelium, like the lining of the intestine. And where those two types of epithelium meet is a very fluid border that moves back and forth, depending on the hormonal influence, how old a woman is, and so on. It is at that junction, where the cells are constantly dividing and changing, that cervical cancer develops. Young teenage girls and pregnant women have very active squamocolumnar junctions. So if those individuals are exposed to multiple partners—or to one partner who has whatever risk factors are necessary—then they are more likely to develop the disease."

CERVICAL CANCER AND SMOKING

Precisely how tobacco impacts on cervical cancer remains a mystery. However, based on population studies, the National Cancer Institute states that the risk appears to increase significantly with the number of cigarettes smoked each day and with the years of smoking. This conclusion, along with the other, well-documented damaging effects of tobacco, should be enough to make anyone give up the habit.

SECONDARY PREVENTION GUIDELINES
FOR CERVICAL CANCER

For Asymptomatic Women with No Special Risk Factors
• Annual physical exam, pelvic exam and Pap test, beginning at age 18 or the onset of first sexual intercourse, if earlier

For Asymptomatic Women at Increased Risk
• Physical exam, pelvic exam and Pap test more than annually if Pap test results are abnormal

Those exposed to diethylstilbestrol (DES) prior to birth:
• Pelvic exam and Pap test at least annually, beginning at age 14 or at onset of menstruation, whichever occurs first

---

PHYSICAL EXAM

Before the exam begins, you are asked to go into the bathroom and give a urine sample. Next you undress, slip on a paper gown, and have your weight and blood pressure taken. If this is your first evaluation, the physician or nurse will record a complete medical history. You will be asked to recount any current symptoms; your menstrual, surgical, reproductive, emotional, social and sexual histories; and any allergies or medications. "We look particularly at a patient's family history," Dr. Hoskins notes. "Is there a pattern of malignancies that would place you at increased risk for gynecologic cancer?" Follow-up visits don't require nearly as detailed information.

As you sit on an examining table, the gynecologist feels your lymph nodes and thyroid gland for enlargement, then palpates your breasts with his fingers (pages 254–55.)

PELVIC EXAM

For the pelvic exam, you lie back on the examining table, spread your legs and place your feet against a pair of stirrups. Given the nature of this procedure, only so much can be done to accommodate a woman's modesty. But most gynecologists drape a sheet over the knees, affording at least a modicum of privacy. The doctor then examines the genitals.

"First we look at the vulva for any kind of infectious diseases or precancerous changes," explains Dr. Hoskins. "We also look for such things as lack of estrogen, atrophy and any kind of genital abnormalities, but that's rarely important except in very young patients or those who are being seen for the first time.

"Then a speculum is inserted into the vagina." This instrument, usually made of plastic and metal, widens the vaginal opening and facilitates visual inspection of the upper vagina and cervix. At most you may feel a fleeting pinching sensation.

"We examine the entire vagina," the doctor continues, "again looking for any kind of infectious lesions or preinvasive cancerous lesions. Then we inspect the cervix, take a Pap smear [explained below], and conduct a bimanual examination, in which we feel the uterus, the fallopian tubes and ovaries." Here the doctor probes for irregularities in shape and size. For example, an ovary large enough to be felt with the fingers might indicate a cyst or tumor.

A rectal-vaginal exam follows. "This provides us with a much better feel for the ovaries and for any kind of masses that are present," Dr. Hoskins says. "It also enables us to feel the cul-de-sac," a recess between the rectum and the uterus.

"And that's basically the pelvic exam. It's like having someone look in your ears, your nose or your mouth. Given your choice, you wouldn't have anybody poking around. But," he emphasizes, "there shouldn't be any pain associated with it, unless some kind of disease is present."

PAP TEST

Dr. George Nicholas Papanicolaou, after whom the Pap test is named, had to wait nearly a quarter-century to see his simple yet immensely valuable procedure fully accepted. In 1925 the Greek-born physician began collecting smears of vaginal fluid from patients at Cornell Medical College as a means for diagnosing cancers of the female genital tract. When magnified under a microscope, cancerous cells appeared distinctly large, dark, dense —easy to identify.

The doctor presented his findings in 1928. "We have a new diagnostic method for certain malignant tumors," he wrote, "especially of the female genital tract." The paper met with a resounding silence, and so Dr. Papanicolaou returned to researching endocrinology, assisted by his wife, Mary.

It wasn't until the 1950s that the rest of the medical community finally caught up with "Dr. Pap," as he would be known until his death at age 78 in 1962. In its 1986 monograph, *Cancer Control Objectives for the Nation: 1985–2000,* the National Cancer Institute estimated that if all women between the ages of 20 and 70 had Pap test screening every three years, as was then prescribed, deaths from cervical cancer could be all but wiped out. The following year the American Cancer Society revamped its guidelines, recommending the test be performed annually.

Schedule your appointment for approximately two weeks after your first day of menstruation. Beginning two days prior to the test, refrain from sexual intercourse; douching; using vaginal medications, jellies or contraception; and do not insert anything into the vagina.

A Pap test can be performed in any setting: office, clinic or hospital. The instrument for obtaining a thin layer of cells from the surface of the cervix and upper vagina varies. "Some people use a plastic or wooden spatula," says Dr. Hoskins. "Others use a spatula and a cotton swab, while still others use a glass rod to aspirate cervical mucus. Here we use two cotton swabs."

A miniature brush called a *cytobrush* may be needed if the gynecologist has difficulty accessing the *os,* the tiny cervical opening that leads to the inch-long canal joining the vagina and the uterine cavity. "We slip it inside the cervix and twirl it," explains the doctor. "Occasionally patients will feel that a little bit, but not enough to be significant." Patient Judith K. describes the sensation as "a bit crampy."

The cells are placed on a slide and sent to pathology for analysis. Most laboratories in the United States use what is called the Bethesda System for reporting Pap smear results. There are three basic categories: normal, low-grade lesion, and high-grade lesion, or carcinoma. Three negative Pap tests in a row may convince your doctor to recommend less-frequent gynecologic exams. Abnormal results, however, would warrant one or more of the following diagnostic measures:

• *Colposcopy.* A binocularlike viewing instrument called a *colposcope* magnifies the cervix 10 to 20 times its actual size, allowing the physician to assess suspicious areas that need to be further biopsied. First a speculum is inserted into the vagina. Then the colposcope, which mounts on a tripod or a metal arm, is positioned. It does not touch the skin, and its bright colored lights generate no heat, so the only discomfort you may feel is a moderate sting from the acetic acid solution painted over the cervix with a cotton swab. In all, expect the procedure to last 10 to 20 minutes.

• *Schiller test.* An iodine stain is swabbed over the cervix and vagina. Normal tissue will turn a deep mahogany brown, explains Dr. Hoskins, whereas "precancerous lesions do not stain" and retain their light-pink color. One drawback to this test, he notes, is that several other conditions cause the stain not to be absorbed. "It's not a very specific test. Some doctors believe it should be used all the time, some never use it and others use it occasionally."

• *Dilation and curettage.* Also referred to as a D&C. Today this procedure is generally called for only if an insufficient number of cells were harvested during the Pap test. After a speculum is gently introduced into the vagina, "We use tiny graduated metal rods to dilate the cervix," says Dr. Hoskins, "then scrape samples from the cervix and the lining of the uterus" with a spoon-shaped *curette.*

Patients are put to sleep for the approximately 15-minute procedure, performed on an outpatient basis in a hospital. Because you may be drowsy afterward, arrange for someone to drive you home. In the days after, mild bleeding or spotting is normal. But

---

SECONDARY PREVENTION GUIDELINES FOR UTERINE CANCER

For Asymptomatic Women with No Special Risk Factors

• No screening recommended at present

The procedures so effective for early detection of cervical cancer have little application in screening for uterine tumors. A cancerous uterus usually retains its normal shape and size, negating the value of the pelvic exam, while the Pap test is only 50 percent accurate in diagnosing malignancies of this organ.

For Asymptomatic Women at Increased Risk

• Annual pelvic exam and uterine aspiration biopsy, beginning at menopause

Although these procedures are made available to women at high risk for uterine cancer, Dr. Hoskins emphasizes that "there has never been a prospective study showing that routine endometrial biopsies are of benefit." Most gynecologists would recommend only an endometrial biopsy if there has been an abnormal biopsy.

heavy bleeding that persists for more than six hours or so should be reported to your doctor at once. Fever, chronic abdominal pain, dizziness or an unusual or foul-smelling vaginal discharge also signals a potentially dangerous condition and needs prompt medical attention.

• Cervical conization, or *cone biopsy*, referred to earlier in this chapter as a therapeutic measure, is also carried out under general anesthesia. Two or three stitches (sutures) are made in the cervix to stem the flow of blood. Next the surgeon uses a knife, scissors or both to excise a cone-shaped tissue sample from the center of the cervix. "The most common way to prevent bleeding afterward," says Dr. Hoskins, "is cautery." The specimen is sent to the lab, where a pathologist looks for evidence of preinvasive or invasive disease.

UTERINE ASPIRATION BIOPSY

In this procedure, usually carried out in a doctor's office, a thin plastic or metal tube is inserted through the vagina into the uterine

---

SECONDARY PREVENTION GUIDELINES FOR OVARIAN CANCER

For Asymptomatic Women with No Special Risk Factors

• Annual pelvic exam

In 1994 a National Institutes of Health panel recommended against routine screening for women at average risk of ovarian cancer, on the grounds that the tests are unreliable and may lead to unnecessary surgery. The Pap smear does not help in diagnosing ovarian cancer. According to Dr. Hoskins, although pelvic examination has not proven to decrease the death rate from ovarian cancer, it can occasionally result in early diagnosis. Likewise, the CA 125 tumor marker and ultrasound are less than perfect, but they are currently the only measures we have for finding ovarian cancer early on. Memorial Sloan-Kettering recommends all women undergo an annual pelvic exam.

For Asymptomatic Women at Increased Risk

• Annual pelvic exam
• CA 125 tumor marker
• Transvaginal or pelvic ultrasound

cavity. The physician then collects tissue by applying suction from a vacuum-type device. Patients sometimes report cramping during the biopsy and afterward. Complications, similar to those described for cervical dilation and curettage of the uterus, can arise and should be brought to your physician's attention at once. If the biopsy is deemed either unsatisfactory or unsuitable, a D&C may be necessary.

CA 125 TUMOR MARKER

CA 125 is a blood test that detects an antigen characteristic of ovarian tumors. According to Dr. Hoskins, "Eighty percent of ovarian epithelial cancers have CA 125 antigen on their cells." A CA 125 antibody will recognize this specific antigen and can be measured by this blood test. Theoretically, the higher a person's *titer,* a measurement used to express the quantity of antigens, the more tumor is present. A normal level is less than 35.

"One of the problems," Dr. Hoskins explains, "is that in one patient almost all the cells may have the antigen," so should a tumor indeed be present, the blood test will yield a high titer. "On the other hand, you may have another patient with the same amount of disease, but only 10 percent of her cells have the CA 125 antigen. And her titer may be much, much lower." *One in two women with early ovarian cancer will not show an elevated CA 125.*

He bluntly admits, "CA 125 is not very good for the early diagnosis of ovarian cancer, and its value as a routine test has not been proven." Memorial Sloan-Kettering recommends against it except for patients like Sylvia A., diagnosed with ovarian cancer in 1990. The mother of three grown children responded extremely well to surgery and chemotherapy, and was soon pronounced in remission. Throughout treatment and the next two years of follow-up exams, she periodically received the CA 125, which provided doctors a means of gauging her level of disease.

"When my tumor was first discovered," says Sylvia, "my CA 125 was around 600 or 800. Then it started to drop considerably, until it was practically down to 7, when the chemo had taken full effect. It just started to go up again in May 1993." Not long after, Sylvia's cancer recurred, forcing her back on chemotherapy. Fortunately, the fact that the malignancy was discovered early on improves her prognosis significantly.

TRANSVAGINAL AND PELVIC ULTRASOUND

Any woman who's given birth in the last decade or so is undoubt-edly familiar with *ultrasound,* an imaging procedure that, not un-like radar, uses high-frequency sound waves to form a picture, the *sonogram,* on a television-type screen.

Based on limited studies, says Dr. Hoskins, "Ultrasound does appear able to diagnose the disease early. However," he cautions, "it can also pick up a lot of things that are not cancer," resulting in an unacceptable number of needless operations. Still, it is an option offered to women at high risk of ovarian cancer, with its shortcomings clearly spelled out.

In a *pelvic ultrasound,* you don a gown and lie on a table. The technologist rubs a special conductive jelly over your lower abdomen, then moves a hand-held probe back and forth across the area. This probe, or *transducer,* pulses ultrasonic beams into the body. Depending on the density of the tissues they strike, some get reflected back to the transducer as echo patterns, which a computer converts into images that a radiologist is specially trained to interpret.

"The probe and the jelly are a little cold," remarks patient Judith K., "but otherwise it's not uncomfortable." You will proba-bly need to empty your bladder afterward: Patients are asked to drink liquids and refrain from urinating the morning of the procedure, as a full bladder better enables the radiologist to distin-guish it onscreen from neighboring organs.

In a *transvaginal ultrasound,* the probe is inserted into the va-gina, facilitating a clearer picture of the uterus, fallopian tubes and ovaries. A full bladder is not necessary for this type of ultrasound.

While patients can usually "see themselves" on the monitor screen, few will be able to discern exactly what they are viewing. We suggest that you resist the temptation to read too much into the technologist's manner or facial expressions during the proce-dure; protocol forbids them from discussing what they see.

Another imaging exam, *computed axial tomography* (CT scan for short), may be used to diagnose ovarian cancer, as well as *laparoscopy* and *laparotomy,* all discussed below.

CT SCAN

This x-ray procedure utilizes a contrast dye to enhance visualiza-tion. At Memorial Sloan-Kettering, patients relax in the soothing waiting area of the Iris Cantor Diagnostic Center and drink two to three cups of citrus-flavored liquid over a period of about 30 minutes. Another method, depending on the organs being examined, is to inject or drip the dye into a vein in the arm.

"As with all intravenous x-rays, patients can have a feeling of warmth," says radiologist Dr. Robert Heelan. Fewer than one in five experience this sensation. "A smaller minority become nauseous, and some vomit." Still less common is a reaction ranging from sneezing to hives. "This is quite rare," he emphasizes, "but it happens enough that we warn patients about the possibility." Patients with a history of severe reactions may receive a cortisone premedication a day or two before the scan, or a different contrast agent may be tried.

Patient Sylvia A. recalls no adverse reactions to the dye. "The CT scan is very simple," she says. "You climb onto a small platform and lie down, then the machine draws you into a large oval-shaped cylinder only as deep as you need to go, which in my case was up to the rib cage or so." A rotating beam then x-rays from the sides, front and back at precise intervals, forming cross-sectional pictures on either a monitor or a paper printout.

According to Dr. Heelan, "CT scans are getting shorter and shorter. It used to be that a standard abdomen and pelvis study would require about fifteen to twenty minutes on the table. With our new scanners we now do an entire study in the space of two and a half minutes."

LAPAROSCOPY AND LAPAROTOMY

Sometimes the only definitive method of diagnosing a cancerous or precancerous condition of the female genital tract is through one or both of these surgical procedures, which are performed in a hospital under general anesthesia.

Laparoscopy is the less extensive. After you are put to sleep, the surgeon prepares for surgery by catheterizing the bladder, if necessary, followed by a pelvic exam. Next gas is injected into the abdomen through a metal tube, to inflate the abdominal cavity. Then he or she makes a one-inch horizontal incision right below the navel, inserts a thin tubular lighted viewing instrument known as a *laparoscope* and inspects the organs for abnormalities.

This procedure takes an average of 30 minutes. Once finished, the surgeon lets the abdomen deflate, gently withdraws the scope and closes the incision with one or two dissolving stitches. Patients

328 PREVENTING THE MAJOR CANCERS

are usually discharged from the hospital's outpatient clinic within four hours of surgery. As with any procedure that requires general anesthesia, you should make plans to be driven home.

About 1 in 120 women encounter complications from laparoscopy, and most feel back to normal within two or three days. However, symptoms such as fever, persistent pain, dizziness, vaginal bleeding, or bleeding or oozing from the incision require your doctor's immediate attention.

One disadvantage to laparoscopy is that it allows for only limited surgical tasks. A doctor who suspects a cancerous tumor in a patient and anticipates an immediate hysterectomy or oophorectomy may select laparotomy instead. Laparotomy, an exploratory surgery, entails a hospital stay of up to one week. Here the surgeon makes an incision in the lower abdomen, right above the pubic hairline. Depending upon the subsequent surgery that will be needed, the incision may be up-and-down rather than across. After the area is sutured, the patient is removed to the surgical recovery room until she regains consciousness; then she is wheeled back to her hospital room.

Women who undergo laparotomy generally find their lives disrupted for anywhere from a month to a month and a half. Driving a car is out of the question until the discomfort from the incision subsides and you no longer need pain medication. Even routine household tasks such as cooking and cleaning are not advisable for a week or two.

After a CT scan revealed an ovarian tumor in 1990, Andrea D., then 55, underwent laparotomy, during which the surgeon confirmed a stage III malignancy and immediately performed a radical hysterectomy. Andrea, an ocean-freight agent for an import-export company and a married mother of three grown children, recalls the agony of the next several months.

"They'd also examined the intestines for cancer inch by inch. Because of that, the abdominal pain was probably more pronounced had it not been done. I would say it was a good three months before the pain disappeared. There was some discomfort thereafter as well, but nothing to the point where I couldn't function normally. But it was a long time before the real pain disappeared. A very long time."

The National Cancer Institute, the American College of Obstetricians and Gynecologists, the American Medical Association, the

American Academy of Family Physicians, the American Medical Women's Association and the American Nurses Association *all* support the American Cancer Society's 1987 stepped-up cervical-cancer screening recommendations of annual pelvic exam and Pap test, both of which have contributed tremendously to the dramatic reduction in cervical cancer both here and in foreign countries where screening is commonplace. Hopefully it won't be long before science develops equally effective techniques for the early detection of uterine and ovarian cancers.

SUGGESTED READING ABOUT GYNECOLOGIC CANCERS

From the National Cancer Institute (800-4-CANCER):

- "What You Need to Know About Cancer of the Cervix"
- "What You Need to Know About Ovarian Cancer"
- "What You Need to Know About Cancer of the Uterus"

KEY WORDS

CA 125 tumor marker: A blood test that measures a substance found in some ovarian malignancies.

Colposcopy: A diagnostic procedure that uses a binocularlike magnifying instrument called a *colposcope*.

Conization: A diagnostic and therapeutic procedure also known as *cone biopsy*. The surgeon uses a knife, scissors or both to excise a cone-shaped tissue sample from the center of the cervix.

Cryosurgery: A virtually painless office procedure for treating early-stage cervical cancer in which intense cold is applied to the affected area.

CT scan (computed axial tomography): A computerized diagnostic x-ray, taken cross-sectionally, which yields countless single-plane images of body tissues.

Diethylstilbestrol (DES): A drug that was once given to expectant mothers to prevent miscarriage and early labor. Women exposed in utero to DES, no longer used for this purpose, are considered at increased risk for both cervical and vaginal cancers, as are their mothers.

Dilation and curettage: Also referred to as a D&C. Cell samples are scraped from the cervix and the lining of the uterus with a spoon-shaped *curette,* then sent to a pathologist for analysis.

Fibroid tumor: Also referred to as *uterine leiomyoma, fibromyoma* or *myoma.* Fibroids, firm, round lumps that often develop in clusters and can range from pea size to cantaloupe size, afflict 1 in 5 women over 30. Fewer than 5 in 1,000 fibroid tumors are malignant.

Gynecologist: A physician who specializes in detecting and treating diseases of the female genital tract.

Gynecologic oncologist: A gynecologist who has additional training in the treatment of gynecologic cancers.

Hysterectomy: Surgery to remove the uterus and cervix (total hysterectomy) or the cervix, uterus, tissue around the uterus and part of the upper vagina (radical hysterectomy).

Laparoscopy: A surgical diagnostic procedure that requires a small incision and a lighted viewing instrument called a *laparoscope.*

Laparotomy: Exploratory surgery that requires a hospital stay and a lengthy convalescence; used to confirm suspicions of gynecologic cancer or to treat gynecologic cancer.

Laser treatment: Treatment for early-stage cervical cancer in which a carbon-dioxide laser evaporates a thin area of surface tissue.

Menopause: The time of life when a woman's menstrual periods cease.

Oophorectomy: Surgical removal of the ovaries.

Salpingo-oophorectomy: Surgical removal of the ovaries and fallopian tubes.

Schiller test: An iodine stain is swabbed over the cervix and vagina. Whereas normal tissue turns brown, precancerous and cancerous lesions retain their light-pink color.

Speculum: An instrument, usually made of metal or plastic, that is inserted into the vagina to facilitate visual inspection of the upper vagina and cervix.

Uterine aspiration biopsy: A method for harvesting tissue samples from the uterus, using a thin tube and a vacuum-type suction device.

Uterine hyperplasia: Hyperplasia, which literally means "excessive growth," is usually benign. But a form called atypical hyperplasia denotes precancerous activity.

CHAPTER

15

Stomach and Esophageal Cancers

Esophagogram · Upper GI Series ·
Upper GI Endoscopy with Biopsy

In the 1930s, with the country mired in the Great Depression, Americans dreaded stomach cancer the way rival mobsters feared Al Capone. Only carcinomas of the uterus and breast stole more women's lives, while among men it reigned as the leading cause of cancer death. But shortly thereafter, the disease began to fade from the American picture along with radio soap operas and boys' knickers. The 24,000 cases reported in 1994 ranked 16th among all cancers.

We attribute this dramatic decline to advances not so much in medicine as in refrigeration. As Norges and Frigidaires found their way into U.S. homes in increasing numbers, food no longer had to be preserved with salt or as many chemicals, both factors in *gastric* cancer. Nevertheless, it remains a pernicious disease, killing 14,000 Americans annually.

Carcinoma of the esophagus, the tube that delivers food and liquid to the stomach, has followed the reverse pattern. From 1958 to 1990 the mortality rate went up 25 percent in women and 23 percent in men. Though relatively rare (1994 brought 11,000 cases), esophageal cancer ends in death 10,400 times a year. Many

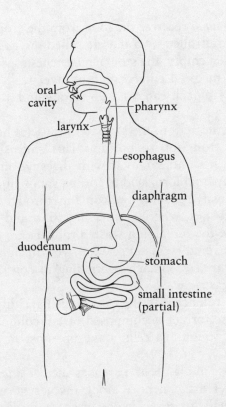

oral cavity

pharynx

larynx

esophagus

diaphragm

duodenum

stomach

small intestine (partial)

Normal Upper Gastrointestinal Tract. The upper GI tract begins at the mouth and ends where the small intestine empties into the colon. In the illustration at left, the small intestine is only partially shown; in an average adult, it is about 20 feet long and is coiled within the abdominal cavity. It is from this organ that nutrients from digested food are absorbed into the body, while waste material and fluid are emptied into the shorter, but much thicker colon.

of those fatalities could be avoided by observing a healthier diet and giving up smoking and excessive alcohol use.

THE STOMACH AND THE ESOPHAGUS

Both of these organs belong to the upper gastrointestinal tract, responsible for processing the food we eat and passing it along to the intestines for digestion and absorption.

The forkful of chicken (skinless, preferably, and baked, not fried!) you place in your mouth gets chewed into smaller pieces. Then three pairs of salivary glands go to work moistening the food, leaving a rounded mass, or alimentary *bolus.*

Once swallowed, the bolus travels down the *esophagus,* or gullet, a hollow tube nestled between the airpipe (trachea) and the spine. Muscles in the esophageal walls automatically contract and relax to propel the food along its approximately 15-inch length, which is lined with mucus-secreting glands for facilitating traffic flow.

The curved, saclike *stomach* receives the food from the esophagus through an opening controlled by a muscle called the *gastroesophageal sphincter*. When empty, the stomach clenches together almost like a fist. But as material enters, its four-layer walls expand. The average adult stomach can hold up to one and a half quarts.

In an agitating, contractile action, the stomach's muscles begin to contract rhythmically from top to bottom. This churns the bolus into smaller fragments and mixes it with digestive juices containing enzymes and hydrochloric acid to form a soupy liquid. The waves gradually intensify, pushing the contents through the *pylorus* and into the intestines, where further digestion and absorption take place before the remaining waste products are disposed of by way of the excretory system. What we call hunger pangs are in reality an emptied stomach continuing to contract, stimulating nerves in the gastric wall.

Though adjoining, the stomach and the esophagus have different cell characteristics. The former is composed of tall columnar cells, while flat, platelike squamous cells make up most of the esophageal epithelium.

Most gastric tumors arise in glands and are classified as *adenocarcinoma*. Stomach cancer may advance along the gastric wall into the esophagus or small intestine. More often, however, it burrows through the wall to infiltrate neighboring organs and tissues such as the liver, pancreas, colon, ovaries and *peritoneum*, the membrane that lines the abdominal and pelvic cavities. Other routes include the lymphatic system and the bloodstream, which can whisk cancerous cells to any organ in the body.

Esophageal cancer presents itself as adenocarcinoma in the lower third of the gullet, near the stomach, but as squamous-cell carcinoma in the upper and middle sections. It too may travel

SIGNS AND SYMPTOMS OF STOMACH CANCER

- Abdominal pain
- Chronic indigestion
- Appetite loss
- A bloated feeling after meals
- Persistent heartburn
- Weight loss
- Fatigue
- Nausea
- Vomiting
- Dark stools from bleeding

through the lymphatic system and bloodstream, affecting other organs.

The warning signs of gastric cancer have remained unchanged since first described in eleventh-century medical records. One reason the disease often escapes notice until it has spread to other organs is that its symptoms—most frequently abdominal pain and indigestion—mirror those of many commonplace ailments. As Dr. Robert Kurtz, a gastroenterologist at Memorial Sloan-Kettering, points out, "Everybody has had abdominal pain, indigestion, nausea or vomiting at one time or another. Usually it's some sort of stomach virus, which subsides in a short time, and the person feels better."

But not always. Early-stage gastric neoplasms typically masquerade as less-serious conditions, and so even when effects such as indigestion linger, most sufferers dismiss it as a mere upset stomach, or, at worst, peptic ulcers, a painful but normally benign malady that strikes 3 out of every 1,000 men and women.

Because gastric tumors are relatively uncommon in the United States, "primary-care physicians themselves will not always investigate patients who are in their fifties and sixties and have a new onset of abdominal complaints," observes Dr. Kurtz. "Instead they'll simply prescribe an antacid or some other medication that will help relieve their symptoms but may in fact mask the warning signs of potentially early and curable cancers." Months may pass before the patient returns to the doctor complaining now of nausea or vomiting.

"And by the time nausea and vomiting occur from gastric cancer," Dr. Kurtz warns, "it's late disease. In the U.S., stomach cancer is almost never identified by screening. The vast majority of gastric cancer patients we see in this country present with advanced and incurable disease—and die from their disease." He strongly recommends informing your doctor of any symptoms that don't subside after two weeks.

As with gastric cancer, "Oftentimes patients who present with

---

SIGNS AND SYMPTOMS OF ESOPHAGEAL CANCER

- Difficult or painful swallowing
- Chronic indigestion
- Persistent heartburn

esophageal cancer have advanced disease," says Dr. Kurtz. The most commonly seen manifestation is *dysphagia,* or difficulty swallowing. "That usually is not acute," he explains, "but becomes severe over a period of time."

At first patients may feel a burning or tightness in the gullet, or the sensation that food is caught behind the breastbone. Initially these problems may be sporadic and noticeable mostly when eating meat, bread or raw vegetables and other coarse foods. But as the malignancy grows, closing off the route to the stomach, softer foods—and eventually even liquids—also become difficult to swallow.

What's more, esophageal cancer can induce heartburn, vomiting, coughing, hoarseness, choking on food and coughing up blood-flecked food. Depending on which organs it infiltrates, potential side effects include chest pain, back pain and anemia. Of course, any of these may indicate a comparatively innocuous disorder. Whether to rid your mind of worry or to arrest a cancer while it's still highly curable, don't delay in seeing your doctor.

STAGING OF STOMACH CANCER AND ESOPHAGEAL CANCER

As with other cancers, the progress of both these diseases is measured from 0 to IV. However, if not treated early, the cure rate drops precipitously. A patient with stage 0 carcinoma of the stomach, in which the cancer affects only the gastric wall's mucosal lining, has a five-year survival rate of greater than 90 percent. But once the tumor invades the second or third layer (stage I), the odds of survival tumble to approximately 58 percent.

Esophageal cancer carries an even bleaker prognosis. The survival rate for stage I disease stands at but 50 percent or higher. By stage II: a discouraging 10 percent to 15 percent.

TREATMENT OF STOMACH CANCER AND ESOPHAGEAL CANCER

Surgery is currently the only successful method for treating gastric cancer, although the usefulness of both chemotherapy and radiation is being investigated in clinical trials. A subtotal *gastrectomy* removes part of the stomach (generally 80 to 85 percent), along with nearby lymph nodes. In a total gastrectomy, the entire stomach is taken out, as well as a section of the esophagus.

If part of the stomach remains, it is connected to a segment of the small intestine; if no stomach is left, the esophagus is then joined directly to the small intestine. Patients can anticipate a hospital stay of ten days to two weeks, and another two to four weeks of convalescence at home. But within two months, says Dr. Murray Brennan, chief of surgery at Memorial Sloan-Kettering, "most of them are back to normal daily living." Because this procedure leaves patients with smaller stomachs, he says, "naturally they'll be more comfortable eating smaller, more frequent meals. But that improves with time, and many people can resume normal eating habits."

One infrequent side effect of this surgery is "dumping," the rapid absorption of nutrients. As Dr. Brennan explains, "Normally the stomach delivers foods at a controlled rate to the small intestine, where it's absorbed. When you have no stomach, and food goes directly from your mouth into the small intestine, you can get rapid absorption in large quantities. And so you experience a rapid increase in your blood glucose and insulin, which can produce palpitations and a feeling of weakness." Most patients can control this condition through learning not to overeat and not to eat large quantities of concentrated food rapidly.

Esophageal cancer patients usually require surgery or radiation therapy. In an operation called an *esophagectomy,* the tumor and all or part of the gullet are removed. "We usually replace that with the stomach," says Dr. Brennan, "so that instead of swallowing from your mouth and into the esophagus, you swallow directly into the stomach. Most of the time, that works very well. However, if the stomach has cancer too, we need to form a new passageway, using tissue from the colon or another digestive-tract organ; they are not as good conduits as the stomach."

WHO IS AT RISK?
STOMACH CANCER

• Men and women age 50 and older

"It's rare to see young people with either gastric or esophageal cancer," says Dr. Kurtz. Stomach cancer strikes nearly twice the number of men as women.

HEREDITARY RISK FACTORS

- Family history of gastric cancer
- Type A blood

Stomach cancer appears to attack a small number of families in clusters. One famous example: Napoleon Bonaparte I and kin, who exhibited a remarkably high incidence of disease. The French emperor-general met his final Waterloo from gastric cancer while living in exile on the British island of St. Helena. It is said that his physician observed the 52-year-old Napoleon's suffering and quietly administered an overdose of mercurous chloride, killing him.

A family history of stomach cancer raises relatives' risk of getting the disease two- to threefold, though whether this is due to genetic inheritance, similar dietary habits or a combination of the two remains a mystery at present.

Likewise, we're still in the process of discovering why having type A blood elevates a person's chances of getting gastric cancer 15 to 20 percent. "It's an association that's been seen repeatedly in various areas of the world," says Dr. William Blot, chief of the biostatistics branch at the National Cancer Institute. "It could be through a genetic mechanism, but what that mechanism is, is unclear."

PERSONAL HEALTH HISTORY RISK FACTORS

- Personal history of pernicious anemia
- Personal history of chronic atrophic gastritis
- Personal history of achlorhydria or hypochlorhydria
- Personal history of partial removal of the stomach to treat a noncancerous condition
- Personal history of *Helicobacter pylori*

The stomach's inner layer, or *mucosa,* contains glands that secrete acid as well as mucus to protect it from abrasive chemicals. Any condition that damages this lining can initiate a chain of events ending in gastric cancer.

For instance, 1 in 10 patients suffering from *pernicious anemia* goes on to develop carcinoma of the stomach. This disorder is caused by the loss of normal stomach glands, resulting in a lack of what we call *intrinsic factor,* a sugar-protein compound, also secreted by the mucosa, that helps regulate the absorption of vitamin B_{12} from the small intestine. When vitamin B_{12} is not absorbed, anemia develops.

In addition, scientists believe that pernicious anemia increases the concentration of nitrite found in the gastric juice. Nitrite, discussed in greater detail later in this chapter, comes from the chemical food preservative nitrate and can turn into potent carcinogens called nitrosamines.

Another disorder, *chronic atrophic gastritis,* appears to unlock the doorway to cancer by destroying the stomach glands and inflaming the gastric lining. "In South America, Japan, China and other areas where stomach cancer rates are high," says Dr. Blot, "there seems to be a fairly consistent pattern of the normal gastric mucosa changing to superficial gastritis, then to chronic atrophic gastritis. This then gives way to precancerous changes in the cells and, finally, to cancer." These stages, in which the cells grow progressively abnormal, are called *metaplasia* and *dysplasia.*

Achlorhydria and *hypochlorhydria* result from either pernicious anemia or atrophic gastritis. In both, the stomach produces less acid than normal, raising the risk of cancer.

"The mechanism there is not clear," says Dr. Blot, "but it could be that bacteria are able to survive in the stomach because they're not killed off by the acid." These bacteria can then go to work on nitrite-laden foods that enter the stomach and act as catalysts in converting the nitrites to harmful nitrosamines.

Helicobacter pylori, the first bacterium cited as a contributor to human cancer, is believed to be a factor in 60 to 80 percent of all gastric malignancies. This microorganism, known to cause gastritis and ulcer disease, may induce carcinoma of the stomach by damaging the organ's lining, then promoting the uncontrolled cell growth that can result in cancer.

One pattern we don't fully understand is why patients who had a portion of their stomach surgically removed as treatment for a nonmalignant disease show a propensity for incurring gastric cancer within 15 to 40 years. It's been suggested the procedure sometimes causes bile from the small intestine to back up into the stomach, where it reacts with nitrites to form cancer-causing nitrosamines. The bile may also stimulate uncontrolled cell growth.

LIFESTYLE RISK FACTORS

- A diet high in salt-cured, smoked and salt-pickled foods

In this chapter we've alluded to nitrates, nitrites and nitrosamines, all key elements in both gastric and esophageal cancers. *Nitrates* are preservatives commonly found in (1) salt-cured foods such as bologna, ham, hot dogs and sausage; (2) smoked foods, including chicken, turkey, salmon and tuna; and (3) salt-pickled tongue, pickles and other salt-pickled meats and vegetables.

When you bite into a hot dog, the nitrates in the meat spontaneously convert to *nitrites* from the normal bacteria in your mouth. In fact, mere exposure to room temperatures brings about the same reaction. Whether or not nitrites possess carcinogenic properties in and of themselves has yet to be determined. However, in the stomach they can merge with other nitrogen-containing compounds, or *amines,* to form *nitrosamines.* "And nitrosamines are known to produce cancer in the laboratory," says Dr. Susan Pilch of the National Cancer Institute's diet and cancer branch. "We can test that."

WHO IS AT RISK?
ESOPHAGEAL CANCER

- Men and women age 50 and older

HEREDITARY RISK FACTORS

- None identified at present

PERSONAL HEALTH HISTORY RISK FACTORS

- Severe, persistent heartburn
- Personal history of Barrett's esophagus
- Untreated achalasia
- Caustic injury to the esophagus

Sometimes, explains Dr. Kurtz, "the acid from the stomach backs up, for whatever reason," and traverses the junction where the esophagus and stomach meet. Patients with this condition, called *reflux esophagitis,* experience a burning sensation in the chest and frequent regurgitation. Medication can usually relieve the symptoms, though some cases may require corrective surgery.

Reflux esophagitis may produce a transformation in the esophageal lining, so that it assumes the cellular characteristics of the stomach. "If it is within three centimeters of the gastroesophageal junction, it's considered normal," says Dr. Kurtz. "But if it goes beyond three centimeters, it's considered *Barrett's esophagus.*"

Barrett's, also referred to as Barrett's syndrome or Barrett's metaplasia, "is an acquired condition believed to develop some time after birth. And there is strong evidence to suggest that people who have Barrett's, probably as a result of reflux esophagitis, are more likely to develop cancer of the lower esophagus." According to the National Cancer Institute, the rate of cancer occurring in this junction has risen recently for men.

Whereas cancer of the esophagus is usually squamous-cell carcinoma, Barrett's induces adenocarcinoma, the form typically found in the stomach, in about 1 in 20 Barrett's patients. Upon diagnosing this disease, most gastroenterologists believe in monitoring the patient on an annual basis, using a fiber-optic instrument called an endoscope.

Achalasia, a disorder that produces progressive difficulty in swallowing, heightens a person's risk of esophageal cancer sevenfold if left untreated. And anyone who suffered caustic trauma to the esophagus (for example, from swallowing a corrosive substance) sees his odds of one day getting esophageal cancer

---

ARE YOU AT RISK FOR STOMACH CANCER?

_____ Men and women age 50 and older

Hereditary Risk Factors

_____ Family history of gastric cancer
_____ Type A blood

Personal Health History Risk Factors

_____ Personal history of pernicious anemia
_____ Personal history of chronic atrophic gastritis
_____ Personal history of achlorhydria or hypochlorhydria
_____ Personal history of the microorganism *Helicobacter pylori*
_____ Personal history of partial gastrectomy

Lifestyle Risk Factors

_____ A diet high in salt-cured, smoked and salt-pickled foods

If one or more of these risk factors applies to you, consult your physician.

skyrocket *1,000* times, according to a study of nearly 400 subjects.

LIFESTYLE RISK FACTORS

- Tobacco use
- Excessive alcohol use
- A diet high in salt-cured, smoked and salt-pickled foods

ARE YOU AT RISK FOR ESOPHAGEAL CANCER?

_____ Men and women age 50 and older

Hereditary Risk Factors

None identified at present

Personal Health History Risk Factors

_____ Severe, persistent heartburn
_____ Barrett's esophagus
_____ Untreated achalasia
_____ Caustic trauma to the esophagus (for example, from swallowing a corrosive substance)

Lifestyle Risk Factors

_____ Excessive alcohol use
_____ Tobacco use
_____ A diet high in salt-cured, smoked and pickled foods

If one or more of these risk factors applies to you, consult your physician.

PRIMARY PREVENTION GUIDELINES FOR BOTH GASTRIC AND ESOPHAGEAL CANCERS

In addition to the general primary prevention steps recommended at the beginning of Chapter 9:

- Cut down on salt-cured, nitrate-cured or smoked foods such as hot dogs, ham and bacon

GASTRIC AND ESOPHAGEAL CANCERS
AND DIET

To find out how vitamins A, C, E and selenium defend against gastric and esophageal cancers, researchers from the National Cancer Institute studied the people of Linxian, China, a rural county plagued by an extraordinarily high rate of fatal esophageal and gastric cancers: 10 times higher than elsewhere in China and 100 times higher than in the United States.

From 1986 to 1991 some 30,000 volunteers were divided into groups and given different combinations of daily vitamin and mineral supplements. While we encourage men and women in this country to get their vitamin intake from food, not supplements, the Linxian diet was glaringly deficient in a number of vitamins and nutrients.

The results, published in 1993, were promising: The group that received a form of vitamin E, the trace mineral selenium and beta-carotene (the plant form of vitamin A) exhibited a 21 percent reduction in mortality from gastric cancer, and a modest 4 percent reduction in deaths from esophageal cancer.

Since the average American is far better nourished than the people of Linxian, "I don't think you can extrapolate directly from China to the United States," cautions Dr. William Blot, one of the study's coauthors. But the report bolstered long-held theories that these and other vitamins could help prevent cancer.

By what mechanism or mechanisms might they work? First, beta-carotene, vitamin E and selenium are all antioxidants, which combine with carcinogens and prevent them from damaging the DNA in the body's cells. And second, wrote the researchers, "beta-carotene, vitamin E and selenium may also possess immunologic and other properties that influence carcinogenesis."

Because it's difficult to identify all the protective compounds in fruits and vegetables, we suggest eating at least five servings a day to cover all the bases, so to speak. "If you follow that diet," Dr. Blot notes, "it is likely that you will reduce your risk of both these cancers. Our study in China, I think, helps support that, because fruits and vegetables provide those nutrients."

Chapter 5 contains extensive lists of foods abundant in vitamins A and E, but here are several fine sources of each, as well as selenium:

Beta-carotene: carrots, squash, yams, peaches, papaya, apricots and broccoli.

Vitamin E: liver, nuts, corn, dried beans, olive oil, wheat germ.

Selenium: seafood, organ meats, lean meats, grains, produce grown in selenium-rich soil. Unlike New Zealand and parts of China and Finland, the average U.S. soil contains sufficient amounts of selenium, so American produce is generally adequate in this mineral.

Though the Linxian study found no significant correlation between vitamin C, another antioxidant, and lowered rates of gastric and esophageal cancers, it has already demonstrated its cancer-fighting value as a natural foe of nitrosamines. "What vitamin C does," explains Dr. Susan Pilch of the National Cancer Institute, "is to prevent nitrite-containing compounds from converting to nitrosamines in the stomach." Vitamin E, too, has shown an ability to thwart nitrosamine-induced esophageal cancer in mice.

SALTED AND/OR CURED FOODS

Japan, Scandinavia and Chile, all among the world leaders in stomach cancer, would appear to share few similarities dietetically. But their respective populations tend to consume an abundance of salt- and nitrate-treated foods.

Nitrates present less of a worry here. In recent years the U.S. Department of Agriculture and the Food and Drug Administration have lowered their acceptable levels of nitrates in prepared meats and fish to the absolute minimum. Furthermore, vitamin C and other nitrosamine-inhibiting substances are now routinely added to these foods.

For most Americans, the idea of having to pass up that hot dog at the ballpark would be tantamount to giving up turkey on Thanksgiving. According to Dr. Kurtz, when it comes to salted, smoked or cured foods high in nitrates, you merely need to exercise restraint.

"I think it would be judicious not to eat large quantities of hot dogs, salami, bologna and other processed meats," he says. "But to say that you can't have a bologna sandwich once in a while doesn't make any sense."

ESOPHAGEAL CANCER AND SMOKING AND ALCOHOL

As you know by now, tobacco smoke contains a number of powerful carcinogens and cocarcinogens. But it also irritates the mucosa of the gullet, which can promote precancerous changes. Half of all deaths from esophageal malignancies can be traced to tobacco use. In an American Cancer Society study of men and women in 25 states, smokers had more than four times the risk of esophageal cancer as nonsmokers.

A French study singled out alcohol as the *primary* cause of esophageal cancer, not tobacco, as had previously been believed. Because heavy drinkers tend to be heavy smokers, scientists had blamed the disease mainly on the latter habit.

"That's why the study in France was so interesting," says Dr. Charles Lieber, director of the alcohol research and treatment center at the Department of Veterans Affairs Medical Center in the Bronx, New York, "because they disassociated drinking from smoking." Participants were split up into three groups: one that drank excessively but smoked moderately; one that exhibited the reverse behavior; and a third that drank and smoked to excess.

"Although both factors were important," says Dr. Lieber, "drinking had twice the impact of smoking. With smoking, there

---

SECONDARY PREVENTION GUIDELINES

For Stomach Cancer

For Asymptomatic Men and Women with No Special Risk Factors
• None recommended at present

For Asymptomatic Men and Women at Increased Risk
• None recommended at present

For Esophageal Cancer

For Asymptomatic Men and Women with No Special Risk Factors
• None recommended at present

For Asymptomatic Men and Women at Increased Risk

For those with Barrett's esophagus:

• Annual upper GI endoscopy with biopsy

was a four- to fivefold increase in the incidence of esophageal cancer; with heavy drinking, a ten- to elevenfold increase. And of course both together had a tremendous impact, effecting a forty-four-fold increase."

Alcohol promotes esophageal cancer by irritating the esophageal lining and triggering the metabolism of cancer-causing agents in the gullet. Furthermore, notes Dr. Kurtz, "People who abuse alcohol often have vitamin deficiencies, particularly of vitamin A."

If you drink at all, do so in moderation, which we define as no more than four alcoholic beverages a week.

SCREENING

No cancer agencies currently recommend routine screening for either esophageal cancer or stomach cancer. It's not that procedures to detect these two diseases have proved ineffective. Quite the contrary, says Dr. Kurtz.

"In Japan, where the gastric cancer rate is very high, they screen everybody who has even minimal symptoms that we in America would toss off as being indigestion," he notes. That country's five-year survival rate after surgery for stomach cancer is nearly double that of the United States. But since gastric and esophageal cancers are relatively rare here, screening asymptomatic patients is not warranted.

Patient Leonard S., a retired real-estate salesman from New Jersey, might not be alive today had he not paid an annual visit to his gastroenterologist. "I'd had ulcers a few years back," says the married grandfather of two, "and was very satisfied with the doctor, so I continued to have yearly examinations with him."

In 1990 his physician decided to perform an endoscopic examination of the esophagus and stomach. "He just felt it was time to do this procedure," explains Leonard, then 73, "and that's when they found I had a problem": abnormal-looking cells in the gullet. "They took a biopsy of it, and it came back that it was precancerous.

"I was startled," he recalls, "because I'd had no symptoms whatsoever." Leonard came for a consultation to Memorial Sloan-Kettering. Upon learning he would have to undergo a partial removal of the esophagus, "I thought, *Gosh, I'm not going to be able to talk anymore*. But they assured me I would be able to.

Within four, five days of the operation I was walking the halls in the hospital, and I was out of there in about two weeks."

Leonard and his wife regularly spend the winter months in the Florida sun. Before heading south, he says, "I have my regular physical checkup and go back to my gastrointestinal man once a year. A lot of friends my age do the same thing."

According to Dr. Kurtz, only a diagnosis of Barrett's esophagus would justify annual screening. "That is the one area where we utilize surveillance endoscopy," he says. "When Barrett's is found because of significant symptoms of reflux esophagitis, patients are routinely followed with endoscopy and biopsies taken on an annual basis looking for severe dysplasia.

"I don't know whether or not long-term studies will demonstrate that this will find early esophageal cancers from Barrett's," he continues, "but endoscopy is available, and I think many gastroenterologists feel uncomfortable not doing regular surveillance endoscopies in patients who have documented Barrett's esophagus."

UPPER GI SERIES

Prior to an upper GI series, an x-ray of the esophagus, the stomach and the upper small intestine, you are asked to swallow a mouthful of barium sulfate, a white, chalky radiopaque contrast solution that coats the inside of hollow organs and shows up on x-ray. In addition to taking x-ray pictures at different stages, the doctor can also use a special x-ray machine called a *fluoroscope* to track the barium as it glides down the gullet.

"With fluoroscopy," explains Dr. Robert Heelan, a radiologist, "we can actually look at the body while it's working and evaluate the swallowing mechanism and the wavelike movement of the GI tract, to see if they're normal. We can also look to see if there's a tumor present, or a narrowing or stricture of the esophagus."

The test lasts anywhere from 15 to 40 minutes and involves no discomfort, although Dr. Heelan notes, "Some people claim not to like the taste of the barium," which is usually peppermint or citrus flavored. "But most find it, if not exactly wonderful tasting, at least palatable."

UPPER GI ENDOSCOPY WITH BIOPSY

In an upper GI endoscopy, the physician examines the entire upper gastrointestinal tract using a fiber-optic viewing device called an *endoscope.*

You will be asked not to eat breakfast the morning of the test. The doctor begins by injecting a sedative into a vein, which makes you feel drowsy; afterward, most patients remember nothing about the procedure. "This is not general anesthesia," clarifies Dr. Kurtz, "where patients are anesthetized to the point of needing breathing assistance."

The flexible scope is passed into the mouth and down the esophagus. "Next we enter the stomach, and look throughout there," says Dr. Kurtz, "and then go into the first portion of the small intestine [the duodenum] and do the same thing.

"There may be some mild gagging," he adds, but due to the sedation, "it's usually not identified as such by the patient." A tiny brush or biopsy forceps can be passed through the scope for removing tissue samples, which are then analyzed by a pathologist. Fifteen to twenty minutes after the beginning of the procedure, the doctor withdraws the scope. Because of the effects of the sedative, expect to spend one to two hours in recovery, and make arrangements for someone to drive you home.

Unless this country should experience an unexpected upsurge in stomach cancer and esophageal cancer, guidelines recommending routine screening tests are not likely. The issue in the United States is really primary-care physicians' heightened awareness of the early symptoms of gastric cancer, which are very nonspecific. The public, too, needs to familiarize itself with the warning signs of stomach cancer, as well as esophageal cancer, and not underestimate the seriousness of these rare but deadly diseases.

SUGGESTED READING ABOUT STOMACH AND ESOPHAGEAL CANCERS

From the National Cancer Institute (800-4-CANCER):

- "What You Need to Know About Cancer of the Esophagus"

KEY WORDS

Achalasia: A neuromuscular disorder of the esophagus that causes difficulty in swallowing. If left untreated, achalasia heightens a person's risk of esophageal cancer sevenfold.

Achlorhydria: Achlorhydria and *hypochlorhydria* reduce production of stomach acid.

Adenocarcinoma: Cancer that arises in glandular tissue or assumes the form of a glandlike structure.

Barrett's esophagus: A condition in which the cells in the lower esophagus assume the characteristics of those in the stomach, due to stomach acid backing up into the gullet. Approximately 1 in 20 Barrett's patients later develop esophageal cancer.

Chronic atrophic gastritis: A risk factor for stomach cancer, this disorder destroys the stomach glands and inflames the gastric lining.

Dysphagia: Difficulty swallowing.

Esophagectomy: Surgery to remove an esophageal tumor and part or all of the esophagus.

Gastrectomy: Surgery to remove part (subtotal) or all (total) of the stomach.

Gastroenterologist: A physician who specializes in diagnosing and treating diseases of the digestive tract.

Helicobacter pylori: The first bacterium cited as a contributor to human cancer, it has been associated with gastric malignancies and is a known cause of gastritis.

Nitrates: Preservatives commonly found in salt-cured, smoked and salt-pickled foods that convert to *nitrites,* which in turn can merge with other nitrogen-containing compounds, or *amines,* to form *nitrosamines,* proven carcinogens.

Pernicious anemia: A disorder that inflames the stomach lining and destroys acid-secreting glands, inhibiting the absorption of vitamin B_{12}. This process is a risk factor for gastric cancer.

CHAPTER

16

Skin Cancers

Basal-Cell Carcinoma •
Squamous-Cell Carcinoma •
Malignant Melanoma •
Safe Sunning Habits •
How to Examine Your Skin

S kin cancer is the most prevalent type of cancer. It is also the easiest to avoid, because the vast majority of these malignancies are caused by overexposure to the sun's ultraviolet rays. Alarmingly, cancers of the skin are on the rise, afflicting 732,000 Americans in 1994. *Malignant melanoma,* the most virulent form, soared 500 percent between 1950 and 1985.

This staggering upsurge can be attributed partly to environmental factors, but especially to the cultural changes that began taking effect around the half-century mark. The aftermath of World War II saw massive migration to the South and Southwest, where the sun's rays are most intense. Around the same time, improved transportation and a booming economy provided Americans unprecedented access to vacation paradises in sunny climes the world over. Add to this today's more casual clothing styles, which leave more areas of the body exposed.

Our modern-day culture promotes tan skin as a barometer of success, well-being and health. Ironic, that last one, in view of the fact that a suntan is actually the visible manifestation of injury to the skin. Although the skin can heal superficial damage, repeated exposure over time impairs its ability to ward off the sun's cancer-causing effects.

It is a fallacy, incidentally, that dry, wrinkled skin is the inevitable badge of aging. In fact, were you to protect yourself completely from sunlight, your skin would remain virtually as soft and smooth as the unexposed skin on your buttocks.

The physical ideal of a golden, lean body is a recent phenomenon. It wasn't so long ago that milky white skin and a well-fed physique were equated with affluence, whereas a tan complexion and thin build identified someone as a member of the lower class, who often toiled outdoors, malnourished.

Despite persistent warnings about the dangers of excessive sunning, sunworshippers' habits have remained largely unchanged. It is presently estimated that nearly half of all men and women to reach age 65 will develop skin cancer in their lifetime.

Dr. Bijan Safai spent 20 years at Memorial Sloan-Kettering, much of that time as head of dermatology. When he started here in 1973, dermatology service didn't even exist. It was under his direction that the center began offering free skin-cancer screenings, an historic event that grew into an annual tradition. According to Dr. Safai, now chairman of the dermatology department at New York Medical College, most Americans do not treat the threat of skin cancer seriously because the disease usually doesn't surface until the later stages of life. But that pattern is changing, he notes ominously, as young people rack up what was once a lifetime's worth of sun exposure in a relatively short time span. Whereas nonmelanoma skin cancer typically struck after age 50, he now sees patients in their twenties and thirties.

"They are much more exposed," he says. "And that's dangerous." Of the 32,000 new cases of melanoma in 1994, one in four involved men and women under 39.

The emotional fallout from skin cancer can be devastating. Patients' realization that they unwittingly contributed to their condition often places on them an added burden of guilt, something that is always painful to witness.

Dr. Safai remarks, "I can tell you story after story of people who suddenly have to face the fact that they are going to die in two to four years because they have melanoma or squamous-cell carcinoma. Or lose part of their nose or ears or eyes to basal-cell carcinoma. All because they were careless. And these are patients who are extremely educated, intelligent and successful. Still, they

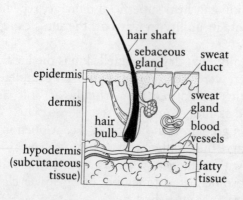

Normal Skin. The skin, which is divided into two main layers, constantly renews itself, with cells from the dermis pushing upward to replace those of the epidermis.

expose themselves to the sun every day. And if there's no sun, they go to a tanning salon."

THE SKIN

You may not think of your skin as an organ, but it happens to be the human body's largest. Skin performs a number of vital functions. Most obvious is protection: from infection, injury, heat, chemicals and sunlight. Nerve endings embedded in the skin speed messages about pain, touch, temperature, pressure and other sensations to the brain. It also governs body temperature, stores water and fat, and assists in manufacturing vitamin D.

The skin consists of two main layers. The thin outer layer, or *epidermis,* contains three main types of cells: *basal cells, squamous cells* and, at its deepest point, *melanocytes.* The latter produce *melanin,* the dark pigment that gives skin its color and protects it from the sun. A tan, very simply, is the skin's response to UV (ultraviolet) rays: Within about 48 hours of sun exposure, the melanocytes transfer melanin to nonpigment-forming cells as a means of safeguarding against further injury.

The thick inner layer, *dermis,* can be likened to a bustling control center. There blood and lymph vessels transport their essential fluids. Sweat glands regulate body temperature by excreting water, urea and other waste products through the pores, while another gland produces sebum, which keeps the skin lubricated. Hair follicles, nerves and fatty tissue also reside in the dermis.

Malignancies of the skin take hold exclusively in the epidermis, due mostly to invisible ultraviolet rays emitted by the sun. Solar radiation is classified according to its wavelength, with UVA the longest and UVC the shortest. Ozone gases in the atmosphere absorb most of the sun's radiation, so that only a small percentage of UVA and UVB radiation reaches the earth's surface. UVB rays burn the skin more easily and are known to have cancer-causing potential. Only after recent animal studies have UVA rays fallen under suspicion as well. These rays don't burn skin as readily, but penetrate tissue more deeply.

BASAL-CELL CARCINOMA

Basal-cell carcinoma, the most common form of skin cancer, affects the tiny, round basal cells. It was first observed in the late nineteenth century among sailors, who spent much of their day under the sun's glare. Scientists named these lesions "sailor's skin" or "*Seamanshaut.*" Turn-of-the-century farmers, too, showed a preponderance of skin cancer.

The disease usually expresses itself as a small, pearly bump on the face, neck or hands, the nose being the most frequent site. Left untreated, basal-cell carcinomas can crust, bleed or ulcerate.

These tumors grow slowly, taking months, even years to measure half an inch in diameter. Although they rarely spread to other parts of the body, basal-cell carcinomas can root under the skin, causing disfigurement and considerable damage to the underlying bone, cartilage and muscle. It is staged as either localized or metastatic and has a cure rate of better than 99 percent if detected early. A *dermatologist,* a physician specializing in diseases of the skin, can treat basal-cell carcinoma a number of ways:

• *Curettage.* In this method, the most common, a local anesthetic is injected into the area; then the doctor uses an instrument called a *curette* to remove the tumor. A second step, *electrodesiccation,* is sometimes necessary to stanch bleeding and destroy any remaining cancer cells by applying an electrical current through a needle electrode. Combined, the two techniques are referred to as curettage and desiccation. One side effect is that this procedure frequently leaves a faint scar.

• *Surgical excision.* Here the malignancy and a small border of normal skin are surgically removed, also under local anesthesia. In some cases the incision is large enough to require a skin graft, in which healthy skin is transferred from one area of the body to another. For example, tissue from behind the ear is often taken and grafted onto the face.

• *Mohs' technique* is generally reserved for difficult-to-treat or recurrent skin cancers, or those located on the eyelid, face or head. This specialized microscopic surgery may also be called on when the extent of the cancer is unclear. It requires utmost precision, for the growth is removed layer by layer and checked under the microscope until only healthy tissue remains.

• For patients who cannot undergo surgery, *cryotherapy* is often the answer. The dermatologist sprays liquid nitrogen onto the lesion, freezing it and killing the abnormal cells, which then thaw and flake off. Like electrosurgery, cryotherapy typically leaves a white scar.

• *Radiation therapy* may be used for especially large or recurrent tumors. Skin cancers of the eyelid, ear and tip of the nose are examples of sites sometimes treated this way.

• In *topical chemotherapy,* 5-fluorouracil (5-FU), an anticancer drug that comes in both cream and lotion form, is applied to the affected area every day for several weeks.

• *Carbon dioxide laser.* Presently considered investigational by many doctors, the carbon dioxide laser vaporizes skin tumors. It is sometimes employed in conjunction with curettage.

Over half a million Americans developed basal-cell carcinoma in 1994. Though it is not fatal, a diagnosis is unnerving nonetheless, especially because the disease can touch those as young as their early 20s. Patricia R., a writer from Long Island, New York, discovered a bump in 1979 at age 23.

"I had really long hair," she recalls, "and one day when I brushed it, I felt something on my neck." She examined it in the mirror. "It was raised and whitish-pinkish—not one color—and it didn't have the smooth feel of a regular mole." Concerned about what it might be, the young woman brought it to the attention of a medical student she knew.

"It just so happened that this friend of mine was talking about his dermatology classes, and I said, 'It's funny you mention that, because I have this thing on my neck. I don't know what it is.' He looked at it and said, 'You should see a doctor right away.' " She still remembers the exact words of the dermatologist after he'd biopsied the growth and prepared to send it to a pathology lab.

"He told me, 'I'm 99.9 percent sure this is benign. You're too young. You're not a sun worshipper.' There was still this idea that only people who baked in the sun got skin cancer." A week later the dermatologist called her at work and with surprise in his voice said, "You have to come to the office. It's cancer."

"I flipped," she says, "because at the time I didn't know the difference between the various types of skin cancer, and my mother had died of pancreatic cancer just six years earlier." The lesion was removed by curettage, required no further treatment and has never returned. Half of all recurrences flare up within five years.

Patricia's brush with skin cancer made her appreciate that there is no such thing as having "just" basal-cell carcinoma. "Even though it's the least dangerous form of skin cancer, it's still very, very scary," she says, "the idea that it can happen to you."

SQUAMOUS-CELL CARCINOMA

The second most frequently seen skin cancer affects more than 130,000 people annually. *Squamous-cell carcinoma,* which forms in the flat, scalelike squamous cells, is also typically found on areas of the body exposed to the sun: face, ears, lips, mouth, neck, hands, arms and back. In extremely rare instances it can occur on the genitals of either sex, as well as in the anal area.

These tumors do not appear markedly different from basal-cell carcinomas. Look for a raised red or pink scaly nodule, or a wart-like growth with an ulcerated center. However, squamous-cell malignancies expand far more rapidly and have the capacity to spread to other organs. It too is staged as either localized or meta-static. The disease claimed more than 2,000 lives in 1994, but with early detection and treatment, squamous-cell carcinoma is 95 percent curable.

A precursor, *actinic keratosis,* identifies itself as a slightly raised tan, red, brownish or grayish hardened patch measuring a quarter inch to half an inch across. About 1 in 20 of these premalignant conditions turn into squamous-cell carcinoma, which can be treated through the same methods outlined above for basal-cell carcinoma.

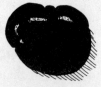

Normal pigmented mole   Growth typical of melanoma

Mole vs. Melanoma. A typical mole has symmetrical borders and even coloration, which can range from pink to dark brown or black, and does not tend to grow. In contrast, a melanoma suddenly begins to grow and is characterized by its Asymmetry, irregular Borders, uneven Coloration and a Diameter of more than a quarter inch. These characteristics are often referred to as the ABCD of melanoma.

MALIGNANT MELANOMA

Dr. Safai uses the term "silent epidemic" to describe melanoma's prodigious increase: 96 percent in the 1980s alone. Three fourths of all skin-cancer mortalities stem from melanoma. Although it

---

SIGNS AND SYMPTOMS OF MELANOMA

Everyone should examine his or her skin periodically for unusual existing moles or new pigmented growths, both of which can be harbingers of melanoma. Among Caucasians, 2 percent to 5 percent have atypical *nevi* (the medical term for moles). Use the following ABCD rule of thumb to gauge whether or not a mole is a potential melanoma:

A = *Asymmetrical:* One half is shaped differently than the other.

B = *Border* is irregular, its edges ragged, blurred or notched.

C = *Color* appears uneven or changes over time. Blemishes usually begin as mottled brown or black, but may eventually assume shades of blue, white or red.

D = *Diameter* exceeds a quarter inch; about the size of a pencil eraser.

A mole manifesting these characteristics should be reported to a dermatologist at once. Not all atypical nevi warrant immediate removal, however. Some people have upward of 100; to eliminate every one would prove expensive and possibly result in cosmetic problems. Many dermatologists prefer to carefully track the progress of these unusual moles and order surgery only for suspicious lesions.

mainly affects the skin, the disease can surface wherever melanocytes exist in the body, including the eye and oral cavity.

Some melanomas emerge as new growths, but others appear in
a preexisting mole. A mole, which varies in size and depth, is
merely a cluster of melanocytes. Most form at birth or before age
20; by adulthood the average person has about 25 moles.

STAGING OF MELANOMA

Unless arrested, melanoma rampages through the following
stages, eventually involving the lymph nodes and, in its most se-

STAGING OF MALIGNANT MELANOMA

STAGE	CHARACTERISTICS	FIVE-YEAR SURVIVAL RATE
0	Cells are precancerous, or in situ.	100%
IA	Melanoma thinner than 0.75 millimeters, or $1/32$ inch.	80%–100%
IB	Growth measures 0.76 millimeters to 1.5 millimeters, or $1/32$ to $1/16$ inch, in thickness.	80%–100%
II	Melanoma 1.51 to 4.0 millimeters ($1/16$ to $1/8$ inch) thick.	Up to 65%
IIIA	Tumor 4.1 millimeters ($1/8$ inch) thick or greater; has metastasized to skin or to *subcutaneous* tissue beneath the skin within 2 centimeters ($3/4$ inch) of primary tumor.	20%–50%
IIIB	Melanoma of any size has spread to a single group of nearby lymph nodes or to skin or subcutaneous tissue more than 2 centimeters from original tumor.	20%–50%
IV	Disease has involved one enlarged and fixed lymph-node group, more than one lymph-node group, or another organ or area of skin.	Less than 10%

vere manifestation, invading vital organs such as the liver and lungs. About 95 percent of all cases are treated surgically, with chemotherapy, radiation therapy and/or biologic therapy sometimes used as well for advanced disease.

WHO IS AT RISK?

- Men and women age 40 and older

The fact that skin cancer generally doesn't occur until relatively late in life shouldn't lead anyone, regardless of age, into thinking she can afford to ignore the primary-prevention steps presented in this chapter. To reiterate a point made earlier, the average age of onset for skin cancer appears to be dropping, a trend directly related to hazardous sunning habits.

HEREDITARY RISK FACTORS

- Fair complexion; many freckles; blond or red hair; blue, green or gray eyes; a greater-than-average number of moles; atypical moles; a large congenital mole
- Family history of xeroderma pigmentosum, albinism, basal-cell nevus syndrome, dysplastic nevus syndrome and/or familial atypical multiple mole melanoma (FAMMM) syndrome
- Family history of melanoma

Predisposition to melanoma can run in families, more than doubling a relative's chances of getting the disease. Several rare genetic skin disorders also place family members at increased risk for it and other skin cancers.

Xeroderma pigmentosum leaves the skin and eyes acutely sensitive to light. People with this condition lack an enzyme that repairs sun damage to the DNA. They tend to develop numerous skin tumors early in life. Albinos (anyone affected with *albinism)* similarly suffer from sunlight intolerance, due to their partial or total lack of protective melanin. Sun exposure exacerbates *basal-cell nevus syndrome,* a genetic propensity to grow malignancies in areas not usually affected, such as the palms of the hands and the soles of the feet.

Another syndrome, *dysplastic nevus syndrome,* affects families plagued by melanoma, heightening relatives' susceptibility to the disease. The same is true of the dominant genetic disorder *familial atypical multiple mole melanoma (FAMMM) syndrome,* which additionally puts family members at risk for cancers of the eye, breast, respiratory tract, gastrointestinal tract and lymphatic system.

It has yet to be shown that basal-cell and squamous-cell carcinomas are inherited. However, genetics play an indirect role in all skin cancers, in that we inherit certain biologic traits that greatly influence our risk. For example, it is known that a fair-complexioned Caucasian is twice as likely to get melanoma as an olive-skinned person. Or that blonds or people with red hair have two to four times the risk of melanoma as brunettes. Other characteristics common to skin cancer patients include freckles; blue, green or gray eyes; a greater-than-average number of moles; atypical moles; and an unusually large congenital mole (one formed at birth).

Dermatologists rely primarily on skin type and the amount of sun exposure to determine who is most at risk for skin cancer. The following table shows the six different classifications established by the American Academy of Dermatology, along with examples of each.

TYPE	EXAMPLE
I: *Extremely sun-sensitive skin:* those who burn easily and never tan	People with red hair, freckles; Celtics, Irish-Scots
II: *Very sun-sensitive skin:* those who burn easily and tan minimally	Fair-skinned, fair-haired, blue-eyed Caucasians
III: *Sun-sensitive skin:* those who sometimes burn and tan gradually to a light brown	Average skin
IV: *Minimally sun-sensitive skin:* those who burn minimally and always tan to a moderate brown	Mediterranean Caucasians
V: *Sun-insensitive skin:* those who rarely burn and tan well	Middle Easterners, some Hispanics, some African-Americans
VI: *Deeply pigmented sun-insensitive skin:* those who never burn and tan darkly	African-Americans and others with dark pigmentation

Types I and II are considered at high risk; type III at average risk; type IV at reduced risk; and types IV, V and VI at little risk. Of course, another extremely important factor—people's behavior—figures into this equation. A type IV person who neglects to follow safe sunning practices may put herself at greater risk for skin cancer than a type I person who wears sunscreen, avoids the midday sun and so on.

African-Americans and other dark-skinned people have less than one tenth the number of skin malignancies that Caucasians do because their skin contains a higher concentration of melanin.

PERSONAL HEALTH HISTORY RISK FACTORS

- Pregnancy
- Personal history of diseases, treatments and/or medical procedures that compromise the immune system
- Exposure to medical x-rays or treatments utilizing artificial UV radiation
- Personal history of skin cancer

Several past or present medical conditions can heighten your risk of skin cancer. You may be surprised to learn that the hormonal changes of pregnancy drive up a woman's sensitivity to sunlight. Accordingly, an expectant mother should avoid the beach, or at the very least wear protective clothing and sunscreen. If normally at reduced risk for skin cancer, she can console herself that this is a temporary state of affairs and dream ahead to next summer.

Because an impaired immune system creates a favorable environment for skin cancer, lymphoma and leukemia patients are considered higher risks for skin tumors. So is anyone who has received chemotherapy and/or radiation, both of which can ravage the immune system response. Immunosuppressive drugs used to prevent the body from rejecting a transplanted kidney may impair the immune system's ability to block the growth of skin malignancies.

Other medical procedures, such as x-rays, can increase your risk of skin cancer. Phototherapy, a method of treating the skin disease psoriasis with artificial UV radiation, has grown in popularity. Sometimes, in addition, the patient is given a drug called psoralen, which makes the skin more sensitive to the ultraviolet light. Men or women undergoing this technique may want to discuss it with their doctor, for according to research published by the National Cancer Institute, "recent studies suggest that these patients are at increased risk of developing nonmelanoma skin cancer."

ENVIRONMENTAL RISK FACTORS

- Working with chemicals such as arsenic and polycyclic aromatic hydrocarbons
- Working outdoors
- Exposure to industrial radiation
- Proximity to the equator and other geographical factors

Various chemicals routinely used in the workplace are known to enhance the risk of skin cancer. For example, polycyclic aromatic hydrocarbons (PAH), typically found in asphalt, coal tars, soot, pitch, creosotes, paraffin waxes, and lubricating and cutting oils, induce squamous-cell carcinoma in animals. Epidemiologic studies of workers exposed to PAH—shale-oil workers, jute workers, wax pressmen and tool setters who run automatic lathes— have revealed a high propensity for the disease. Naturally highway asphalters, roofers and anyone else who works with PAH under the sun's glare raises his or her odds of developing a skin malignancy.

Chapter 7, on carcinogens in the workplace and the home, offers recommendations on how to protect yourself on the job, not only by observing safety regulations and wearing protective gear, but, if necessary, by alerting the appropriate government agencies to an employer's health and safety violations.

Where you work and live also affects your level of risk. In the 1970s the National Cancer Institute set up solar-radiation meters in cities scattered across the United States. Comparing those readings with the skin cancer rates in four of the cities confirmed that proximity to the equator elevates the likelihood of skin tumors. Indeed, southerners have double the rate of skin cancer as compared with northerners.

However, latitude isn't the only geographical factor; altitude and cloud cover also have an influence. Consider that Atlanta, Georgia, and El Paso, Texas, sit on the same parallel, approximately 32 degrees latitude north. Yet on account of El Paso's drier climate and higher elevation, it has a 38 percent higher UVB count than Atlanta.

LIFESTYLE RISK FACTORS

- Excessive sun exposure during the first 10 to 15 years of life
- Blistering sunburns

One or more severe sunburns received during childhood or adolescence increases your chance of getting melanoma.

ARE YOU AT RISK FOR SKIN CANCERS?

Basal-cell Carcinoma   *   Squamous-cell Carcinoma   *   Melanoma

_____ Men and women age 40 and older

Hereditary Risk Factors

Any of the following traits:
_____ Fair complexion
_____ Red or blond hair
_____ Many freckles
_____ Blue, green or gray eyes
_____ A greater-than-average number of moles
_____ Atypical moles
_____ A large congenital mole (one present at birth)

_____ Family history of xeroderma pigmentosum
_____ Family history of albinism
_____ Family history of basal-cell nevus syndrome
_____ Family history of dysplastic nevus syndrome
_____ Family history of familial atypical multiple mole melanoma (FAMMM) syndrome
_____ Family history of melanoma

Personal Health History Risk Factors

_____ Pregnancy
_____ Personal history of leukemia
_____ Personal history of lymphoma
_____ Any medical condition that required chemotherapy or radiation therapy
_____ Personal history of kidney transplant
_____ Exposure to medical x-rays or treatments utilizing artificial ultraviolet radiation
_____ Personal history of skin cancer

Environmental Risk Factors

_____ Working with chemicals such as arsenic and polycyclic aromatic hydrocarbons
_____ Working outdoors
_____ Exposure to industrial radiation
_____ Close proximity to the equator

Lifestyle Risk Factors

_____ Excessive sun exposure during the first 10 to 15 years of life
_____ One or more blistering sunburns during childhood or adolescence

If one or more of these risk factors applies to you, consult your physician.

WAYS TO REDUCE YOUR RISK

GUIDELINES FOR PRIMARY PREVENTION

- Avoid the midday sun.
- Wear protective clothing.
- Apply sunscreen to unprotected skin.
- Avoid tanning parlors.
- Especially avoid the sun if you are taking medications containing Retin-A, tetracycline, sulfa drugs, thiazide diuretic or indomethacin.

Taking precautions against solar radiation doesn't require living like a hermit, or cloaking yourself from head to toe like one of the Jedi from the movie *Star Wars*. It merely calls for moderation and preparation.

Awareness of safe-sunning habits truly entered the public consciousness only within the past two decades. Patricia R., the young woman who got basal-cell carcinoma in her early twenties, recalls that while growing up in Key West, Florida, in the mid-1960s, "I don't think anybody really knew about sunscreen. And if you got a sunburn, it was part of the normal course of events, like a kid scraping his knee."

Today Patricia applies sunscreen before any activity that may expose her to the sun. She wisely does the same for her two-year-old son. "It's the parents' responsibility to prevent their child from being in the sun too much and getting sunburned," says Dr. Safai, noting that the seeds of skin cancer are usually planted before adulthood. About 80 percent of a person's lifetime sun exposure comes in the first 18 years of life. The Skin Cancer Foundation recommends that children begin wearing sunscreen at six months. Just as important, they should be taught the guidelines to sun safety, the same way they learn other safety habits.

Some parents believe that youngsters need plenty of sun in order to stay healthy. While it is true that sunlight helps to produce vitamin D in the skin, a well-rounded diet high in milk and milk products can supply a more than adequate amount of this vitamin. Infants age six months and younger should be kept out of the midday sun or at least be well covered by clothing and a wide-brimmed hat.

SAFE SUNNING

The sun's ultraviolet rays are harshest from 10 A.M. to 2 P.M. (11 A.M. to 3 P.M. during daylight savings time). Just avoiding solar radiation between 11 A.M. and 1 P.M. (12 P.M. and 2 P.M. DST) can reduce your exposure by *half*. But as Dr. Safai points out, "This really depends where you are on the earth's surface. If you're near the equator, the sun can be very strong even at nine o'clock in the morning."

The National Cancer Institute has come up with a "shadow method" that is applicable anywhere, any season. Very simply, if your shadow is shorter than you are, stay indoors, for this indicates the sun is overhead, and its UV rays are at their strongest.

When out in the sun, cover up. Nine of ten skin cancers form on areas uncovered by clothing. That is why women have more skin cancers of the leg than do men. "Wear a hat, a long-sleeved shirt and pants or a skirt," advises Dr. Safai. Tightly woven garments are best; white fabrics, though a fashion favorite in summertime, can actually act as a conduit for solar radiation. The same is true of wet clothes that cling to the body. Since shorts and sleeveless tops are more comfortable in hot weather, be certain to rub sunblock on any and all bare skin.

SUNSCREENS

Sunscreens are classified in strength according to their Sun Protection Factor, or SPF, which ranges from 2 to 50. Dr. Safai explains: "If someone burns in 10 minutes, and he puts on sunscreen number 10, it will take him 150 minutes to burn. In other words, sunscreen delays the skin-burning effect of sun exposure; the higher the SPF number, the longer it will take you to burn."

In determining the grade of protection you need, you must take into account your skin type. "Generally speaking, a fair-skinned person who burns easily needs a sunscreen with a higher SPF," Dr. Safai says, "while for someone who tans easily a lower number will suffice." *Even when using an appropriate sunscreen, prolonged sun exposure is still discouraged.*

Both the American Academy of Dermatology and the Skin Cancer Foundation recommend using sunblocks with an SPF of at least 15, no matter what your skin type. SPF 15 screens out 93 percent of the sun's burning rays. Using it for the first 18 years of life can lower a person's skin cancer risk by an impressive 80 percent. As a point of comparison, SPF 2 provides only 50 percent protection; and SPF 34, 97 percent.

These ratings refer exclusively to UVB rays, incidentally; the Food and Drug Administration (FDA) has yet to set standards measuring protection against UVA rays. The major ingredient in most absorbent sunscreens, PABA (para-aminobenzoic acid), is highly effective against UVB rays, but not UVA rays. Therefore, we advise using so-called "broad-spectrum" sunscreens. Scan the label for beneficial ingredients such as:

- benzophenones
- oxybenzone
- sulisobenzone
- Parsol 1789 (butyl methoxydibenzoylmethane, also known as avobenzone)
- titanium dioxide
- zinc oxide

The latter two are usually found in the opaque-cream sunblocks, which are excellent for masking the nose, lips, shoulders and other sensitive areas. Because some people have allergic reactions to PABA, almost all drugstores carry sunscreens containing some of the aforementioned alternatives.

The general rule is to apply sunblock to your dry skin roughly twenty minutes before going out in the sun, then reapply it at least once every two hours while you're outside. (One ounce should cover your entire body.) But Dr. Safai emphasizes that once again skin type, time of day and location must all be considered.

"Most physicians," he goes on to say, "recommend you put sunscreen on your skin every morning, so it builds up." Sunscreens rub off and wash away, however, even brands claiming to be water-resistant. "If you are swimming, each time you come out of the water, put it on. If you're perspiring, and it gets washed away by sweat, then you must apply it again."

Some other important tips concerning sunscreens:

- Oil sunscreens typically offer only minimal protection, SPF 2, while gel types wash off easily.
- Wear sunscreen even on overcast days. Though the sun may be obscured by clouds, 80 percent of its harmful rays still reach your skin.
- Skiers should dab sunscreen on exposed skin, for snow can reflect 80 percent of the sun onto your face, especially at high altitudes. Other reflective surfaces include concrete, sand, water, snow and ice.
- Be careful to avoid your eyes, and wash your hands thoroughly after applying.
- Protect your eyes by wearing sunglasses.

TANNING BOOTHS

It's a common misconception that tanning booths are safer than sunning outdoors. "Tanning booths are not safe," warns Dr. Safai. "One, they intensify the ultraviolet rays. And two, they make tanning *available*." Each day one million Americans, mainly young people, frequent tanning parlors. Believing that UVA rays were safer than UVB rays, most of these establishments have switched from UVB sunlamps to models that emit 95 percent UVA rays and 5 percent UVB rays. But as we've pointed out, UVA radiation is now presumed to promote nonmelanoma skin cancers. Furthermore, a mere 1 percent of UVB radiation can increase skin cancer risk. The FDA, charged with regulating the labeling of tanning devices, insists that the long-term effects from sunlamps may be no different than those from solar radiation. Yet another factor: Tanning parlors aren't always carefully monitored, so that customers may use the equipment without proper calibration supervision or protective eyewear.

SKIN CANCER AND DIET

Dr. Safai advises his patients to eat a well-rounded diet rich in vitamins A, C and E, all antioxidants. No conclusive reports of their value yet exist, he says, "but there is some anecdotal evidence that these vitamins are a way to prevent skin cancer." In addition, it has recently been reported that a low-fat diet can help protect against skin cancer.

SKIN CANCER AND MEDICATIONS

Medications containing Retin-A, tetracycline, sulfa drugs, thiazide diuretics or indomethacin may make the skin more sensitive to sunlight and more apt to burn. If you are taking any of these medications, consult your doctor before going sunning, whether the light source is natural or artificial.

GUIDELINES FOR SECONDARY PREVENTION

For Asymptomatic Men and Women with No Special Risk Factors

- Periodic self-examination
- Annual dermatologic exam, beginning at age 40

For Asymptomatic Men and Women at Increased Risk

- Periodic self-examination
- Exam by a dermatologist at least once a year, depending on individual circumstances

---

For someone at high risk for melanoma, says Dr. Safai, examination "twice a year may not be enough; every three to four months may be necessary." Mary V., who has a familial predisposition to melanoma, sees her dermatologist at least every six months. "I have fair skin and lots of odd little patches on my skin now that I'm over 40," she explains, "and I have them looked at routinely—because I've seen what melanoma does to people. It's not a joke. I see people out there getting suntans, and it makes me crazy.

"My uncle had it on his nose and had surgery, and my father had to have disfiguring operations on his face and hand." Her father's first surgery was what convinced Mary, then in her mid-twenties, to abandon the sun. "Unfortunately," she says, "it had

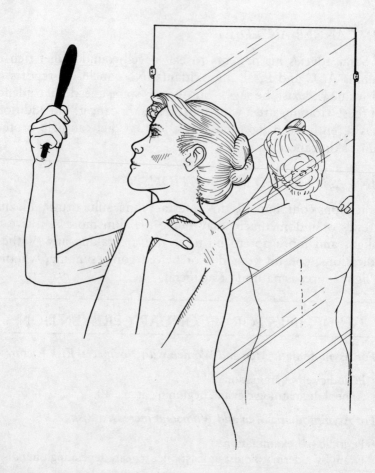

Skin Self-examination. Dermatologists recommend that you carefully examine your skin periodically, using a hand mirror to view your back, scalp and other hard-to-see places. See a doctor promptly if you find a new mole or one that appears to be growing or undergoing other suspicious changes.

done a lot of damage in the ten years prior to that. And I want to point out that my uncle was not fair-skinned. He was very dark-haired, dark-skinned, a Mediterranean-looking person. And he got melanoma."

SKIN SELF-EXAMINATION

Anyone can visually inspect the body for signs of skin cancer. Dr. Safai recalls a patient who came to his office claiming she had a malignant melanoma on one arm.

"How do you know?" he asked.

"My husband said so," she replied.

"Is your husband a doctor?"

"No, he runs a grocery store."

The woman explained that she and her husband had been listening to a New York talk-radio station. As a dermatologist described to the program's host what melanoma looked like, her husband glanced at her arm and blurted out, "Honey, you have melanoma. We have to go see the doctor!" His amateur diagnosis proved correct; the biopsy came back positive, though fortunately the disease hadn't metastasized and was still curable. A sidenote: The dermatologist heard over the airwaves? None other than Dr. Safai.

In instructing men and women on how to examine their bodies, he tells them, "Become aware. Get to know your skin." All you need is a brightly lit room, a full-length mirror and a hand-held mirror. "You need to check *all* the skin," he emphasizes. "The scalp, inside the mouth, between the toes, the bottom of the feet —everywhere."

Begin by gazing at your front in the full-length mirror. Do you spot any lesions? If so, analyze their appearance. Are they dark? Light? "You don't have to be compulsive and go crazy," explains Dr. Safai, "just take account of what is present."

After examining your front, inspect the rest of your body in this order, to ensure that nothing gets overlooked:

- Check your back.
- Then look at your right and left sides, arms raised.
- Next bend your elbows and carefully check your forearms, upper arms, underarms and the palms of your hands.
- Sit on the floor and look at the backs of your legs and feet, the soles and between your toes, too.
- Now pick up the hand-held mirror. Standing, examine the back of your neck and your scalp. Part your hair with your fingers, a brush or a blow dryer.
- Finally, check your buttocks—and your back once again— using the hand mirror.

"Every three or four months, do it again," says Dr. Safai, "and see what is there. Is the mole the same? Is there something different? Did you develop new moles?" Moles change for a number of reasons, some as innocent as gaining or losing weight. "There are a lot of changes that are normal," he explains. "But there are some that are not." Based on the symptoms of skin cancer listed earlier, report any suspicious growths to a dermatologist. Also, any skin condition that persists for longer than two weeks should be brought to a doctor's attention.

DERMATOLOGIC EXAM

Dermatologists have a saying: Have your birthday suit examined on your birthday. It's not meant literally, but, says Dr. Safai, "Everyone age 40 and older should have the skin examined at least once a year by a physician." The dermatologist, trained to visually identify maladies of the skin, will examine you from head to toe, biopsying anything considered potentially cancerous.

SKIN BIOPSY

In a biopsy, a local anesthetic is injected into the skin. Dr. Safai describes the feeling as similar to "a mosquito bite—very quick, with some burning sensation." Once the area is numb, a small sample of tissue is cut out using one of two instruments: a surgical knife (scalpel) or a punch. "Either the site is sutured closed," he explains, "or if it's very superficial, we cauterize it." The procedure lasts 10 to 20 minutes. The biopsy is then sent to a pathology lab for analysis, with results available usually within three days.

Skin cancer rates are expected to climb further due largely to the depletion of the earth's stratospheric ozone, which filters out most of the sun's harmful rays. The main culprits in this environmental tragedy are chlorofluorocarbons (CFCs), chemical compounds developed in the 1930s as nontoxic, nonflammable refrigerants.

The United States Environmental Protection Agency and the Food and Drug Administration banned the use of CFCs as spray-can propellants in 1978. Yet they still can be found in everything from air conditioners to refrigerators to cleaners to foamers. In 1987 more than 40 countries mutually agreed to reduce CFC emissions by half in the next decade, with a total ban to take effect in the year 2000. But considerable damage has already been done. Over Antarctica, a hole blanketing the entire continent has sent the ozone level there plummeting by 60 percent. According to scientists at the National Aeronautics and Space Administration (NASA), responsible for monitoring ozone, levels fell to an all-time low in 1993.

The outgrowth from this isn't expected to unfold until the twenty-first century. The Environmental Protection Agency estimates that each 1 percent drop in ozone will heighten the risk of skin cancer by 5 percent.

Would you twirl a pistol with the safety off? Carry gasoline in one hand and a lit match in the other? As the dangers rise steadily, basking in the sun minus protective clothing and sunscreen is no less foolhardy.

SUGGESTED READING ABOUT SKIN CANCERS

From the National Cancer Institute (800-4-CANCER):

- "What You Need to Know About Melanoma"
- "What You Need to Know About Skin Cancer"

From the Skin Cancer Foundation (212-725-5176):

- "For Every Child Under the Sun"

From the American Institute for Cancer Research (800-843-8114):

- "Reducing Your Risk of Skin Cancer"

KEY WORDS

Actinic keratosis: A precursor to squamous-cell carcinoma; symptoms include scaly, thick patches of skin.

Basal-cell carcinoma: The most common form of skin cancer, it arises in the round *basal cells* of the skin's surface layer, or *epidermis*.

Curretage: The most common method for treating basal-cell carcinoma. After injecting a local anesthetic into the area, the physician removes the tumor using an instrument called a *curette*.

Dermatologist: A physician who specializes in diagnosing and treating diseases of the skin.

Electrodesiccation: A method of killing remaining nonmelanoma skin-cancer cells and controlling bleeding through electrical current.

Melanin: The skin pigment found in the melanocytes.

Melanocytes: The cells that form and store melanin.

Melanoma: The least common but deadliest skin cancer, melanoma originates in the melanocytes and can spread to internal organs.

Mohs' technique: Specialized microscopic surgery in which malignant growths are removed layer by layer until only healthy tissue remains.

Nevi: The medical term for moles. Atypical moles may be harbingers of melanoma.

Skin biopsy: Under local anesthesia, a scalpel or punch tool is used to cut out a small sample of tissue. This is then analyzed by a pathologist, with results typically available within three days.

Squamous-cell carcinoma: Cancer arising from the flat squamous cells found in the epidermis.

Subcutaneous tissue: The layer of tissue beneath the skin.

Surgical excision: Treatment method in which the malignancy and a small border of normal skin are surgically removed under local anesthesia.

Topical chemotherapy: Another skin cancer treatment. Here an anticancer drug is applied to the affected area every day for several weeks.

PART FOUR

The Future of Cancer Prevention

CHAPTER

17

New Methods, New Hope

Testing for Genetic Susceptibility to Cancer • Chemoprevention

We are closing in on cancer from both sides: Improved methods of treatment have nudged the survival rate steadily upward, while we are hopeful that new frontiers in cancer prevention will one day enable us to halt the disease before it takes hold. The research being waged on three fronts is very promising.

IMAGING TECHNOLOGY

Technologic advances in CT scanning and MRI (magnetic resonance imaging) may provide new noninvasive approaches to early detection of a number of cancers. Currently these techniques are used mainly for diagnosis and follow-up. MRI holds two advantages over computerized axial tomography in that it provides a more detailed cross-sectional image and exposes patients to no radiation, for the machine generates its computer pictures through a huge, powerful electromagnet.

GENETIC TESTING

As we've seen, defective genes can predispose to cancer. The defects may have been inherited or, for reasons that remain a mystery, occurred at some point after birth. Altered *BRCA1* genes, for example, are believed to account for half of all hereditary breast cancers, while up to half of all colorectal cancer patients are believed to carry a defective K-*ras* oncogene. According to Dr. John Mendelsohn, chairman of Memorial Sloan-Kettering's department of medicine, these biologic markers may one day help us to save lives.

"We can envision the possibility," he says, "of testing patients' blood samples, looking at the genes in the white blood cells and predicting the cancers they have a high risk of developing during their lifetimes, and then conducting preventive screening."

Another promising method, *monoclonal antibodies,* may also act as an early-warning system and allow for early diagnosis. These scientifically tailored proteins can locate and bind to cancer cells long before the onset of symptoms. While they are not known to destroy malignant cells by themselves, monoclonal antibodies could be used as biologic smart bombs that deliver anticancer agents directly to the tumor.

CHEMOPREVENTION

A third tier of research involves identifying cancer-preventive compounds that could be administered like vaccines to patients deemed at increased risk. A vaccination against the hepatitis B virus, a major cause of liver cancer, is already widely in use, and as of 1994, approximately 40 clinical trials were under way to test an array of compounds (see box).

Dr. Peter Greenwald, director of cancer prevention and control for the National Cancer Institute, explains that the chemoprevention studies can be loosely divided into four categories, each aimed at a particular segment of the population.

"The ultimate aim is to benefit the population at large," he says. "In the best-known study, 22,000 doctors are taking either a beta-carotene pill or a placebo, a pill that looks and tastes like beta-carotene but it's not. They're being followed to see if their frequency of new cancers is lowered.

CHEMOPREVENTIVE COMPOUNDS CURRENTLY UNDER INVESTIGATION

CHEMO-PREVENTIVE AGENT	DESCRIPTION	BEING STUDIED FOR EFFECTIVENESS AGAINST
Beta-carotene	A precursor of vitamin A	Oral premalignancy Lung cancer Cervical cancer and dysplasia Skin cancer Colon polyps
Retinoids	A synthetic form of vitamin A	Oral premalignancy Skin cancer Lung cancer
13-*cis*-retinoic acid	A synthetic form of vitamin A	Skin cancer Cancers of the head and neck Lung cancer Oral premalignancy
Beta-*trans*-retinoic acid	A synthetic form of beta-carotene	Cervical dysplasia
Ascorbic acid	Vitamin C	Colon polyps
Alpha-tocopherol	A natural or synthetic form of vitamin E	Oral premalignancy Colon polyps
DFMO (difluoro-methylornithine)	Synthetic enzyme inhibitor	Colorectal cancer Cervical neoplasms
Aspirin	Common drug used to relieve pain and reduce fever	Colon polyps
Wheat bran	Fiber	Colon cancer

(continued)

CHEMO-PREVENTIVE AGENT	DESCRIPTION	BEING STUDIED FOR EFFECTIVENESS AGAINST
Calcium carbonate (antacid)	Most abundant mineral in the body	Colon cancer Neoplastic polyps
Piroxicam	An antiinflammatory agent commonly used to treat arthritis	Colon cancer
Omega-3 fatty acids	A polyunsaturated fatty acid found in certain fish	Colorectal cancer
4-HPR (hydroxy-phenylretinamide)	A nuclear effector that affects the nuclear receptors in cancer cells	Skin cancer Bladder cancer Prostate cancer Breast cancer Cervical neoplasms
Sulindac	An antiinflammatory agent commonly used to treat arthritis	Colorectal cancer and polyps
Tamoxifen	Antiestrogen, currently used to treat breast cancer	Breast disease
Acarbose	A complex sugar compound that destroys or inhibits the bacterial flora in the colon	Colon cancer

"The second group has a high risk of cancer because of a previous exposure but doesn't have the cancer at this point." As an example, he names a Seattle clinical trial currently tracking 18,000 workers, some of them heavy smokers, others heavy smokers exposed to asbestos. "So they have a tremendously high risk of getting lung cancer," says Dr. Greenwald. "The scientists running this study are trying to intervene after the exposure and prevent the cancer from occurring, using beta-carotene and retinol [vitamin A].

"A third type of study concerns people who have a precancerous lesion. They are being given a chemopreventive agent to see if we can prevent the lesion from progressing to cancer or reverse the precancerous lesion.

"And the fourth group is those who've had one cancer and are at high risk of a second, new cancer. We have a large breast-cancer prevention trial under way to study tamoxifen, an antiestrogen used in breast-cancer therapy. It has shown a reduction in cancers in the opposite breast by about 40 percent." Some chemopreventive agents, such as tamoxifen, produce side effects, against which benefits must be carefully weighed.

NOW FOR THE TRULY EXCITING PART

Once we've perfected genetic testing and chemoprevention, we merge the two areas of research, says Dr. Daniel Nixon of the American Cancer Society, so that "we'll be able to test a person for malignant potential, then give them something to stop it. A pill or a shot."

These innovations are still some years away. But by following the guidelines outlined in these pages, we have the ability to prevent a vast number of cancers right now—*we* meaning patients and physicians, working together in partnership.

KEY WORDS

Chemoprevention: Using various agents to suppress cancer development before the disease takes hold.

Monoclonal antibodies: Scientifically tailored proteins that can locate and bind to cancer cells long before the onset of symptoms. In the future they may be used to deliver anticancer agents directly to a tumor.

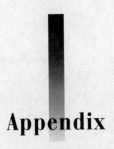

Appendix

RESOURCES

With just a few toll-free phone calls, you can receive these highly recommended booklets free. They are clear, concise, extremely informative and updated regularly. Except where noted, all are from the National Cancer Institute Office of Cancer Communications, Building 31, Room 10A24, Bethesda, MD 20892 (800-4-CANCER), Monday through Friday, 9 A.M. to 7 P.M. EST. In Oahu, Hawaii: 524-1234; call collect from other Hawaiian islands.

GENERAL INFORMATION ABOUT CANCER

- "Cancer Prevention"
- "Cancer Tests You Should Know About: A Guide for People 65 and Over"
- "What You Need to Know About Cancer"
- "Everything Doesn't Cause Cancer"

ON SPECIFIC CANCERS

Bladder Cancer
- "What You Need to Know About Bladder Cancer"

Bone Cancer
- "What You Need to Know About Cancer of the Bone"

Brain Cancers
- "What You Need to Know About Brain Cancers"

Breast Cancer
- "Breast Exams: What You Should Know"
- "Questions and Answers About Breast Lumps"
- "What You Need to Know About Breast Cancer"

From the American Institute for Cancer Research, 1759 R Street, N.W., Washington, DC 20069 (800-843-8114):

- "Questions and Answers About Breast Lumps and Breast Cancer"

For more on breast cancer, see Chapter 11.

Cervical Cancer
- "What You Need to Know About Cancer of the Cervix"

For more on cervical cancer, see Chapter 14.

Colorectal Cancer
- "What You Need to Know About Cancer of the Colon and Rectum"

For more on colorectal cancer, see Chapter 13.

Esophageal Cancer
- "What You Need to Know About Cancer of the Esophagus"

For more on esophageal cancer, see Chapter 15.

Hodgkin's Disease
- "What You Need to Know About Hodgkin's Disease"

From the Leukemia Society of America, 600 Third Avenue, New York, NY 10016 (212-573-8484):

- "Hodgkin's Disease and the Non-Hodgkin's Lymphomas"

Kidney Cancer
- "What You Need to Know About Kidney Cancer"

Laryngeal Cancer (Cancer of the Larynx)
- "What You Need to Know About Cancer of the Larynx"

Leukemia
- "What You Need to Know About Adult Leukemia"

From the Leukemia Society of America, 600 Third Avenue, New York, NY 10016 (212-573-8484):

- "Acute Lymphocytic Leukemia"
- "Acute Myelogenous Leukemia"
- "Chronic Lymphocytic Leukemia"
- "Chronic Myelogenous Leukemia"

Lung Cancer
- "What You Need to Know About Lung Cancer"

For more on lung cancer, see Chapter 12.

Multiple Myeloma
- "What You Need to Know About Multiple Myeloma"

From the Leukemia Society of America, 600 Third Avenue, New York, NY 10016 (212-573-8484):

- "Multiple Myeloma (MM)"

Non-Hodgkin's Lymphomas
- "What You Need to Know About Non-Hodgkin's Lymphomas"

From the Leukemia Society of America, 600 Third Avenue, New York, NY 10016 (212-573-8484):

- "Hodgkin's Disease and the Non-Hodgkin's Lymphomas"

Oral Cancers
- "What You Need to Know About Oral Cancers"

Ovarian Cancer
- "What You Need to Know About Ovarian Cancer"

For more on ovarian cancer, see Chapter 14.

Pancreatic Cancer
- "What You Need to Know About Cancer of the Pancreas"

Prostate Cancer
- "What You Need to Know About Prostate Cancer"

For more on prostate cancer, see Chapter 10.

Skin Cancers
- "What You Need to Know About Melanoma"
- "What You Need to Know About Skin Cancer"

From the Skin Cancer Foundation, 245 Fifth Avenue, Suite 2402, New York, NY 10016 (212-725-5176):

- "For Every Child Under the Sun"

From the American Institute for Cancer Research, 1759 R Street, N.W., Washington, DC 20069 (800-843-8114):

- "Reducing Your Risk of Skin Cancer"

For more on skin cancer, see Chapter 16.

Soft-Tissue Sarcomas
- "Soft Tissue Sarcomas in Adults and Children"

Testicular Cancer
- "What You Need to Know About Testicular Cancer"

For more on testicular cancer, see Chapter 10.

Uterine Cancer
- "Cancer of the Uterus: Endometrial Cancer Research Report"
- "What You Need to Know About Cancer of the Uterus"

For more on uterine cancer, see Chapter 14.

ON CANCER-PREVENTIVE NUTRITION

- "Diet, Nutrition & Cancer Prevention: A Guide for Food Choices"
- "Diet, Nutrition & Cancer Prevention: The Good News"

From the American Institute for Cancer Research, 1759 R Street, N.W., Washington, DC 20069 (800-843-8114):

- "Be Your Best: Nutrition After Fifty"
- "Celebrate Good Health"
- "Cooking Solo"
- "Cook's Day Off"
- "Dietary Fiber to Lower Cancer Risk"
- "Dietary Guidelines to Lower Cancer Risk"
- "Get Fit, Trim Down"
- "Menus and Recipes to Lower Cancer Risk"
- "No Time to Cook"
- "Sneak Health into Your Snacks"

For more on nutrition, see Chapter 5.

ON HOW TO QUIT SMOKING

- "Clearing the Air: How to Quit Smoking . . . and Quit for Keeps"

From the American Cancer Society, 1599 Clifton Road, N.E., Atlanta, GA 30329 (404-320-3333); regional offices: (800-ACS-2345), Monday through Friday, 9 A.M. to 5 P.M.:

- "How to Stay Quit over the Holidays"
- "Smart Move! A Stop Smoking Guide"

STOP-SMOKING PROGRAMS

Cancer Information Service
(800-4-CANCER), Monday through Friday, 9 A.M. to 4:30 P.M. In Oahu, Hawaii: 524-1234; call collect from other Hawaiian islands.
CIS counselors can refer you to programs in your area.

- Freedom from Smoking, American Lung Association, 1740 Broadway, New York, NY 10019 (212-315-8700). Cost: $60.
- Fresh Start, sponsored by the American Cancer Society. To learn more, contact ACS headquarters or your local chapter (800-ACS-2345). Cost: $25.

Many local hospitals also run stop-smoking programs.

For more on the dangers of tobacco and how to quit smoking, see Chapter 6.

ON HOW TO PROTECT YOU AND YOUR FAMILY FROM RADON

From the U.S. Environmental Protection Agency Information Access Branch, Public Information Center, 401 M Street, S.W., Washington, DC 20460 (202-260-2080):

- "A Citizen's Guide to Radon"
- "Home Buyer's and Seller's Guide to Radon"
- "How to Reduce Radon Levels in Your Home"

FOR REFERRALS TO RADON TESTERS AND RADON-REMOVAL CONTRACTORS WHO MEET EPA STANDARDS

Call your state radon contact:

Alabama	(800) 582-1866	Idaho	(800) 445-8647
Alaska	(800) 478-4845	Illinois	(800) 325-1245
Arizona	(602) 225-4845	Indiana	(800) 272-9723
Arkansas	(501) 661-2301	Iowa	(800) 383-5992
California	(800) 745-7236	Kansas	(913) 296-1560
Colorado	(800) 846-3986	Kentucky	(502) 564-3700
Connecticut	(203) 566-3122	Louisiana	(800) 256-2494
Delaware	(800) 554-4636	Maine	(800) 232-0842
District of		Maryland	(800) 872-3666
Columbia	(202) 727-5728	Massachusetts	(413) 586-7525
Florida	(800) 543-8279	Michigan	(517) 335-8190
Georgia	(800) 745-0037	Minnesota	(800) 798-9050
Hawaii	(808) 586-4700	Mississippi	(800) 626-7739

Missouri	(800) 669-7236	Oregon	(503) 731-4014
Montana	(406) 444-3671	Pennsylvania	(800) 237-2366
Nebraska	(800) 334-9491	Rhode Island	(401) 277-2438
Nevada	(702) 687-5394	South Carolina	(800) 768-0362
New		South Dakota	(605) 773-3351
Hampshire	(800) 825-3345,	Tennessee	(800) 232-1139
	ext. 4674	Texas	(512) 834-6688
New Jersey	(800) 648-0394	Utah	(801) 538-6734
New Mexico	(505) 827-4300	Vermont	(800) 640-0601
New York	(800) 458-1158	Virginia	(800) 468-0138
North Carolina	(919) 571-4141	Washington	(800) 323-9727
North Dakota	(701) 221-5188	West Virginia	(900) 922-1255
Ohio	(800) 523-4439	Wisconsin	(608) 267-4795
Oklahoma	(405) 271-5221	Wyoming	(800) 458-5847

For more on radon and cancer, see Chapter 7.

FOR ANSWERS TO QUESTIONS ABOUT THE HEALTH AND ENVIRONMENTAL EFFECTS OF PESTICIDES

National Pesticide Telecommunications Network
(800-858-PEST), Monday through Friday, 8 A.M. to 6 P.M. CST

FOR INFORMATION ON HOW TO PROPERLY DISPOSE OF HAZARDOUS PESTICIDES

Call your state pesticide agency:

Alabama	(205) 242-2631	Iowa	(515) 281-8591
Alaska	(907) 465-2609	Kansas	(913) 296-2263
Arizona	(602) 542-4373	Kentucky	(502) 564-7274
Arkansas	(501) 225-1598	Louisiana	(504) 925-3763
California	(916) 322-6315	Maine	(207) 289-2731
Colorado	(303) 866-2838	Maryland	(301) 841-5710
Connecticut	(203) 566-5148	Massachusetts	(617) 727-3020
Delaware	(302) 739-4811	Michigan	(517) 373-1087
District of		Minnesota	(612) 296-1161
Columbia	(202) 404-1167	Mississippi	(601) 325-3390
Florida	(904) 487-0532	Missouri	(314) 751-2462
Georgia	(404) 656-4958	Montana	(406) 444-2944
Hawaii	(808) 548-7119	Nebraska	(402) 471-2341
Idaho	(208) 334-3243	Nevada	(702) 688-1180
Illinois	(217) 785-2427	New Hampshire	(603) 271-3550
	or (217) 782-4674	New Jersey	(609) 530-4123
Indiana	(317) 494-1492	New Mexico	(505) 545-2133

New York	(518) 457-7482	Tennessee	(615) 360-0130
North Carolina	(919) 733-3556	Texas	(512) 483-7534
North Dakota	(701) 224-4756	Utah	(801) 538-7123
Ohio	(614) 866-6361	Vermont	(802) 828-2431
Oklahoma	(405) 521-3864	Virginia	(804) 371-6558
Oregon	(503) 378-3776	Washington	(206) 753-5062
Pennsylvania	(717) 787-4843	West Virginia	(304) 348-2212
Rhode Island	(401) 277-2781	Wisconsin	(608) 266-9459
South Carolina	(803) 656-3171	Wyoming	(307) 777-6590
South Dakota	(605) 773-3724		

TO LEARN IF YOUR DRINKING WATER CONTAINS CARCINOGENS

U.S. Environmental Protection Agency Safe Drinking Water Hotline
(800) 426-4791

FOR REFERRALS TO WATER-ANALYSIS LABORATORIES

American Council of Independent Laboratories
(202) 887-5872
Also, check the Yellow Pages under "Water Analysis."

For more about drinking-water safety, see Chapter 7.

FOR ANSWERS TO QUESTIONS ABOUT ASBESTOS, INCLUDING HOW TO REMOVE IT SAFELY FROM YOUR HOME OR BUSINESS

Toxic Substance Control Act Assistance Office
401 M Street, S.W., Washington, DC 20460 (202-554-1404), Monday through Friday, 8:30 A.M. to 5 P.M.

For more on the dangers of asbestos, see Chapter 7.

FOR ANSWERS TO QUESTIONS, AS WELL AS TIPS ON HOW TO REDUCE YOUR RISK OF CANCER, CALL THESE HOTLINES

American Cancer Society
(800-ACS-2345), Monday through Friday, 9 A.M. to 5 P.M.

American Institute for Cancer Research Nutrition Hotline
(800-843-8114), Monday through Friday, 9 A.M. to 5 P.M. EST
A registered dietitian will answer your questions about diet, nutrition and cancer.

Cancer Information Service
(800-4-CANCER), Monday through Friday, 9 A.M. to 4:30 P.M. In Oahu, Hawaii: 524-1234; call collect from other Hawaiian islands.

Leukemia Society of America Hotline
(800) 955-4LSA

FOR REFERRALS TO SUBSTANCE- AND ALCOHOL-ABUSE TREATMENT PROGRAMS

Alcoholics Anonymous
475 Riverside Drive, New York, NY 10115 (212-870-3400)
Locate the AA fellowship nearest you by looking in the White Pages.

Center for Substance Abuse Treatment Referral Hotline
11426 Rockville Pike, Suite 410, Rockville, MD 20852 (800-662-HELP)

National Council on Alcoholism and Drug Dependence
12 West 21 Street, New York, NY 10010 (800-NCA-CALL)

National Drug Abuse Treatment Referral and Information Service
Provided by National Medical Enterprises
PO Box 100, Summit, NJ 07902-0100 (800-COC-AINE)

For more on drugs and alcohol and their relation to cancer, see Chapter 6.

TO OBTAIN A COPY OF A FAMILY MEMBER'S DEATH CERTIFICATE

Write the department or office of vital records for the state in which you believe the relative died. You must include the following information: (1) the deceased's full name as it would have appeared on the certificate; (2) the city, town or village in which he or she died; (3) the date of death; (4) your relationship to this person; (5) and your reason for requesting a copy of the death certificate. A small fee is charged for this service.

TO LOCATE A GENETIC COUNSELOR NEAR YOU

Cancer Information Service
   (800-4-CANCER), Monday through Friday, 9 A.M. to 4:30 P.M. In
   Oahu, Hawaii: 524-1234; call collect from other Hawaiian islands.
   CIS counselors can refer you to medical centers in your area that have
genetic-counseling departments.

Hereditary Cancer Institute
   Creighton University, Department of Preventive Medicine, 2500 California Plaza, Omaha, NE 68178 (800-648-8133)

Memorial Sloan-Kettering Cancer Center Clinical-Genetics Service
   1275 York Avenue, New York, NY 10021 (212-639-7099)

Both Memorial Sloan-Kettering and the Hereditary Cancer Institute offer
free genetic counseling to families that appear to have a significant cancer
history.

For more on cancer and heredity, see Chapter 4.

TO LEARN OF MAMMOGRAM FACILITIES CERTIFIED BY THE AMERICAN COLLEGE OF RADIOLOGY

American College of Radiology
   1891 Preston White Drive, Reston, VA 22091 (800-ACR-LINE)

Cancer Information Service
   Regional offices: (800-4-CANCER), Monday through Friday, 9 A.M.
   to 4:30 P.M. In Oahu, Hawaii: 524-1234; call collect from other
   Hawaiian islands

For more on mammograms, see Chapter 11.

TO LEARN OF X-RAY FACILITIES CERTIFIED BY THE AMERICAN COLLEGE OF RADIOLOGY

American College of Radiology
   1891 Preston White Drive, Reston, VA 22091 (800-ACR-LINE)

For more on chest x-rays, see Chapter 12.

FOR A FREE CYTO-SPUTUM TEST KIT (TO TEST FOR LUNG CANCER)

National Cancer Cytology Center
   88 Sunnyside Boulevard, Suite 307, Plainview, NY 11803 (516-349-
   0610)

For more on the sputum cytology test, see Chapter 12.

FOR REFERRALS TO TRAINED HYPNOTHERAPISTS

American Society of Clinical Hypnosis
2200 East Devon Avenue, Suite 291, Des Plaines, IL 60018 (708-297-3317)

For a list of hypnotists in your area, send an SASE, or call for a few referrals.

Society for Clinical and Experimental Hypnosis
6728 Old McLean Village Drive, McLean, VA 22101 (703-556-9222)

For a list of hypnotists in your area, send an SASE, or call for a few referrals.

For more on hypnosis, see Chapter 8.

FOR REFERRALS TO TRAINED BIOFEEDBACK PROFESSIONALS

Biofeedback Society of America, 10200 West 44 Avenue, Wheat Ridge, CO 80033 (303-422-8436)

For more on biofeedback, see Chapter 8.

FOR REFERRALS TO VARIOUS STRESS REDUCTION TECHNIQUES

American Institute of Stress
124 Park Avenue, Yonkers, NY 10703 (914-963-1200)

FOR REFERRALS TO ACUPUNCTURISTS

National Commission for the Certification of Acupuncturists
1424 16th Street, N.W., Suite 501, Washington, DC 20036 (202-232-1404)

To receive a list of acupuncturists in your state, send a check or money order for $3.

For more on acupuncture, see Chapter 8.

IF YOU SUSPECT YOUR EMPLOYER OF COMMITTING A HEALTH OR SAFETY VIOLATION AND WISH TO FILE A COMPLAINT

U.S. Department of Labor Occupational Safety and Health Administration (OSHA)

200 Constitution Avenue, N.W., Washington, DC 20210 (202-219-9308)
Call the OSHA regional office nearest you:

Atlanta	(404) 347-3573	Kansas City	(816) 426-5861
Boston	(617) 565-7164	New York	(212) 337-2378
Chicago	(312) 353-2220	Philadelphia	(215) 596-1201
Dallas	(214) 767-4731	San Francisco	(415) 995-5672
Denver	(303) 844-3061	Seattle	(206) 442-5930

National Institute for Occupational Safety and Health (NIOSH)
  4676 Columbia Parkway, Cincinnati, OH 45226 (800-356-4674)

NIOSH requires the signatures of three or more employees, but all complaints are kept confidential.

For more on carcinogens commonly found in the workplace and what you can do about them, see Chapter 7.

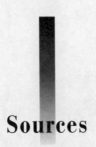

Sources

The authors are especially grateful to the patients who so generously shared their experiences with us. The case examples presented in this book are based on their experiences, but we have changed names and other details to protect the anonymity of the patients and their families.

We would also like to express our deep appreciation to the many health-care professionals, patients and others who kindly took the time to speak to us. Alphabetically they are: Ann Beigel (Fresh Start), Dr. Aaron Blair (National Cancer Institute), Dr. William Blot (National Cancer Institute), Dr. William Farland (Environmental Protection Agency), Dr. Valdis Goncarovs (Environmental Protection Agency), Dr. Peter Greenwald (National Cancer Institute), Dr. Curtis Harris (National Cancer Institute), Al Heier (Environmental Protection Agency), William Hoffman (American Society of Clinical Hypnosis), Dr. Peter Infante (Occupational Safety and Health Administration), Dr. Bruce Johnson (National Cancer Institute), Dr. I-Min Lee (Harvard University School of Public Health), Dr. Lawrence LeShan, Dr. Charles Lieber (Department of Veterans Affairs Medical Center, Bronx, New York), Dr. Henry T. Lynch (Creighton Hereditary Institute), Dr. Marc Manley (National Cancer Institute), Dr. Daniel Nixon (American Cancer Society), Dr. Susan Pilch (National Cancer Institute), Dr. Paul Rosch (American Institute of Stress), Dave Rowson (Environmental Protection Agency), Dr. David Schottenfeld (University of Michigan), Dr. Charles Sharp (National Institute on Drug Abuse), Margaret Stasikowski (Environmental Protection Agency), Vanessa Vu (Environmental Protection Agency), Anthony Wolbarst (Environmental Protection Agency) and Stephen Young (Health Insurance Association of America).

From Memorial Sloan-Kettering Cancer Center: colleagues Rachel Barcia-Morse, Abby Bloch, Dr. Murray Brennan, Karen Brown, Lori Cohen, Dr. William Fair, Dr. Hans Gerdes, Lynn M. Gossfeld, R.N.C., Kathryn Hamilton, Dr. Robert Heelan, Dr. Jimmie Holland, Dr. William J. Hoskins, Dr. Robert Kurtz, Dr. Paul A. Marks, Dr. Mary Jane Massie, Dr. John Mendelsohn, Dr. Michael P. Moore, Dr. Kenneth Offit, Dr. Bijan Safai, Dr. Joseph V. Simone, Dr. Diane E. Stover, Amalia Vallance and Dr. Willet F. Whitmore Jr.

Selected Bibliography

BOOKS

Dreher, Henry. *Your Defense Against Cancer.* New York: Harper & Row, 1988.

Eddy, David M., M.D. *Common Screening Tests.* Philadelphia: American College of Physicians, 1991.

Fink, John M. *Third Opinion.* Garden City, New York: Avery Publishing Group, Inc., 1988.

Goleman, D., and J. Gurin, eds. *Mind-Body Medicine.* Yonkers, NY: Consumer Reports Books, 1993.

Holleb, Arthur I., M.D., Diane J. Fink, M.D., and Gerald P. Murphy, M.D. *American Cancer Society Textbook of Clinical Oncology.* Atlanta: The American Cancer Society, Inc., 1991.

Krause, Carol. *How Healthy Is Your Family Tree?* New York: Macmillan Publishing Co., 1994.

McAllister, Robert M., M.D., Sylvia Teich Horowitz, Ph.D., and Raymond V. Gilden, Ph.D. *Cancer.* New York: Basic Books, 1993.

Miller, Benjamin F., M.D., and Claire Brackman Keane. *Encyclopedia and Dictionary of Medicine, Nursing, and Allied Health.* Philadelphia: W. B. Saunders Company, 1987.

Shils, Maurice, Jim Olsen, and Moshe Shike. *Modern Nutrition in Health and Disease,* eighth edition. Philadelphia: Lea and Febiger, 1994.

Stewart, Felicia, M.D., et al. *Understanding Your Body.* New York: Bantam Books, 1987.

Tapley, Donald F., M.D., et al. *The Columbia University College of Physicians and Surgeons Complete Home Medical Guide,* revised third edition. New York: Crown Publishers, Inc., 1995.

Varmus, Harold, and Robert A. Weinberg. *Genes and the Biology of Cancer.* New York: Scientific American Library, 1993.

Winawer, Sidney J. *Management of Gastrointestinal Diseases.* New York: Gower Medical Publishers, 1992.

NEWSPAPERS, PERIODICALS, MEDICAL
JOURNALS, REPORTS AND OTHER SOURCES

"A Citizen's Guide to Radon." United States Environmental Protection Agency, 1992.

"Acute Lymphocytic Leukemia." Leukemia Society of America, 1991.

"Alcohol and Cancer Risk: Make the Choice for Health." American Institute for Cancer Research, 1989.

Andersen, Barbara L., and Peter M. Jochinsen. "Sexual Functioning Among Breast Cancer, Gynecologic Cancer, and Healthy Women." *Journal of Consulting and Clinical Psychology,* Vol. 53, No. 1, pp. 25–32, 1985.

Antman, Karen H., M.D. "Natural History and Epidemiology of Malignant Mesothelioma." *Chest,* Vol. 103, No. 4, April 1993.

"Application of Radon Reduction Methods." United States Environmental Protection Agency, 1988.

Arraiz, Gustavo A., Donald T. Wigle, and Yang Mao. "Risk Assessment of Physical Activity and Physical Fitness in the Canada Health Survey Mortality Follow-up Study." *Journal of Clinical Epidemiology,* Vol. 45, No. 4, 1992.

Arria, Amelia M., B.S., and David H. Van Thiel, M.D. "The Epidemiology of Alcohol-Related Chronic Disease." *Alcohol Health & Research World,* Vol. 16, No. 3, 1992.

"Asbestos Exposure: What It Means, What to Do." U.S. Department of Health and Human Services, 1989.

"Asbestos in Your Home." United States Environmental Protection Agency.

Beckett, William S., M.D., M.P.H., "Epidemiology and Etiology of Lung Cancer." *Clinics in Chest Medicine,* Vol. 14, No. 1, March 1993.

Blair, S. N., et al. "How Much Physical Activity Is Good for Health?" *Annu. Rev. Public Health.* Vol. 13, pp. 99–126, 1992.

Blot, William J., et al. "Nutrition Intervention Trials in Linxian, China: Supplementation with Specific Vitamin/Mineral Combinations, Cancer Incidence, and Disease-Specific Mortality in the General Population." *Journal of the National Cancer Institute,* Vol. 85, No. 18, September 15, 1993.

"Breast Biopsy: What You Should Know." U.S. Department of Health and Human Services, 1990.

"Breast Exams: What You Should Know." U.S. Department of Health and Human Services, 1992.

Brody, Jane. "Does a Bout of Exercise a Day Keep the Doctor Away?" *The New York Times,* July 7, 1993.

Butterworth, C. E., Jr., M.D., et al. "Folate Deficiency and Cervical

Dysplasia." *Journal of the American Medical Association*, Vol. 267, No. 4, January 22–29, 1992.

"Cancer and the Immune System: The Vital Connection." Cancer Research Institute.

Cancer Control Objectives for the Nation: 1985–2000. NCI Monographs, No. 2, 1986.

"Cancer Facts and Figures—1993." American Cancer Society, 1993.

"Cancer of the Lung Research Report." U.S. Department of Health and Human Services, 1993.

"Cancer Prevention." U.S. Department of Health and Human Services, 1984.

"Cancer Process, The." American Institute for Cancer Research, 1991.

"Cancer Rates and Risks." U.S. Department of Health and Human Services, 1985.

"Cancer of the Stomach Research Report." U.S. Department of Health and Human Services, 1988.

"Cancer Tests You Should Know About: A Guide for People 65 and Over." U.S. Department of Health and Human Services, 1992.

"Cancer of the Uterus: Endometrial Cancer Research Report." U.S. Department of Health and Human Services, 1991.

"Chemical Hazard Communication." U.S. Department of Labor, Occupational Safety and Health Administration, 1992.

"Chronic Lymphocytic Leukemia." Leukemia Society of America, 1992.

"Chronic Myelogenous Leukemia." Leukemia Society of America, 1991.

"Citizen's Guide to Pesticides." United States Environmental Protection Agency, 1991.

"Clearing the Air: How to Quit Smoking . . . and Quit for Keeps." U.S. Department of Health and Human Services, 1992.

Clifford, Carolyn, Ph.D., and Barnett Kramer, M.D., M.P.H. "Diet as Risk and Therapy for Cancer." *Medical Clinics of North America*, Vol. 77, No. 4, July 1993.

"Consumer's Guide to Radon Reduction." United States Environmental Protection Agency, 1992.

Dantzer, Robert, and Keith W. Kelley. "Stress and Immunity: An Integrated View of Relationships Between the Brain and the Immune System." *Life Sciences*, Vol. 44, pp. 1995–2008. New York: Pergamon Press, 1989.

Davis, Lisa. "One in Nine." *Health*, January-February 1993.

"Decline in Smoking Levels Off and Officials Urge a Tax Rise." *The New York Times*, April 2, 1993.

"Diet, Nutrition, and Cancers of the Colon and Rectum." American Institute for Cancer Research, 1992.

"Diet, Nutrition, and Prostate Cancer." American Institute for Cancer Research, 1991.

Doll, Sir Richard. "Progress Against Cancer: An Epidemiologic Assessment." *American Journal of Epidemiology,* Vol. 134, No. 7, October 1, 1991.

"EMF in Your Environment." United States Environmental Protection Agency, 1992.

"Everything Doesn't Cause Cancer." U.S. Department of Health and Human Services, 1990.

Fackelmann, Kathy A. "Family Ties and Risk of Breast Cancer." *Science News,* Vol. 144, July 24, 1993.

—— "Refiguring the Odds." *Science News,* Vol. 144, July 31, 1993.

"Facts About Asbestos." American Lung Association, 1990.

Fink, Diane J., M.D. "Guidelines for the Cancer Related Checkup." American Cancer Society, 1991.

Fletcher, Suzanne W., M.D. "Breast Cancer Detection and Mortality." *ACP Journal Club,* March–April 1993.

Gorman, Genevieve A., R.N., M.S.N., O.C.N., and Joseph Treat, M.D. "Lung Cancer: Taxol Appears to Be the Most Effective Drug in Non Small Cell Lung Cancer." *Cope,* Vol. 9, No. 4, July–August 1993.

"Healthy Lawn, Healthy Environment." United States Environmental Protection Agency.

Henderson, Brian E., Ronald K. Ross, and Malcolm C. Pike. "Hormonal Chemoprevention of Cancer in Women." *Science,* Vol. 259, January 29, 1993.

"Hodgkin's Disease and the Non-Hodgkin's Lymphomas." Leukemia Society of America, 1991.

"Home Buyer's and Seller's Guide to Radon." United States Environmental Protection Agency, 1993.

"How to Help Your Patients Stop Smoking: A National Cancer Institute Manual for Physicians," U.S. Department of Health and Human Services, 1992.

"How to Prepare for a Colonoscopy." Memorial Sloan-Kettering Cancer Center, 1992.

"How to Prepare for a Flexible Sigmoidoscopy." Memorial Sloan-Kettering Cancer Center, 1992.

"How to Stay Quit Over the Holidays." American Cancer Society, 1985.

"Insurance Linked to Early Diagnosis." *The New York Times,* July 29, 1993.

Jaret, Peter. "Mind Over Malady." *Health,* November–December 1992.

Johnson, Bruce E., M.D., and Michael J. Kelley, M.D. "Overview of Genetic and Molecular Events in the Pathogenesis of Lung Cancer." *Chest,* Vol. 103, No. 1, January 1993.

Kern, Jeffrey A., M.D., and Andrew E. Filderman, M.D. *Clinics in Chest Medicine,* Vol. 14, No. 1, March 1993.

Kowal, Samuel J., M.D. "Emotions as a Cause of Cancer." *The Psychoanalytic Review,* Vol. 42, No. 3, July 1955.

Krontiris, Theodore G., M.D., et al. "An Association Between the Risk of Cancer and Mutations in the HRAS1 Minisatellite Locus." *The New England Journal of Medicine,* Vol. 329, No. 8, August 19, 1993.

Lauffer, R. B. "Exercise as Prevention: Do the Health Benefits Derive in Part from Lower Iron Levels?" *Medical Hypotheses,* Vol. 35, pp. 103–107, 1991.

"Lawn Care Pesticides: Reregistration Falls Further Behind and Exposed Effects Are Uncertain." United States General Accounting Office, 1993.

Leary, Warren E. "If You Can't Run for Health, a Walk Will Do, Experts Say." *The New York Times,* July 30, 1993.

Lee, I-Min, and Ralph S. Paffenbarger Jr. "Quetlet's Index and Risk of Colon Cancer in College Alumni." *Journal of the National Cancer Institute,* Vol. 84, No. 17, September 2, 1992.

LeShan, Lawrence, Ph.D. "Psychological States as Factors in the Development of Malignant Disease: A Critical Review." *Journal of the National Cancer Institute,* Vol. 22, No. 1, January 1959.

Li, Jun-Yao, et al. "Nutrition Intervention Trials in Linxian, China: Multiple Vitamin/Mineral Supplementation, Cancer Incidence, and Disease-Specific Mortality Among Adults with Esophageal Dysplasia." *Journal of the National Cancer Institute,* Vol. 85, No. 18, September 15, 1993.

Lippman, Scott M., M.D., Steven E. Benner, M.D., and Waun Ki Hong, M.D. "Chemoprevention Strategies in Lung Carcinogenesis." *Chest,* Vol. 103, No. 1, January 1993.

Longnecker, Matthew P., M.D., Sc.D. "Alcohol Consumption in Relation to Risk of Cancers of the Breast and Large Bowel." *Alcohol Health & Research World,* Vol. 16, No. 3, 1992.

Lusky, Karen, and Hiroshi Takahashi, M.D., Ph.D. "Targeting Colon Cancer with Biological Smart Bombs." *Cope,* Vol. 9, No. 4, July–August 1993.

Maisel, Alan S., et al. "ß-Adrenergic Receptors in Lymphocyte Subsets After Exercise." *Circulation,* Vol. 82, No. 6, December 1990.

"Mastectomy: A Treatment for Breast Cancer." U.S. Department of Health and Human Services, 1990.

McGinnis, J. Michael, M.D., et al. "Health Progress in the United States." *Journal of the American Medical Association,* Vol. 268, No. 18, November 11, 1992.

Mehta, Atul. C., M.D., F.C.C.P., F.A.C.P., Jerry J. Marty, M.D., and Francis Y. W. Lee, M.D., M.B.B.S. "Sputum Cytology." *Clinics in Chest Medicine,* Vol. 14, No. 1, March 1993.

"Melanoma Research Report." U.S. Department of Health and Human Services, 1992.

"Mesothelioma Research Report." U.S. Department of Health and Human Services, 1988.

Mulshine, James L., M.D., et al. "Initiators and Promoters of Lung Cancer." *Chest,* Vol. 103, No. 1, January 1993.

"Multiple Myeloma (MM)." Leukemia Society of America, 1992.

"National Household Survey on Drug Abuse." U.S. Department of Health and Human Services, 1993.

"NCI to Advise Women in 40s to Ask Doctor About Mammography, End Routine Screening." *The Cancer Letter,* Vol. 19, No. 37, November 5, 1993.

"NCI Fact Book." U.S. Department of Health and Human Services, 1992.

"NCI Official Says Public Health Issue As Important As Data in Mammography." *The Cancer Letter,* Vol. 19, No. 14, April 2, 1993.

"Occupational Risk of Cancer from Pesticides: Farmer Studies." National Cancer Institute, 1991.

Perera, Frederica. "Green-Bashing: A Health Hazard." *The New York Times,* July 29, 1993.

Petrek, Jeanne A., M.D., et al. "Is Body Fat Topography a Risk Factor for Breast Cancer?" *Annals of Internal Medicine,* Vol. 118, No. 5, March 1, 1993.

"Q&A: Questions People Ask About the Prevention and Early Detection of Colon Cancer." Memorial Sloan-Kettering Cancer Center, 1992.

"Questions and Answers About Breast Lumps." U.S. Department of Health and Human Services, 1992.

"Questions and Answers About Electric and Magnetic Fields (EMFs)." United States Environmental Protection Agency, 1992.

"Radon Reduction Techniques in Schools." United States Environmental Protection Agency, 1989.

"Radon-Resistant Construction Techniques for New Residential Construction." United States Environmental Protection Agency, 1991.

"Recognition and Management of Pesticide Poisonings," 4th edition. United States Environmental Protection Agency, 1989.

Redd, William H., Ph.D., and Paul B. Jacobsen, Ph.D. "Emotions and Cancer." *Cancer,* Vol. 62, October 15, 1988.

"Reducing Radon Risks." United States Environmental Protection Agency, 1992.

"Reducing Your Risk of Skin Cancer." American Institute for Cancer Research, 1992.

"Restaurant Smoking as Threat to Waiters." *The New York Times,* July 28, 1993.

"Review and Evaluation of Smoking Cessation Methods: The United

States and Canada, 1978–1985." U.S. Department of Health and Human Services, 1987.

Richert-Boe, Kathryn E., M.D., and Linda L. Humphrey, M.D., M.P.H. "Screening for Cancers of the Cervix and Breast." *Archives of Internal Medicine,* Vol. 152, December 1992.

———. "Screening for Cancers of the Lung and Colon." *Archives of Internal Medicine,* Vol. 152, December 1992.

Samet, Jonathan M., M.D. "The Epidemiology of Lung Cancer." *Chest,* Vol. 103, No. 1, January 1993.

Schapira, David V., M.B.Ch.B., F.R.C.P.C, et al. "Upper-Body Fat Distribution and Endometrial Cancer Risk." *Journal of the American Medical Association,* Vol. 266, No. 13, October 2, 1991.

Severson, Richard K., et al. "A Prospective Analysis of Physical Activity and Cancer." *American Journal of Epidemiology,* Vol. 130, No. 3, 1989.

"Skin Cancer Fact Sheet." American Academy of Dermatology, 1993.

"Skin Cancers: Basal Cell and Squamous Cell Carcinomas Research Report." U.S. Department of Health and Human Services, 1990.

"Smart Move! A Stop Smoking Guide." American Cancer Society, 1988.

"Smoking Policy: Questions and Answers." U.S. Department of Health and Human Services.

Strauss, Gary M., M.D., Ray E. Gleason, Ph.D, and David J. Sugarbaker, M.D., F.C.C.P. "Screening for Lung Cancer Re-examined," *Chest,* Vol. 103, No. 4, April 1993.

"Suspended, Cancelled, and Restricted Pesticides." United States Environmental Protection Agency, 1990.

"Testicular Cancer Research Report." U.S. Department of Health and Human Services, 1990.

Thun, Michael J., M.D., Mohan M. Namboodiri, B.S., and Clark W. Heath Jr., M.D. "Aspirin Use and Reduced Risk of Fatal Colon Cancer." *The New England Journal of Medicine,* Vol. 235, No. 23, December 5, 1991.

Thun, Michael J., M.D., et al. "Risk Factors for Fatal Colon Cancer in a Large Prospective Study." *Journal of the National Cancer Institute,* Vol. 84, No. 19, October 7, 1992.

"Vitamin A and Breast Cancer Risk." *The New York Times,* July 27, 1993.

Wallis, Claudia, Janice M. Horowitz, Elaine Lafferty, and Eugene Linden. "Why New Age Medicine Is Catching On." *Time,* November 4, 1991.

Watson, Charles G., and Donald Schuld. "Psychosomatic Factors in the Etiology of Neoplasms." *Journal of Consulting and Clinical Psychology,* Vol. 45, No. 3, 1977.

"What You Need to Know About Bladder Cancer." U.S. Department of Health and Human Services, 1992.

"What You Need to Know About Brain Cancers." U.S. Department of Health and Human Services, 1992.

"What You Need to Know About Breast Cancer." U.S. Department of Health and Human Services, 1990.

Whittemore, Alice S., et al. "Diet, Physical Activity, and Colorectal Cancer Among Chinese in North America and China." *Journal of the National Cancer Institute,* Vol. 82, No. 11, June 6, 1990.

"Why Mammography Scares Women Off." *Health,* November–December 1992.

Winawer, Sidney J., M.D., and Lynn Hornsby-Lewis, M.D. "What You Should Know About Colon Polyps." New York: Gower Medical Publishing, 1991.

Winawer, Sidney J., M.D., David Schottenfeld, and Betty J. Flehinger. "Colorectal Cancer Screening." *Journal of the National Cancer Institute,* Vol. 83, No. 4, February 20, 1991.

Winawer, Sidney J., M.D., et al. "The Natural History of Colorectal Cancer." *Cancer,* Vol. 67, No. 4, February 1, 1991.

Winawer, Sidney J., M.D. "Prevention of Colon Cancer by Colonoscopic Polypectomy." *The New England Journal of Medicine,* Vol. 329, December 30, 1993.

Yesner, Raymond, M.D. "Pathogenesis and Pathology." *Clinics in Chest Medicine,* Vol. 14, No. 1, March 1993.

Index